MOVING MOUNTAINS

MOVING MOUNTAINS

The Race to Treat Global AIDS

◆

ANNE-CHRISTINE D'ADESKY

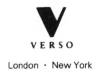

VERSO

London · New York

First published by Verso 2004

1 3 5 7 9 10 8 6 4 2

Verso
UK: 6 Meard Street, London W1F 0EG
USA: 180 Varick Street, New York, NY 10014–4606
www.versobooks.com

Verso is the imprint of New Left Books

ISBN 1–84467–002–3

British Library Cataloguing in Publication Data
A catalogue record for this book is available from the British Library

Library of Congress Cataloging-in-Publication Data
A catalog record for this book is available from the Library of Congress

Typeset in Garamond 3 by Servis Filmsetting Ltd, Manchester
Printed in the USA by R.R. Donnelley & Sons

CONTENTS

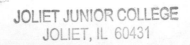

PART I

Introducing the Global Perspective

I

MOVING MOUNTAINS

I

In 1991, during the Lenten Carnival season in Port-au-Prince, Haiti, I drove up to Delmas, a densely populated shantytown of dirt streets and brightly painted one-room shacks that cling to the edge of the hills above the capital, threatening to slide into garbage-filled ravines full of snakes. I'd come to the island for a short visit to report on political affairs and see family and journalistic colleagues.

It was a rare afternoon of political stability on the island. It was extremely humid. On the radio, different Carnival bands were competing to have their song declared the best. Back downtown near the National Palace I'd left several friends from New York whom I'd met through the activist network ACT UP – the AIDS Coalition to Unleash Power.

For my generation, ACT UP served as a crash-course on activism. By taking to the streets to risk arrest, ACT UP had achieved many victories related to access to life-saving medicines. It launched its first protests against the high price of AZT, a former cancer drug approved for AIDS in March 1987 – at a cost of $10,000 a year. Ronald Reagan was in office then, and 20,000 Americans had already died of AIDS. ACT UP had helped focus my activism, while the politics and science of AIDS shaped my personal and professional life. I shifted from international reporting about politics and human rights in Haiti and elsewhere to covering gay issues and AIDS in America, and related social justice battles. Now and then, I reported on the

Haitian AIDS crisis, which was generally ignored by the mainstream US media, as was Africa's, until the late 1990s.

In Haiti, the death toll from AIDS in 1987 can only be guessed at, but no one was getting AZT, unless they were the wealthy children of the elite who'd gotten their hands on a few months' supply of the drug. I'd begun tracking the epidemic there in 1984, and, to this day, Haiti remains my lens for viewing the global epidemic. My father was born there and the family's roots go far back; my extended family still lives there. I spent many childhood summers in Haiti and grew up with an acute awareness of the repressive political climate of terror that existed under "President for Life" François "Papa Doc" and his political goons, the infamous Tontons Macoutes militia, and his successor-son, Jean-Claude or "Baby Doc" Duvalier.

I did my first reporting in Haiti, covering political events and the grassroots pro-democracy movement. In 1987, Haiti began a long *dechoukaj* – or uprooting – of the thirty-year Duvalier dictatorship. Baby Doc and his wife were sent packing to exile in France, having looted the national coffers. The streets and shantytowns were filled with the victims of political violence. AIDS might have been killing more people, but they were hidden.

By then, a handful of Haitian doctors I knew were doing their best to treat severe cases of pneumonia, diarrhea and skin cancers that, in a matter of months, laid waste to young men and women already weak from malnourishment and chronic diseases like malaria, tuberculosis and waterborne parasites. I recall how hard it was to spot AIDS cases among the emaciated, sweaty patients batting away flies in the public hospital. Whenever I was in town, I'd stop by the AIDS clinic on Rue Berne, where my doctor friends would decry the silent epidemic they were battling with limited medicine and almost no support.

Outside of their clinic, the hospital and the morgue, the epidemic was not on the global or domestic radar. AIDS was something whispered about, *la maladi katrach* – the four H's – for the four groups first identified as targets: homosexuals, hemophiliacs, heroin users and Haitians. It was linked with prostitutes and *masisis* – queers – two stigmatized groups. There was little government talk of AIDS. Families turned their sick children out, husbands blamed their wives, and many AIDS patients died alone in hospitals, shunned even by fearful hospital staff, according the Haitian doctors treating the early epidemic.

Today, the taboos surrounding discussions of sexuality continue to shroud AIDS in Haiti, a country steeped in catholicism and voudon, an animist religion. It's common for gay and bisexual men to live closeted lives, to marry and have children in order to fulfill parental expectations. Stigma prevents those who are ill from risking disclosure to seek HIV testing and care until they are quite ill.

That was the reason I was driving up away from the pre-Carnival party downtown to a quiet house in Delmas, where a human rights worker I'd never met, a friend of a friend, was sick. As someone working in AIDS, I'd been asked by a colleague to stop by, to see what I could do.

What I found there is seared in my memory. His wife, an intelligent, composed young woman, led me to the dark inner bedroom of a small house where her husband was dying of AIDS, though no one uttered the word. A half-dozen people from the neighborhood were sitting beside his small bed on stools and overturned buckets, praying softly and chanting.

The man was standing up in bed, semi-naked, wild-eyed and delirious. He eyed me with suspicion and fear. Who was I?, he asked his wife, confused. Was I Legba – the voudon guardian of doorways and barriers? I was wearing a straw hat, a Carnival souvenir. Was I Baron Samedi in my hat – a symbol of the dead (and not coincidentally, of the elder dictator François "Papa Doc" Duvalier)? The people in the room smiled, embarrassed.

The wife calmed her husband down. She introduced me as someone from America, from a Haitian family, who knew about medicine, who wasn't a doctor but might be able to help them. She made me feel his head: he had a very high fever and was trembling, he was hotter than the sweltering room. She explained that he'd already been hospitalized for weeks. There was little the doctors could do for him besides relieve his pain, she'd been told; they had no more medicine. He was *kondane* – condemned. Her husband's family, peasants from the interior, didn't like being at the hospital. If he was going to die, she wanted him home.

Away from the scene, I told her what I knew about the treatment of late-stage brain infections linked to AIDS. I'd come empty handed, with no warning of what to expect. I left her with the name of another doctor who promised to come up as soon as he could to see this man. The next day, I dropped off vitamins, strong painkillers and, at the insistence of my friend Jon Greenberg, a believer in holistic therapy, ampoules of injectable liquid vitamin B-12 that ACT UP friends with HIV thought helped brain function. Jon was using this experimentally to boost his own depleted immune system. I promised to send better medicine back as quickly as I could. But it was too late. The man died seventy-two hours later.

II

What I encountered in 1991 continues today, on a global scale that is hard to imagine. The headlines have been trumpeting these statistics for years now: 25 million already dead of AIDS, 42 million affected with the virus, including 35 million in less-developed countries. By almost any measure – human, social, cultural, economic, financial, political – the scope and impact of the pandemic makes it almost unfathomable, a many-headed Hydra.

Today, the great majority of people living with HIV and AIDS – 28 million – live in sub-Saharan Africa, the world's poorest region. In some countries – like South Africa, the hardest-hit nation – infection rates top 70 percent among some groups of young women. In Botswana, where 40 percent of adults are affected, adult life expectancy has fallen from seventy-three to thirty-seven years. AIDS has wiped out entire families and villages, and left no sector of society untouched. The epidemic has so depleted the workforce of southern Africa that several countries are headed into negative economic growth due to a decline in productivity.

These are numbing, staggering statistics; the numbers become abstractions. But each one is a life, a member of a family. Whenever it gets too big, I break it down, think of this person I met or that one. With drugs, they could be alive, they could be pulled back from madness or blindness – another symptom of untreated late-stage AIDS.

III

Let me offer another portrait. In 1999 I met Chatinkha Nkhoma, a dynamic, newly minted AIDS activist from Malawi. We met at a virology conference in Baltimore, where, in her inimitable way, she'd wangled an invitation to sit among the leading AIDS scientists to learn more about the virus and newer treatments. Over thirty years old, she was good-natured, yet very angry with the big drug companies, a mother and woman living with HIV in a kind of exile, on borrowed time and money. She'd gotten to

Baltimore via a contact in Malawi and was accessing AIDS drugs free by participating in a US federal clinical drug trial. Against crazy odds, she'd reached the land of treatment – the United States of America.

Life wasn't great for her in Baltimore. Back in Malawi, she'd worked in a government ministry, been relatively well paid, and supported others. Now she had no money and couldn't legally work. It was painful to accept charity, she said, but she'd done it to survive. She lived in a small apartment with her son. She was lonely and she worried daily about her relatives back home. Several had died; others were battling the virus. None had treatment. Years back in Malawi, she'd been given up for dead; they'd planned her funeral. By luck, she'd gotten her hands on some recycled antiretroviral medicine, a few weeks' supply. Two drugs at first, then three. It did the trick. It got her on her feet. She later ran out, then got more. It wasn't the prescribed way to take AIDS medicine, it wasn't the way Western doctors recommended to avoid resistance or drug failure, she knew, but she'd done it and she'd recovered. Her son, now college age, was not an orphan – yet.

When I later saw her walking with a cane, suffering from early deterioration of her hip joints – a serious drug-related side-effect emerging in some patients after years of therapy – she waved away my concern. HIV was no picnic, she reminded me, nor were the medicines. Eventually, she might need a hip replacement. But she was undaunted. She'd walk again, go back to Malawi, soon, start a treatment access program there.

In her wheelchair, she attended the Thirteenth International AIDS Conference in Durban, South Africa in 2000, a turning point in the global fight to access medicine. At a protest rally organized by South Africa's Treatment Action Campaign and ACT UP – the first major AIDS protest on African soil – she grabbed the microphone, pointed to a building behind her where World Bank officials and drug company experts were discussing the cost-effectiveness of global AIDS treatment, and shouted to a sea of African faces like hers: "There is a crime being committed here! You cannot have 42 million people dying and have the issue be about money!"

IV

The crime Chatinkha is referring to is the lack of affordable AIDS medicines for the world, and the huge gap in access that has allowed people in rich countries to live and those in poorer countries to die. While many people in the United States and Western Europe have had access to AZT and other antiretroviral drugs for fifteen years, these drugs have been too highly priced for the rest of the world. A three-drug HIV regimens costs $10,000 in the US. Compare that with a $5-a-year per capita health budget for citizens in the poorest countries in sub-Saharan Africa, and the treatment gap becomes very clear.

In truth, the drugs are too costly for many US patients, too, and there are waiting lists on the federal programs that provide these drugs for those who lack insurance. Most people get the drugs through their employee insurance policies, but many don't. HIV causes disability, and that can lead to unemployment. One thread that connects the access issue in rich and poor countries is poverty, which is linked to AIDS and other diseases of the poor like tuberculosis, and in Africa and Asia to malaria and sleeping sickness.

Scratch the surface and the AIDS access battle reveals a single, ugly motive: profit. That's what has led the big drug companies to charge so much for their drugs, yet block competitors from selling generic alternatives at a fraction of that cost. There are billions to be made. Patents and international trade laws are the instruments used to keep AIDS and other essential medicines from reaching Africa. It's important, then, to see AIDS as not merely a medical or public health issue, but fundamentally a social and political one. That's why AIDS activists adopt the language of human rights and social justice to discuss the access battle.

V

This book is about the global challenge to provide HIV treatment and care to people living in resource-poor settings. It examines the feasibility of that effort in light of existing and emerging obstacles that lie ahead for governments and affected communities. Given the complexity of the AIDS epidemic, the challenges are immense. Each step forward reveals a new layer of complexity.

I began this reporting after the 2000 street protests in Durban, which put the issue of global AIDS center-stage in the world's consciousness – where it has remained. At that time, the question of whether to treat was still being hotly debated. Many skeptics were demanding concrete proof – hard clinical data – that such a monumental project could work. They worried about the negative consequences of failing, of starting to treat then stopping due to lack of funds, and of the possibility of causing an epidemic of drug resistance to occur – something that is on the rise in the US and Western Europe. These remain concerns for some critics, who have openly doubted the ability of Africans and Haitians and other people living in developing countries to manage the rigors of a lifetime of antiretroviral therapy.

This book focuses on the frontline efforts of pioneering groups who established pilot programs in the months following Durban. I wanted to chronicle the first steps – and missteps – of these groups in order to identify some of the key ingredients of their success or failure. By looking at what was happening in rural hospitals and community clinics, in the field, in prisons, in the halls of government, in classrooms, and in the bedroom, I hoped to offer an early litmus test of our collective progress so far.

I was particularly interested in efforts to educate and mobilize communities around treatment, and whether this would in fact help break down stigma. I wanted to see how treatment was impacting on the lives of the first lucky few, like Chatinkha, who accessed drugs. I wanted to focus on where the gaps existed between blueprints and funding promises versus concrete action and commitment, where the hurdles were proving greater or smaller than expected.

This book does not aim be a comprehensive survey of the global AIDS epidemic. It looks more narrowly at the myriad challenges – political, social, medical, technical, cultural – to delivering therapy, and to issues related to disease control and the capacity of nations to mobilize their civil societies and health sectors to deliver accelerated access to AIDS medicines.

The management of HIV is complex in wealthy countries with state-of-the-art tools. It is far more difficult in impoverished Africa where HIV rides on the coat-tails of endemic co-diseases like tuberculosis and malaria. How would doctors cope with fewer resources and without tools such as HIV diagnostic tests? Would new, simpler daily drug regimens and alternative treatment guidelines for managing HIV in limited-resource settings prove useful to patients and doctors in the field?

Each chapter reflects this unfolding story at a particular time and place, offering a multifaceted view of the fast-changing landscape of global treatment. I visit projects in a range of countries and different geographic settings. I compare public and private programs, urban and rural programs, government and community-based programs. I also look at how treatment programs are linked to prevention, vaccine and research efforts.

In each country I focus on a specific issue, angle or obstacle that is critical to HIV treatment there. In Mexico, for example, I look at the issue of infrastructure, as well as the challenge of delivering treatment and care in urban versus rural settings. In Haiti, I also look at the infrastructure question, but focus on an innovative strategy being used to help poor villagers adhere to their daily regimens – Directly Observed Therapy. In Uganda, which has attracted attention for national prevention efforts, I study mother-to-child transmission, trying to gauge whether MTCT prevention programs will indeed provide stepping stones to treatment in adults. In India, I look at the emerging generic AIDS drug industry, and the issues that underlie the bitter competition between multinational drug companies and the Indian upstarts.

I am also interested in the experiences and needs of women, sexual minorities, drug users, prisoners, youths, and other vulnerable groups. Russia provides a close look at a fast-moving epidemic that is crossing over from high-risk groups to the general population. I also examine the frontiers of HIV science and research, to determine the potential impact of future threats on developing countries.

With new money pouring into the international AIDS arena, it seems like everyone is beginning to chase research and treatment dollars – be they scientists, public health officials, agencies, physician groups, non-profit organizations, community and activist groups. What matters most is how new programs will directly benefit those living with HIV and AIDS, and those very ill or dying in hospitals or bedrooms, desperately waiting for medicine. With new groups at all levels entering this fast-growing arena, I want to know who they are and what role they may play. I am concerned that while the expanding field of global AIDS offers fresh opportunities – funding, programs, jobs, influence – to established and new groups, it will inevitably lead to negative competition and lack of cooperation between frontline groups. This could easily lead to a duplication of efforts and a squandering of precious resources rather than the unified action that is needed. That scenario has played itself out in richer countries, and it would be foolish to expect anything different in much poorer ones, where the fight for resources is even more intense.

For now, provision of the money and resources needed to carry out the monumental task of the global treatment rollout is growing, but remains completely inadequate. That makes the odds of achieving an overall victory impossibly high. It also makes it unrealistic to hope to predict accurately the long-term outcome of the global effort. But a close look at the money, groups and agendas can give a rough picture of what we can expect in the short term.

VI

As I write, in the fall of 2003, the number of people actually receiving anti-retroviral (ARV) drugs for HIV has more than doubled in the developing world, and increased by over two-thirds in Africa, since 2000. But it remains minuscule – only 1 percent of the 4 million people in southern Africa who need drugs today actually get them. At the start of this year, official figures show that, of the 300,000 people in developing countries on ARV therapy, half were Brazilians who receive free HIV drugs through Brazil's much-lauded universal health system. Globally, the World Health Organization estimates that 6 million people require treatment now and will die without it in the near future. The agency has now dedicated itself to having 3 million people on antiretrovirals by 2005 – the "3 × 5 plan" – though the agency will not actually be providing the treatment.

How quickly this commitment translates into action, into medicine getting into bodies through sustainable, effective national programs, remains the burning question. Much will depend on the openness and ability of political leaders and health officials who are developing comprehensive AIDS programs to learn from each other's mistakes; and on their national commitment to medical treatment and a range of steps that will help assure greater access for citizens.

VII

If the global effort succeeds, it will radically alter what our world will look like in the future. With so many lives hanging in the balance, the most important questions are: How many can be saved? How quickly? For how long? By then, how many more will have contracted the virus? Will the push to treat bolster prevention and vaccine efforts, as hoped? Will it help hard-hit nations to rebuild their basic health infrastructure? To fight other diseases? To reverse the economic devastation wreaked by AIDS?

And what about those with HIV? How will poor rural Haitians and Mexicans and Ugandans and others in developing countries manage HIV treatment-for-life? How well will they adhere to simplified regimens? Will we see a global version of what occurred in the US and Western Europe, where ARV drugs quickly cut the AIDS death rate and extended survival to patients? Or will the chronic lack of basic life resources – food, water, shelter, jobs – prevent such miracles from being repeated in poorer countries?

There are also problems associated with long-term use of potent but toxic AIDS therapies in richer countries, including drug resistance and serious side-effects. These side-effects include lipid and metabolic problems that cause damage to major organs like the liver, pancreas, heart, and kidneys. Studies show the risk of developing drug side-effects is linked to the length of time on therapy. So we may not see such problems in Africa for a few years, but what about down the line? Will people there also develop resistance to new simplified regimens being introduced, and then require alternatives? What if substitutes aren't available?

In a later section, I'll look at the myriad treatment challenges that physicians and individuals encounter in poor settings. As my field reports illustrate, these offer a glimpse of what new problems could crop up, and what life on HAART – highly active antiretroviral therapy – may be like in these countries.

If treatment-for-life is going to succeed, we need to develop and implement such plans and programs soon to ensure that the initial benefits of therapy are not short-lived. That means looking squarely at the potential global downside of treatment, not just the miracles.

In other words, what if the grand plan fails? Or the big money doesn't fully materialize? Or begins to flow, then is delayed or stopped, as frequently happens when programs rely on outside funding? What if treatment succeeds in some places, but not as well in others (a likely scenario)? How well can any region contain HIV, if the epidemic is poorly controlled in neighboring countries?

As the recent lessons of SARS remind us, viruses know no borders in a world of globalization and fast travel. What occurs in Dar es Salaam can affect what happens in Bangkok or Moscow. Looking ahead, will ever-wily

HIV – with its proven ability to quickly mutate, recombine into new sub-strains, and lie dormant in the body for a lifetime – gain the global upper hand? Instead of disappearing or being controlled by drugs, will HIV eventually follow the path of other global diseases of the poor like tuberculosis and malaria, and in time become resistant to the current drug arsenal? By then, will new weapons be available in Africa or Haiti?

Compared with AIDS, there is little social stigma attached to SARS, perhaps because SARS is not viewed as a sexually-transmitted disease. There is fear of contagion and illness, but it is not linked to a moral judgement of human behavior. It is striking to note the difference in the world's response to these two global threats. Although Chinese officials initially covered up the SARS epidemic, global health officials issued an emergency call for all nations to respond to what they viewed as a threat to global public health. SARS was a matter of concern to all citizens, while AIDS is still viewed by many as a disease that is punishment for a sexual or other transgression from the social norm.

As we look to the future, no one can predict which new doomsday scenarios may emerge with AIDS or HIV, or where they will occur. But it's safe to assume that if funding or programs are started then abandoned, if political and civic leaders fail to unite or act responsibly, if stigma continues to prevent people from accessing testing and care, if drug companies block generic manufacturers, if privatization weakens public health systems, then such scenarios present a considerable risk.

VIII

One obstacle common to all developing countries is weak infrastructure, including public health systems. This issue is often cited by skeptics as a justifiable reason not to offer AIDS drugs to the world's poor. But as we learn from Brazil's example, AIDS treatment programs provide an opportunity to develop infrastructure, to introduce education and testing, to prepare communities for vaccine trials. Infrastructure – or lack of it – is not an acceptable reason to withhold, delay or scale back treatment.

To quote Paul Farmer, a pioneer of AIDS treatment in Haiti, "You'll always find people looking for excuses not to act, and AIDS is no exception. I find they're usually the people holding the purse strings. That doesn't make them right in my book, it just makes them greedy." Farmer was speaking to me in 2001, when his own project was just beginning to get global recognition. Like many in the trenches, he casts the access issue in moral terms of justice and health equity.

Yet Farmer is the first to acknowledge that it's harder to treat HIV in poor settings than rich ones. The extreme poverty of people in some countries makes the task of fighting and controlling any disease a complex endeavor, one linked to issues of national, regional and local development. How can one ask individuals to take AIDS medicines when they don't have enough food or clean water to swallow their pills? That's a question I wanted to ask in Haiti, where I know people don't eat every day.

As Farmer and others argue, infrastructure can indeed be developed, but it requires money, materials and human resources. In many countries there are resource gaps of all kinds across the board: not enough hospitals, clinics, trained doctors, nurses, basic medicine, affordable tests to deliver care to those living far from cities; not enough roads, warehouses, trained patent officials, pharmacists to procure, register, store and deliver drugs; not enough telephones, dependable electricity, refrigerators, computers, and other physical infrastructure to test thousands of blood samples and provide immediate results to patients; not enough of an industrial base or trained engineers or chemists to embark on local manufacturing of generic HIV drugs and make it cost-effective; not enough teachers, educators, lay counselors, and community organizers to take on the urgent task of educating and mobilizing local communities to take charge of their own care.

Instead, sub-Saharan Africa has been, and remains, under siege. So do parts of Asia and Eastern Europe, where the degree of overall poverty and development may be less severe, but still leads to limited or low-quality health and HIV services for the poorest citizens. In the hardest-hit countries of southern Africa, like Botswana and South Africa, a critical percentage of the very workforce needed to administer AIDS programs, deliver care or educate people about HIV has died or is ill: civil servants, doctors, nurses, technicians, midwives, teachers. Time and money are lacking to quickly replace and train a new generation of professionals. That spells a diminished human capacity to carry out the national AIDS effort.

Treatment education and literacy – including cultural literacy – are also critical factors in developing a national response to AIDS. This is challenging due to the diversity of populations, with so many languages spoken. It's not enough to provide information about HIV and drugs, but to make sure the information can be understood, is culturally sensitive, and addresses the educational needs of target groups. AIDS requires a discussion of the body, sexuality, identity, social attitudes toward healing and illness. Here again, the experience and resources of the West require translation, adoption, and redefinition to fit an African, Asian or other cultural model.

IX

What are experts doing to prepare communities around the world for these challenges? It's one thing to roll out treatment, quite another to sustain programs for decades. Doing so requires much more than a steady supply of drugs, food and clean water to take pills. It demands long-term emotional support for individuals facing not only a life-threatening illness, but daily battles with nausea, fatigue and other common drug side-effects; with depression and suicidal thoughts; with worries that HIV will win the upper hand despite treatment; with failure to take exactly the right pills on time to avoid resistance. We know from the experiences and testimonies of US and other patients that life with HIV is very hard, and life on therapy is no picnic. All of this is likely to be even more challenging for individuals trying to cope with far fewer resources.

There are myriad challenges in maintaining good health, particularly in settings where daily survival is the name of the game. But many of the supportive elements that are taken for granted in rich countries are missing for patients in the poorest settings. The denial of AIDS has affected mainstream society. HIV is not talked about openly. Instead people are stigmatized and face fear, hostility, violence and overt discrimination. Those on treatment are likely to hide this aspect of their lives from neighbors and even loved ones to avoid being stigmatized. Right now, there aren't support groups for those with HIV in many countries, and relatively few mental health services have been developed with AIDS and HIV-positive individuals in mind. Along with drug therapy, the provision of mental health needs to be introduced into the formula. What it looks like will reflect social and cultural practices in different communities.

Ethics present yet another challenge. Up to now, people with AIDS who are receiving treatment have often been excluded from the decision-making processes that greatly affect them. A far greater effort is needed now to bring their voices into the discussion, at all levels of planning and administration. I knew this from the experience in the US, where people with HIV had to fight to get onto the review boards of clinical trials, and inside closed-door meetings to discuss drug development with manufacturers.

Right now, those with the most at stake in relation to treatment are individuals at death's door and their loved ones. After a few weeks on therapy, they are likely to regain their health, and then they need jobs, training, housing and other services – just like other citizens, except that HIV provides an extra challenge. Without housing or work, it becomes that much harder to care for yourself. Are governments and NGOs prepared for that challenge? Are they taking into consideration housing, mental health services, such as rape counseling for women, family planning services, or school programs for HIV-positive children?

Care providers and institutions need long-term support too. In some countries, there are few non-governmental organizations (NGOs) or community-based groups with experience in rolling out comprehensive AIDS programs. As we saw in the US and Western Europe, the learning curve can be steep. Given the dearth of resources and funding in the poorest countries, there will be problems of mismanagement, of funds being squandered, of corruption – all problems seen in richer countries. Given that outside donors and agencies are funding treatment programs, how prepared are they for the difficult road ahead? What about scientists, health professionals, medical schools? How prepared are they for the long-term test of controlling HIV?

The upside of all these challenges is the many opportunities they present for creating capacity, for providing resources, jobs, and solutions. HIV treatment is related to the challenge of development, of providing these resources in such a way that individuals, groups, institutions, governments and societies become self-sufficient. Here again, there is no simple blueprint. Instead, politics and economics are big factors that threaten to derail the best-laid plans of political and health leaders or communities.

X

The ability of affected communities to shape national treatment efforts is linked to their status in society. The effective treatment and control of AIDS also requires laws and policies that do not discriminate, but instead offer protection and support to vulnerable groups. The explosion of AIDS among women worldwide, for example, is directly linked to issues of gender, to the physical, social, economic and sexual vulnerability of women and girls in decision-making, to their decreased access to education, work and health-care, to their exposure to domestic violence and rape. Getting drugs into bodies is a hard enough task, but getting a woman into a clinic may be equally difficult if her husband refuses to allow it, or will beat her or divorce her if she gets tested.

Today, many developing countries also have strict laws outlawing homo-sexuality, prostitution, and recreational drug use. The criminalization of such behaviors makes it harder to reach out to closeted gay men, sex workers, and drug addicts who need access to testing, support, treatment and care. Changes in law and policy are thus integral to supporting the goals of global AIDS treatment.

Immigrants are another vulnerable group. On a global level, there is an important question – a contradiction – that is being ignored by global leaders and activists alike. In pushing for treatment, we are asking millions of people to come forward for testing, to risk disclosure. Yet almost every nation has laws that track those with HIV, and that prevent their easy passage across borders. By advocating access to treatment, are we also asking people to risk the loss of their civil rights? Little of this discussion has made its way into media coverage, but I imagine it has taken place among individuals and groups contemplating treatment. Or has it? How much information do communities have about the implications of starting HIV treatment, beyond their immediate need to survive?

XI

This book opens with the case of Brazil, widely considered the model for a global scaling up of treatment. I went there after visiting many other coun-tries. I wanted to look at how far Brazil had come, and what the limits of its program might be now. How well does its model apply to the explod-ing epidemics in Lagos, Addis Ababa, Kiev, or the Henan province of China? Will it prove a global exception, or the rule for the developing world?

Looking beyond AIDS to the greater revolution in global health-care and policy, will the gains of the access movement extend to other arenas? Will medicine for life-threatening diseases be removed from the realm of commercial profits? Will the battle over AIDS drugs and patents lead to wider use of generics globally? Will the anti-globalization battle lead to a reconsideration of proposed international forums like the World Trade Organization (WTO) and Free Trade of the Americas Agreement (FTAA), which stand to have a profound effect on our health in the future?

As I crossed the globe, all these questions and more informed my travels. Then and now, what seems most important is to ask a lot of questions, look hard at the numbers, read the plans, note what is and isn't getting included and why; to talk with people with HIV and their family members, with activists and doctors, researchers and policy makers, with health and trade officials, with drug manufacturers on both sides of the drug war – all in an effort to gain insight into this unfolding epic challenge.

2

AIDS AND EMPIRE I:
A BRIEF CHRONOLOGY OF RECENT EVENTS

The global treatment revolution that began in the fall of 1998 has quickly transformed apocalyptic despair into cautious hope and accelerated action. By revolution, I don't mean a single catalyst or event, but a series of extraordinary steps and counter-steps taken by different actors at many levels. But these steps followed almost two decades of frustrated, small-scale actions and projects by disparate grassroots groups in the global south who allied themselves with activists in the US and Western Europe in an effort to highlight the global pandemic.

The push to provide AIDS drugs has existed as an urgent demand since the mid 1980s, when what was called Slim Disease – AIDS – began ravaging cities like Kinshasa, Dar es Salaam, and other African hotspots. To this day, we really don't know how many Africans died of AIDS, because the disease was barely named and so many died of what looked like hunger – wasting – or familiar illnesses like tuberculosis. During these years, the words of the few activists from developing countries who could attend annual international AIDS conferences, pleading the case of Africa, fell on largely deaf ears. Their domestic protests rarely got global media attention. The international movement gained momentum only after protease drugs had become widely available in the US and Western Europe in the early 1990s, providing immediate proof that AIDS combination therapy could turn the epidemic around. By then, many of the early and pioneering activists from Africa and Asia and other developing regions were dead.

In the United States, small groups of HIV-positive treatment activists, many with ties to developing countries, formed alliances with groups in Africa and Haiti and Latin America and began small-scale AIDS drug donation projects. These community-based projects, often involving physicians, would collect leftover but unexpired AIDS drugs and other medicines from US hospitals, clinical trials, and individual patients. After carefully sorting and repackaging them, they would work with physicians in developing countries to provide a continuous supply of this "recycled" medicine to individual patients. These largely volunteer projects operated on shoestring budgets, but managed to keep dozens of people alive for years. Others in Africa or Haiti or Thailand had relatives living in Europe or the US who would send short-term supplies of AZT or other drugs. As in the early days of the US AIDS epidemic, people were desperate and went to extreme ends to get their hands on any medicine they could.

Over the years, sporadic protests took place in the US to demand attention to the plight of people living with HIV/AIDS (PLWHAs), in Africa and other poor countries. In 1992, AIDS activists joined Haitian protesters to demand the release of HIV-positive Haitian refugees detained at the US navy base in Guantánamo, Cuba. A year later, a federal judge shut down the camp. Other joint protests were held with other groups against the US immigration policy that bans entry by HIV-positive individuals.

At the start of what is now referred to as the global treatment movement, nearly 40 million people had HIV, and that number was expected to double by 2010. Some 8,000–10,000 people were dying of AIDS every day due to lack of access to life-saving medicines. Thousands were and continue to be exposed daily.

One of the first actions around access for Africa was taken was by French president Jacques Chirac. At a December 1997 Conference on AIDS and STDs in France, Chirac launched the French International Therapeutic Solidarity Fund (FSTI), to begin funding pilot treatment projects in Francophone Africa. A year later, UN officials established the Drug Access Initiative, a tiered-pricing program that sought to provide discounted brand-name drugs to poor nations.

Much of the early victory can be credited to grassroots AIDS activists from Thailand, Brazil and South Africa, who formed alliances with US ACT UP chapters in Philadelphia, New York and Paris. In the early 1990s, gay and AIDS activists in Brazil risked arrest in street protests to demand access to antiretrovirals. In 1998 and 1999, Thai protesters took aim at their government, as well as the multinational drug companies, which they accused of gross profiteering on AIDS drugs; so did South Africans. In the US, AIDS activists began targeting the Clinton White House, demanding that politicians intervene to help sub-Saharan Africa combat AIDS. On Capitol Hill in 1998, a fierce legislative fight began between African-American groups over competing trade bills that would address Africa's plight. The Black Congressional Caucus and leaders like Jesse Jackson backed a Hope for Africa bill that would allow African countries to use trade provisions to access cheap, generic AIDS drugs. An opposing bill, the Africa Growth and Opportunity Act, sponsored by House members Philip Crane (R-IL) and Charles Rangel (D-NY) upheld US patent laws.

While Congress fought, gay activists from Fed Up Queers in New York and AIDS activists from ACT UP chapters on the east coast began hounding Vice-President Al Gore during his fall presidential campaign, highlighting his role as a spokesperson for big pharmaceutical companies. They demanded that the Clinton administration and United States Trade Representative Charlene Barshefsky stop allying themselves with multinational drug companies in a legal battle to block South Africa from accessing generic AIDS drugs. They also denounced similar USTR actions against India, Thailand, Brazil and Argentina.

Taking this message to the media, AIDS activists formed Health GAP – the Health Global Access Project. They began focusing on trade issues and AIDS, and on how drug patents and international trade bodies like the World Trade Organization were being used to advance corporate agendas at the expense of public health in developing countries. Health GAP demanded that global leaders make an exception to the WTO's Trade Related Aspects of Intellectual Property (TRIPs) law, which requires all countries to adhere to US patent laws by 2005. It gives companies twenty-year monopolies on patents. Health GAP's slogan was simple: AIDS Drugs for Africa!

By then, US watchdog groups like Ralph Nader's Consumer Project on Technology were providing AIDS activists with data to support the push for access to cheaper generic medicines. James Love of CPT educated members of Congress about the profits being made by AIDS drug patent holders. In May 1999, CPT joined Doctors Without Borders (Médecins Sans Frontières, or MSF), and Health Action International to issue the "Amsterdam Statement," a seminal text calling on nations to take emergency measures such as compulsory licensing in order to access affordable generic AIDS drugs. When the AGOA bill passed, Clinton signed an Executive Order banning US agencies from doing anything, including threatening WTO action, to discourage African nations from pursuing a generic alternative. In Thailand, and later in South Africa, AIDS activists pushed health officials to access generic drugs for opportunistic infections.

In October 1999, MSF was awarded the Nobel Peace Prize, and became an early, vocal leader in demanding AIDS treatment for the world. A month later, AIDS activists joined anti-globalization protesters at the "Battle for Seattle," the outcome of a ministerial meeting of the then 134-member WTO which led to violent clashes and grabbed more international headlines. In November 1999 Mark Schoofs, a *Village Voice* reporter, began publishing a series on AIDS in Africa that later won a Pulitzer Prize, increasing public awareness of the devastation the epidemic was wreaking.[1] Then US Health Secretary Sandra Thurman also toured Africa with US journalists in tow, raising domestic awareness of the global epidemic.

Other activists launched Jubilee 2000, a "Drop the Debt" campaign that demanded a cancellation of Africa's $300 billion foreign debt to rich country creditors. Africa's debt, they pointed out, totals $15 billion annually – far surpassing the $10 million global leaders say is needed today to pay for global AIDS treatment. Debt activists argue that many foreign loans were made to Cold War-era dictators like former Zaire's Mobutu Sese Seko, or to the illegitimate apartheid regime in South Africa, and used to repress citizens or line the pockets of those in power. This money did little to develop Africa, and now impoverishes it.[2]

In response, the multinational drugs companies – "big pharma" – began offering the first of a series of charitable drug programs, including Bristol-Myers Squibb's "Secure the Future" program. In May 2000 the Accelerating Access Initiative was started, an alliance between five UN organizations and five big pharma companies (later six). The AAI began providing steeply discounted drugs to the Least Developed Countries (LDCs), based on country GNP. That same month they backed a WTO complaint to prevent Brazil from acquiring and making generics, and two months later revived their lawsuit against South Africa.

The Durban AIDS conference in June 2000 proved a watershed event. There, Harvard economist Jeffrey Sachs used the global pulpit to make an impassioned plea for a "war chest" to pay for treatments in Africa and other poor countries. Scientists and global leaders responded with a standing ovation. The debate began focusing on the cost-effectiveness and viability of treatment, given the high global price-tag.

To many, the turning point in the global battle was the pioneering decision by Cipla, a leading Indian generic drug manufacturer, to offer its copycat AIDS drugs to frontline groups like MSF for $360 a year. Overnight, the single biggest obstacle to global access fell away, setting the stage for what has become the era of treatment.[3]

Here the Treatment Action Campaign of South Africa showed its muscle for the first time. Zackie Achmat, one of its early leaders, publicly defied government authorities and drug companies by declaring his intention to illegally import generic fluconazole from India. MSF also allied itself with TAC, and pushed other NGOs such as Oxfam to declare their alliance with poor countries seeking access to low-cost generics.

As big pharma and the Indian upstarts battled, drug prices began to fall. In early 2001, reporter Tina Rosenberg published a *New York Times Magazine* cover story trumpeting Brazil's success at curbing its AIDS epidemic by opting to manufacture generics.[4] Days later Bush was elected, with the help of the big drug companies who had generously backed his candidacy. He later surprised and angered his big pharma supporters when he left in place the Clinton Executive Order that would allow other countries to use generic AIDS drugs. By then, United Nations officials were admitting the Accelerating Access Initiative had failed to deliver enough treatment to Africans. New sources of funding were needed, said UN Secretary General Kofi Annan, who began strongly pushing world leaders to fund treatment of AIDS.

That March, South African President Thabo Mbeki toured Cuba, and accepted Fidel Castro's offer of technological help to produce generic AIDS drugs – something Cuba had achieved. Facing a torrent of negative publicity, some forty multinational drug companies dropped their lawsuit against South Africa on April 19, a remarkable victory for TAC. By mid June, GlaxoSmithKline had dropped the price of its drugs in sixty-three countries to what they called the "cost of production" – a considerable discount. Yet generic manufacturers were still beating GSK's prices. The debate over generics dominated discussions at the historic UN General Assembly Special Summit on AIDS – UNGASS – held June 25, 2001. So did a debate over the merits of investing in prevention versus treatment programs. The consensus was that these were inseparable, and that treatment could be used to bolster prevention efforts, since people need to be tested in order to receive care.

At UNGASS, amid more protests led by Health GAP, world leaders signed a Declaration of Commitment that serves as a roadmap for the current global rollout. It reflects a newfound political commitment by nations to AIDS treatment as an issue of human rights. Under the leadership of Kofi Annan, the Global Fund for Tuberculosis, AIDS and Malaria was launched to fund nascent national AIDS programs.[5]

In South Africa, the door to generics – and all treatment – was closed. Mbeki emerged as a denier of HIV as the cause of AIDS, and refused to provide or distribute AZT to HIV-positive pregnant women, or adult treatment to millions of citizens there. His actions spurred TAC to broaden its civil disobedience campaign and drew more attention to the raging epicenter of the epidemic.

In November 2001 came another critical juncture. In Doha, Qatar, the then 142-member WTO (today it has 146 members) issued a ruling allowing the poorest countries to use compulsory licensing and other trade mechanisms to access generic drugs in cases of public health emergencies, such as AIDS, TB and malaria. But the fine print betrayed a major obstacle: generic drugs could only be produced for "predominantly" domestic consumption. The so-called Doha Declaration requires developing countries to have or acquire the local capacity to make the drugs, something most lack. And it made no provision for exports – shutting the door to promising generics, not opening it. In 2002 and early 2003, WTO ministers tried to resolve the issue, as mandated by the WHO's own rules. But they failed, blocked by US vetoes.[6]

To its credit, the Global Fund initially moved quickly to disperse seed grants to a growing number of needy nations, though funding for the Global Fund remained rocky. Activists continued to assail G-8 leaders at global economic forums, accusing them of backpedaling on UNGASS pledges to support the multilateral Global Fund. They have lately grown critical of the Global Fund's executive director, Richard Feacham, deeming him too acquiescent to political pressures put on Global Fund's board by the Bush administration and its allies in big pharma.

More money has come in from private foundations like the Bill and Melinda Gates Foundation, The Rockefeller Foundation, and most recently the William Jefferson Clinton Foundation. The Gates Foundation has been a real maverick in the arena of prevention, providing major funding to launch new initiatives to develop an HIV vaccine and a topical microbicide (a product to block sexual transmission of the virus), and has funded a major pilot treatment project in Botswana. It also funds research into developing world diseases like malaria and dengue fever. The Rockefeller Foundation has concentrated on maternal and pediatric HIV prevention. The big actor in treatment has been Bill Clinton, who has used his presidential experience and contacts to help governments develop comprehensive AIDS plans that involve private–public alliances. His Foundation focuses on the issue of infrastructure, including logistical details of drug procurement and the delivery of medicines by the public health sector.

In mid 2002, world leaders met again in Barcelona for another international AIDS conference, and there saw the first results from pilot studies of treatment by groups like MSF in South Africa and Partners In Health in Haiti. AIDS activists there targeted the Bush administration, drowning out a prepared speech by its representative, US Health and Human Services Secretary Tommy Thompson, to demand the US fulfill its pledged contribution to the Global Fund. ACT UP also targeted Coca-Cola, demanding that it extend a new workplace treatment program to all its African employees, not only managers. At Barcelona, the World Health Organization also announced a plan to treat 3 million people by 2005 – dubbed the "3×5" program. The International Treatment Access Coalition was also formed between large technical agencies, private groups and front-line players to push the 3×5 envelope.

In 2003 the Bush administration raised world hopes by pledging $15 billion in new money to global AIDS, which would be given to fund prevention and treatment programs in twelve African nations, Haiti and Guyana. Only $1 million was channeled into the Global Fund. Activists quickly did the math, and found that some of the money was not new; it was merely being shifted from other programs. Others noted that Bush put his global AIDS project under the umbrella of a bilateral agency, the US Agency for International Development, and the State Department, which is a political, not health agency. This was a clear sign that AIDS was being treated as a matter of US foreign policy and security by the Bush administration.

In fact, the Bush initiative seems to be a thinly-disguised unilateral move designed to sabotage the multilateral UN-backed Global Fund. It also allows the administration to promote a religiously conservative agenda and directs funds to faith-based groups to implement it. The Bush money favors prevention programs that support sexual abstinence over the use of condoms, and opposes funding groups that support family planning services that even indirectly allow abortion. Shortly after his narrow election Bush resurrected the Mexico City Policy as one of his first political acts. It is known as the global gag rule, and bars US international funding for family planning organizations that support abortion – even when abortion is legal in a given country. The Mexico City Policy was first passed in 1984 by Ronald Reagan, but retracted by Clinton.[7]

The Bush initiative also provides an opening for big pharma companies to market their discounted brand-name AIDS drugs to the developing world.[8] Media reports revealed that multinational drug companies paid some $25,000 each to join working groups to back the Bush Africa plan, an initiative the companies assumed would secure developing country markets for their higher-priced AIDS drugs.[9] The multinationals were reportedly shocked when, in his State of the Union address, Bush suggested his global AIDS plan would use foreign generic drugs. They have also opposed other administration efforts to increase access to generic drugs for US consumers.[10] Since then, big pharma lobbyists have worked overtime to get that decision changed or simply ignored, according to Bill Haddad, a spokesman for the US generic lobby and CEO of Biogenerics, a US company. Haddad has represented Cipla and other Indian generic producers at various meetings with health officials in the past year, and says, "The multinationals are doing everything they can to prevent generics from gaining further entry. They have a lot of money to spend and they're letting people in Congress know it."[11]

The Bush plan can also be seen as part of a larger US economic agenda aimed at facilitating entry for other US products into African markets. One example is the last-minute inclusion in the Bush $15 billion AIDS bill of a provision calling for the use of genetically modified food in US food-aid programs. The move was made by Senate Majority Leader Bill Frist, a Republican and religious conservative who often lobbies on behalf of US agribusiness. But it's hardly a secret that the US and the Bush administration are trying hard to open up new markets to US agribusiness. Instead, they have publicly vowed to help producers of genetically modified food break into developing world markets. Nor it is a surprise that, in this field too, the issue of patents is being hotly debated within the WTO.[12]

As I write, all eyes are on the upcoming Cancún Ministerial WTO meeting, where the issue of generics will again be debated (see Chapter 3). If there is a positive resolution on the Doha Declaration, the poorest countries will be given a green light to import generics, though activists caution that there will be conditions that will make it hard for these countries to do so, regardless of the legality of the WTO ruling. What's unclear is who will supply these countries and whether there will be new hurdles facing potential exporters like Brazil or Canada.

For now, what's needed by poor countries is more political muscle to confront the US and its economic interests. But most countries are too dependent on US foreign aid to risk accessing generics and angering the Bush administration.

The larger economic issue concerns the 2005 TRIPs deadline, which may cripple even Brazil's future ability to access cheap medicines – and India's ability to offer them. So could new free-trade agreements like the upcoming Free Trade of the Americas (FTAA) in late November, another seething battleground where the fight over access to drugs will play itself out.

Moving ahead, the economics of AIDS remains the critical issue that may derail the global AIDS treatment effort. Even as the Bush administration backs certain treatment programs, it has threatened countries that are pushing for revisions of the WTO TRIPs rules.[13] Other countries are also engaged in contradictory actions and double-speak around AIDS, trade and money; G-8 leaders have called for major increases in funding for the Global Fund, but have continually failed to invest at levels they have promised.

In spite of these under-the-table fights and competing agendas, the fact remains that, within a space of three years, the essential ingredients for a global response have coalesced: cheaper drugs, high-level political will, new money to pay for treatment and growing grassroots muscle to push governments to follow through on their promises. But AIDS activists will have to maintain pressure on the Bush administration at each step along the way.

3

BRAZIL'S AIDS MODEL:
A GLOBAL BLUEPRINT?

In the mid 1990s, AIDS was spreading so quickly in Brazil that health ana-lysts were predicting catastrophe for the South American giant. The epidemic there rivaled South Africa's, which was also exploding. The difference between the two countries today is dramatic: Brazil has gained a degree of control over its runaway epidemic, while South Africa has the greatest number of people with HIV, and faces collapse within two decades.[1] The key for Brazil has been use of generic antiretroviral drugs that it began importing from Indian suppliers in 1996, and then learned to make. Today, Brazil is the success story of global AIDS, having proved that it's possible for a developing country with a fast-moving epidemic to gain a degree of control over it. Although HIV continues to increase in Brazil, the rate of new infections there has plateaued since 1996 – the start of generic manufacturing there.

Brazil's early success was trumpeted in a New York Times Magazine *cover story that, overnight, seemed to change world opinion away from despair to hope.[2] In the ensuing three-year period, world leaders have flocked to Brazil and its state manufacturing plants to see the miracle up close. Brazil's greater success, to many, lies not only in its technical prowess at making cheap, high-quality drugs, but its commitment to universal health-care; and the chutzpah of its progressive leaders in taking on the big powers, namely the United States government and its allies in big pharma, as well as the legal hawks at the World Trade Organization. Brazil is a member of the WTO, and has played a critical role in rallying other developing nations into a powerful voting bloc. In May 2003,*

Brazil won the $1 million Gates Award for Global Health for its national AIDS program.[3]

I went to Brazil shortly after this latest accolade. I wanted to see for myself how well the miracle was really working. I'd heard from activist friends that, despite many positive aspects, there were problems. What was hype and what was hopeful? Most importantly, was Brazil's model something less-developed countries could copy? What were its main ingredients? Could the model work for countries with different health systems? Political systems? On a global scale, did Brazil represent the exception or the rule?

In June 2003, an historic agreement took place in Washington between two odd allies: President Bush and President Luiz Ignacio Lula da Silva, Brazil's charismatic, radical former labor leader, known as "Lula." The duo agreed to assist in rolling out a national AIDS treatment program in two Portuguese-speaking African countries – first Mozambique, then Angola. The effort will rely on new partnerships among US, Brazilian and Lusophone African groups and institutions.[4]

Because of Brazil's success in pioneering AIDS treatment at home, it will oversee many details of these programs, including a transfer of technical knowledge in manufacturing generic antiretrovirals and overseeing their use in countries whose populace lacks adequate health-care. The programs are part of Bush's effort to spearhead AIDS treatment to the hardest-hit nations of Africa and the Caribbean through his five-year, $15 billion Presidential Emergency Plan for AIDS Relief (PEPFAR), announced in early 2003.

For Brazilians, the joint agreement is the sweetest victory to date in the ongoing global effort to provide universal access to AIDS care and anti-retrovirals, affecting some 30 million people living in Africa and other developing regions.

Until now, the US has been strongly allied with big pharma in a tooth-and-nail fight with Brazilian officials to prevent generic competition in the AIDS drug arena. In February 2001, the US government, under the Clinton administration, filed a complaint with the WHO to stop Brazil from making generic antiretrovirals from Indian raw materials, and threatened it with trade sanctions.[5] It made a similar move to try to stop South Africa. Before then, few knew the true cost of making AIDS drugs, priced at $10,000 annually in the US for a three-drug combination. Brazil's move

revealed this to be much more than the market price. After failing to negotiate drug discounts from multinational patent holders, Brazil, Thailand
and Cuba opted to manufacture generics.

For big pharma, what was at stake wasn't really the tiny AIDS market
in Africa – which represents only 1 percent of the billion-dollar AIDS
market – but the larger patent system. Makers of new products or processes
are now guaranteed a twenty-year market monopoly under a WTO
Agreement on Trade Related Aspects of Intellectual Property and Public
Health, or TRIPs. US trade officials feared that softening TRIPs' rules for
lifesaving HIV medicines in a pandemic would usher in generic competition for other products as well.[6] Undeterred, Brazil fought back, arguing
that Article 68 of Brazil's 1997 patent law allowed it to make generics to
address its national emergency.[7] These drugs are designed only for its
national AIDS program, not for export, and therefore do not break patents.

In 1990, Brazil, the second-most populous country in the western hemisphere, had an exploding AIDS epidemic – average survival period was less
than six months after a clinical diagnosis. Most citizens lacked access to
HIV tests and drugs. In 1993, the private Brazilian company Microbiologics began making generic AZT, and in 1994 the state did the same,
providing AZT free through its public health system. By 1997, public
laboratories were making ddC and d4T[8] and within two years other nucleosides were available. In 2000, indinavir – a protease inhibitor – was added
to the state mix, then nevirapine.

Brazil's estimated savings on these last two drugs alone are $80 million,
or 30 percent of total drug costs for that year. By the time of the US WTO
challenge in 2001, drug prices in Brazil had fallen by 70 percent. So had
AIDS deaths. The health system had saved $677 million, and freed up hos-
pital beds. Armed with such positive, cost-effective results, Brazil was cast
as a fiery David against the Goliath of greedy big pharma companies.

Four months after filing the complaint, the US dropped it.[9] Brazil continued to up the ante, threatening compulsory licensing to negotiate sharp
40 percent and 65 percent discounts on patented antiretrovirals from
Switzerland's Roche and US-based Merck. Then, in November, Brazil
helped broker a victory for developing countries at the then 142-nation
WTO Ministerial Conference in Doha, Qatar. A new ruling guaranteed
poorer nations facing national emergencies the right to practice parallel
importing or issue compulsory licenses to import or make generic drugs.

But the Doha agreement was only a partial victory, because of a clause that banned exports and required countries to develop the capacity to manufacture their own generics – something they all lack. In 2002 WTO members again failed to resolve the country-capacity issue. Although thirty-one countries have adopted Brazil's treatment and prevention guidelines, the Doha clause has effectively prevented the world from following its lead on generics.

Before Doha, world leaders were converging almost weekly on Brazil's state-run generics factory, Far-Manguinhos in Rio de Janeiro, eager to discuss technology and how to apply the model back home. But aside from Thailand's and Cuba's state programs, not a single country, other than tiny neighboring Guyana, has moved to adopt Brazil's model of generic production, though they still hope to. A major barrier, claim Brazilian officials, is the threat of US trade sanctions.

"Why has no country adopted this? We need the agreement of countries," said Paolo Teixeira, the outspoken head of the Brazilian Ministry of Health's AIDS program, in June 2003. [At that time, Teixeira was preparing to join the WHO and was in line for the job of directing the agency's global 3×5 effort, a position he assumed months later.[10]] "We can only say that some countries have tried to consider this and stopped with fear of pressure from the United States." Threatening to withhold foreign aid is an effective weapon against very poor countries, he noted.

It's not an idle threat either. The Bush administration has shown itself willing to cut both critics and allies off when they challenge its policies. In July, the Bush administration suspended military assistance to thirty-five countries because they refused to exempt Americans from prosecution before the International Criminal Court.[11]

The Pressure to Export

US opposition isn't the only reason for the global reluctance to produce generics. The reality is that making quality antiretrovirals is neither cheap nor easy, even for richer countries. It requires a substantial investment, an industrial manufacturing base, and technical manpower. Aside from Brazil, Thailand and Cuba's state programs, only a half-dozen private companies in India and China have this capacity. And very few are producers of the raw materials or "active pharmaceutical ingredients" used to make antiretroviral pills.[12]

Subsequently there's been a growing international demand on Brazil to export not just its technical knowhow, but its high-quality drugs. But even with possible approval from the WTO, that won't be easy. Brazil still imports 80 percent of its raw materials from India, which is costly. "Many drugs could be produced in Brazil and a large number are not under patents," said Dr. Norberto Rech,[13] head of the government technology division, which oversees drug development for the public sector. "The problem here is the absence in investment in the basic chemistry industry that would generate these raw materials." Current domestic antiretroviral production, he said, "is insufficient to meet national needs."[14]

Six of seventeen public laboratories now produce fifteen AIDS drugs, and Brazil hopes to add four more by 2005, including new "fixed-dose" combinations,[15] and soon, new fixed-dose combination pills for TB and malaria. There are four production plants, including Far Manguinhos, which produces 40 percent of Brazil's generics, including nine different antiretroviral combinations.

As of July 2003, Brazil was buying thirteen other antiretrovirals from private companies, nine of which were imported. A single imported brand-name drug – Roche's Viracept (nelfinavir) – consumed 27 percent of the AIDS drug budget. Together with Merck's Sustiva (efavirenz) and Abbott's Kaletra (lopinavir), these three drugs accounted for almost two thirds of the budget.[16] Brazil has developed generic versions of these drugs and has threatened to produce them if the companies do not lower their prices for the brand-name products. "If we don't reach a deal, we will use the licenses in a compulsory way," declared Health Minister Humberto Costa.[17] Negotiations began in August to determine the outcome. Ironically, Abbott is also the biggest maker of local generics in Brazil, according to Brazilian sources. Private companies are also stepping up their activities. Aside from Microbiologica, both Labogen and Cristalia produce antiretrovirals.

Scaling Up Manufacturing

At Far-Manguinhos, there is a lot of activity. The now-famous state manufacturing plant is located in an odd place: smack in the middle of a forested park, surrounded by other buildings that belong to Fio Cruz, the biggest Latin American producer of pharmaceuticals. Fio Cruz is often compared with the National Institutes of Health, and has two hospitals (one that delivers health-care, the other devoted to research) and units devoted to biologics, organic synthesis, medicines, natural products and pharmacology, a vaccine factory, and Far-Manguinhos, its technical unit. Far-Manguinhos has a production branch and a research and development branch, but only produces for the Ministry of Health. A new director, Nubia Boechat Andrade, MD, recently came on board from the development department at GlaxoSmithKline. She has quickly lured many private industry talents to the public system, partly because wages are now equal in both sectors.

Like all drug manufacturers, Far-Manguinhos is regulated by MVISA, Brazil's federal regulatory agency. Its antiretrovirals have also been evaluated by the Pan American Health Organization, which gave its approval of their quality.

Brazil's domestic regulatory drug agency has approved the quality of its state-produced antiretrovirals. But to date the WHO has not conducted any quality-control inspections of the public factories or laboratories, a critical step for a drug to be included on that agency's list of approved drugs. Right now, Far-Manguinhos officials are busy repeating bioequivalancy tests on existing antiretrovirals – a move mandated by the government – and they anticipated a WHO inspection in late 2003. The bioequivalency tests show how well a generic drug compares to a brand-name drug. Although Rech and Teixeira dismiss talk of pill exports, to an outsider it looks like Brazil is getting ready should the global call come.

"We will not break patents," insisted Teixeira in an interview in June 2003.

> We are focusing on the transfer of technology. Our question now is concentrated on how to solve the Doha resolution for developing countries without capacity or production. We are trying to get the WTO to adopt one resolution, for example, where Paraguay can adopt compulsory licensing and ask Brazil to produce, as a way of overcoming these barriers.

With Bush pushing his new international AIDS agenda, Teixeira said, there are hints the US may now accept such a ruling. But critics say even that revision won't do the trick, since countries would still lack political muscle to issue compulsory licenses for generic imports.

While awaiting the WTO's decision, Brazil has invested $1 million to set up ten pilot national antiretroviral production plants – five in Latin America and the Caribbean and five in Africa. It is working closely with the WHO to develop these proof-of-concept projects. Teixeira, a tough negotiator, is also helping the WHO's new Director General, Dr. Jong Wook Lee, in the agency's goal of treating 3 million people by 2005. In May 2003, Teixeira began drafting a global treatment blueprint modeled after Brazil's example. Two months later, Lee named him officially to head the agency's 3×5 effort. By then, Brazil was moving to transfer technology and send teams from Far-Manguinhos to train technicians in Guyana and Mozambique. The new Bush–Lula agreement is part of this new era of cooperation.

"We will use this as a kind of approval of the Brazilian policy," said Teixeira of the joint US–Brazil venture.

> We are putting this out publicly as a sign from the WHO, the new administration, and officially the American government – after some hesitation – that they have presented their support to me. We are going to use it, because we understand it is not easy to spend this money [$15 billion]. They will need help from WHO, from Brazil, from the NGOs.[18]

Mobilizing Civil Society

With the spotlight on Brazil, the question remains: How useful is its much-vaunted AIDS model for poorer countries? After all, generics are only part of its successful formula. The national AIDS program was built upon a decentralized, unified health system that offers free drugs and care to all Brazilians. It links prevention to care and treatment, and favors innovative campaigns and strategies. The government not only distributes condoms widely, but helps finance a condom factory in the Amazon rainforest using latex harvested from live rubber trees. It backs explicit safer sex campaigns in the media and has extended AIDS education to primary public schools, within a general health and sex education curriculum. Although Brazil has tough laws against illegal drug use, the government supports harm reduction and rehabilitation programs for addicts. Such progressive policies reflect a general openness in Brazilian society to subjects like sexuality and hard drug use that are more taboo elsewhere. Across Brazil today, AIDS awareness is high.

According to Teixeira, the national program reflects the mobilization of a broad sector of civil society and NGOs, who, from early on, viewed the AIDS battle through a civil and human-rights lens. These rights are important to a society that has recently undergone re-democratization. In 1988, Brazilians ousted a twenty-year military dictatorship and drafted a new constitution, then adopted a universal health system. In 1991, universal access to antiretrovirals began. A year later, Brazilians got rid of another president accused of dipping into the national coffers. Political engagement by gay activists and civil society spilled over to AIDS. Today, a handful of early activists, including Teixeira, hold key positions in the government AIDS programs.

"The AIDS program as a whole works very well, and I'm very supportive of that, but I always like to repeat, it is so because we were there first," explained Ezio Tavora dos Santos Filho, director of Grupo Pela Vidda (For Life), an AIDS NGO in Rio de Janeiro. He met me at the organization's small but bright office, and quickly provided a thumbnail history of the AIDS movement, in which he has played a very active role. An openly gay, HIV-positive man in his early forties, Dos Santos Filho can testify to a difficult battle: "The community activists were there before to push the government to do something. People were dying like flies," he told me, his voice still angry. "We just hated the government. If I went to any hospital to say I had AIDS, they would put me out the door." Homophobia, he and other activists assert, was behind Brazil's initially slow response to the epidemic, and drove them to seek legal means to address discrimination.

The role played by the church is also different in Brazil than elsewhere in Latin America. Around 75 percent of Brazilians are Catholics, but many belong to a progressive wing of the church that includes radical liberation theologians dedicated to helping the poor. This progressive wing has openly supported the government's AIDS prevention efforts, and countered the opposition of a minority of conservative Catholics and evangelical Protestant groups who have sought to block sex education aimed at gay men, condom distribution or needle exchange programs for drug users – all hallmarks of prevention programs targeted at high-risk communities.

An Encouraging Picture

As of July 2003, there were 600,000 Brazilians with HIV – half the number predicted a decade earlier. Of these, 250,000 were receiving care, and 130,000 got antiretrovirals – most of them three-drug regimens. Nationally, seventy diagnostic laboratories are used to measure viral load and T-cell tests three times a year, for those on therapy. Officially, anyone who tests positive and registers with the public health system qualifies for free drugs and care. The program also provides prophylactic antiretrovirals for pregnant women and health workers in case of accidental exposure to HIV.

The latest national results remain very positive, showing Brazilians with AIDS continue to benefit from therapy with quickly restored health and a return to productivity. Most patients on therapy are now treated on an out-patient basis, boosting their quality of life and saving the health system money.

A recent study documented the dramatic increased survival rate of adult AIDS patients in Brazil due to treatment.[19] "Median survival was five months for cases diagnosed in the 1980s, 18 months for those diagnosed in 1995, and 58 months for those diagnosed in 1996," reported Jose Ricardo Pio Marins, MD, and colleagues from the University of Campinas in Sorocaba, Brazil. The study tracked 3,930 randomly selected adult AIDS patients from Brazil's seven regions who were diagnosed in 1995 and 1996, as antiretrovirals were being introduced, and followed them for five years. Treatment was the main predictor of survival. "It is the first time a study has demonstrated that universal free access to triple antiretroviral therapy in a developing country can produce benefits on the same scale as in richer countries," Marin said.[20] He noted, however, that too few Brazilians had been tested.

Also, most adhere very well to their regimens. An April 2003 survey reported a 6.6 percent rate of resistance among newly diagnosed HIV cases in Brazil – far lower than similar figures for resistance in the US (15 percent–26 percent), Britain (14 percent), Spain (23 percent–26 percent) or neighboring Argentina (15.4 percent).[21] Some resistance was expected in Brazil, since suboptimal AZT monotherapy and dual-nuke regimens were used there before 1995 and 1996, when protease inhibitors were introduced. But it's good news because it shows that poverty or lack of infrastructure – which critics still cite as reasons to withhold treatment from poor countries – don't automatically spell drug resistance.

On the downside, drug side-effects such as lipodystrophy, a metabolic disorder that causes a disfiguring redistribution of body fat, are a growing problem. The rates are not as high as in the US or Western Europe, but are still a cause for concern, said Teixeira. Yet here again, Brazil has shown its humane side, helping those with severe lipodystrophy regain an appearance of health by covering the costs of facial cosmetic surgery or liposuction.

Unfinished Business

The generally rosy picture in Brazil tends to obscure the gaps. But there are limits to the programs' success, and they reflect serious challenges to this huge country, where so many live in poverty, particularly those in rural areas, and indigenous groups in the Amazon. "It's very important to remember that we made a lot of progress but we didn't solve the situation absolutely," stated Teixeira. "I can say we have some major problems considering access and prevention. I fear they will not be solved in five years, particular those dependent on the economic situation of the country."

Another challenge is testing. About 20 percent of Brazil's population has now been tested for HIV – an impressive achievement in a country of 170 million. But that still leaves four out of five citizens who don't know their serostatus. The government is pushing to increase voluntary testing rates, particularly in pregnant women; only half now get tested. As Teixeira admitted, "That's unacceptable."[22]

"There's a general impression that there is a lag of access to care for [HIV-positive] women," said Bettina Durovni, a physician in charge of transmissible diseases at the city department of health in Rio de Janeiro.[23] Some 20,000 HIV patients access drugs and care from sixty-one public clinics in the city. "Some of this impression comes from mortality data, since the impact of antiretrovirals on mortality was sharper in men," added Durovni. "It's a mix of things, including underdiagnosis, because not everybody thinks of AIDS in women as easily as they do in men. This is something that we are trying to overcome with prevention and counseling projects, giving special attention to pregnant women."[24] In her clinic, pregnant women offered HIV testing often accept it. Those who test positive are usually given prophylactic AZT, though other drugs like nevirapine may be offered to women with severe anemia, since AZT can cause anemia.

"The main problem is that the health attention for women is not good as a whole," she explained. "We still have high mortality rates for pregnancy because of other causes like bleeding, and complications from C-sections." Although a high percentage of pregnant women do access health services, they don't get the care they need. "I would say that coverage is good, like 85 percent to 90 percent in Rio," she added of the percentage of city women accessing services. "The thing is not the coverage, but the quality. We have some studies that showed even if a woman has six visits, she still has syphilis at the end of the pregnancy." Although she views the national AIDS program as very strong, the quality of care may falter when HIV patients are referred to other programs or branches of the municipal health system. "This is a complex issue," she admitted, adding that physicians need training to better respond to women's health needs.

That said, she feels there is a high level of awareness of HIV among women in Brazil. "Many surveys have shown that. But between knowledge and attitude – that is where we have to work." She noted that although women are aware of the risks of contracting HIV, they still might not be able to negotiate condom use – a universal problem for women worldwide. "Many women can't protect themselves," Durovni stated. The AIDS program does distribute female condoms to specific populations, including commercial sex workers, but distribution is limited. Few women use them, "because they are expensive," she explained.

"The main population who are not getting treatment are those people who don't know they are HIV-positive," explained Durovni. "So it's important that we extend testing for people. Of course it is still difficult to reach some populations like drug users. They are very poor people who can't leave their communities because of violence or drug trafficking. So we are starting special programs with outreach workers."

Prisoners are another group lagging behind in access to testing and treatment. An estimated 15 percent to 20 percent of the total prisoner population of 200,000 is HIV-positive. But conditions inside are terrible, said Teixeira. There is severe overcrowding and inadequate facilities to provide care and drugs for inmates with HIV or AIDS. Meanwhile, violence and male rape are serious problems that also spread HIV inside the prisons.

Dr. Estevao Portelo Nunes is an infectologist (infectious disease specialist) and one of three doctors who follow 1,500 HIV patients at the Botafogo public clinic in Copacabana, a Rio suburb. The clinic is among the largest in the state for HIV clients. Half the clients are gay men, a quarter are women; there are few drug users. Another 1,500 HIV patients attend the clinic to pick up their medicine but are followed by private doctors. Around twenty to thirty patients attend the clinic each day. Generally, it takes only a week for a patient to obtain a clinic appointment.

Like Durovni, he praises the national AIDS program, but admits there are gaps when patients must be referred to other programs for services. His clinic, for example, has enough medicine to treat most HIV-related illnesses, but sometimes a referral is needed to a specialist or hospital. "The public hospitals are very deficient these days," he acknowledged. "This is hard because they are full most of the time, there is no room for patients — even the emergency room is not easy. So the patients come to the door and they can't enter. If they get in, they can get free medication."

According to Dr. Nunes, the AIDS program is working well, but adherence is an area where there is a continued need for counseling and follow-up.

> When we start antiretroviral therapy we always have the discussion about adherence and we schedule the patient for the next two weeks to make sure everything is okay with the [drug] schedule. It's important for them to understand that if they don't take the drugs correctly, it will fail and other antiretroviral therapies will be less efficient.

Unfortunately, they lack enough staff to send someone to a patient's home if they don't show up for a follow-up appointment. Patients miss follow-up appointments for a variety of reasons, he said, including "social problems, psychological reasons, a lack of money, or perhaps they are living too far away from here and they don't have the money to travel." A number of patients come from small towns some distance from Copacabana. "They can get drugs where they are but they don't like to," Nunes added, saying patients feared disclosure of their HIV status back home.

To date, the main opportunistic infection in patients at the Botafogo clinic is PCP pneumonia, with a high number of cases of toxoplasmosis. The latter is common in patients with later-stage HIV illness.

Nunes also noted a new problem in Brazilian patients: Kaposi's sarcoma (KS), the purplish skin lesions that became the hallmark of AIDS in US patients during the early years of the epidemic. "A few years ago, KS stopped and we weren't dealing with it anymore," Nunes explained. "We are seeing a surprising number of cases of KS, which is beginning to reappear even with a CD4 T-cell count that is not so low – above 200." In his clinic, three patients have turned up with KS in the last six months. "I talked to some other doctors here in Brazil and they agreed [they are seeing it too]."

The reason for a resurgence of KS there isn't known, he added. It is a cancer linked to human herpesvirus 8, or HHV-8, and is generally associated with immunosuppression in HIV patients. Although it appears on the skin, it also affects internal organs, and can lead to death if untreated.

A Rural Gap

For their part, AIDS activists contend that universal access to care exists on paper, but in reality varies depending on geography. "Officially, what the government says is that everybody who needs medicine is on therapy – it's not true," said Dos Santos Filho.[25] "If you are sick and you are not in Rio or São Paolo or a major city, it will take a while to get your drugs. There is no medicine on the shelf of the pharmacy of the public health center; there is medicine for a number of people who are registered. For new cases, it can take months."

For rural residents, Brazil's vast size can be fatal. "The only AIDS reference hospital in the state of Amazon is Manaus," stated Dos Santos Filho. "We saw cases of people who had to travel ten days to go to Manaus to get their treatment."

Finally, the decentralized funding structure of the health system has its limits. It has become easier to get antiretrovirals, but not other state-funded drugs for opportunistic infections, malaria, or hepatitis. "It's very inconsistent, because the majority of the twenty-seven states don't put a penny in," claimed Dos Santos Filho. "Malaria in this country is horrible. I met people who had malaria twelve times in Manaus, a city of 4 million people in the middle of the Amazon jungle. In February, there were 40,000 cases in an urban area."[26]

AIDS NGOs are now beginning to work with groups fighting TB and other diseases to bridge this gap. "For a long time, AIDS was seen as the rich cousin among diseases," said Ana Paola Prado of Arco Iris (Rainbow), an AIDS NGO in Brasilia. "Today, we are beginning the opposite movement – a true movement for social control of health as a whole."

Though imperfect, then, the Brazil model is a useful compass for others. It illustrates how spending money now can save money for governments later. Although increased HIV testing leads to a greater demand for treatment, Brazil's government estimates its AIDS program is helping the economy by saving hospital costs and loss of wages. While not all countries have universal health-care, or a comparable health infrastructure, its core tenets are available to all societies: a commitment to health as a civil right, and to upholding or passing laws that protect the most vulnerable citizens – gays, drug users, sex workers, street children – from discrimination. In Brazil, pro-democracy and AIDS activists, progressive church groups, bold congressional leaders, and talented health officials all played important roles. But the initial fight for life came from those who represent the biggest potential weapon in this battle: people with HIV and AIDS who took their battle to the streets and halls of justice and government, and made it universal.

That is the principal global lesson of the Brazil model. "The success of the Brazilian experience is because it was built by many hands," emphasized Prado. "We do not have the best model in the world, but our model answers the demands from Brazil."

PART II

All Around the World

4

TIPPING THE SCALES:
INDIA AND GENERIC DRUGS

Across Asia, the HIV epidemic has exploded quickly in many countries, including India, the most populous country in the world after China. The national government estimates that 4 million Indians have HIV, but the frontline doctors mock that figure, placing it closer to 10 or 12 million*. Unlike Thailand, where leaders acted quickly in the early 1990s to mount an effective national prevention campaign, one aimed especially at sex workers, India's nationalist Hindu government has been slow to respond. So have leaders in other Asian and western Pacific nations. Based on the rise of other sexually-transmitted diseases, WHO experts have warned political leaders in Burma, Laos, Vietnam, Malaysia, China, and the Philippines that, unless they act quickly, they may see the kind of catastrophe now facing India.[1] In many of these countries, HIV is linked to prostitution and to illegal drug use.

I went to India to visit the Indian generic companies that make antiretroviral drugs. I also wanted to meet with activists I knew who worked for the Lawyers Collective in Bombay, a leading NGO in the treatment access battle.[2] During the week I was there, political tensions were escalating across India between Hindu nationalists and Muslims, a recurring conflict.[3] These events demonstrate how the issue of religion still tears at the democratic fabric of secular India. In recent months, several bombings have rocked Mumbai and other cities, some attributed to Muslim extremist groups who are critical of India's close alliance with the Bush administration's War on Terror.[4]

---

*Information given throughout Part II is accurate as of December 30, 2003.

This was my first trip to India and a relatively brief one. So my observations about the epidemic in southern India represent only a snapshot from a country that is vast. One thing I observed immediately in Mumbai was the connection between social vulnerability, class status and HIV. A number of HIV-positive female sex workers I met identified themselves as "untouchables." Similarly, India has 500,000 to 1 million hijras, or eunuchs – transgendered individuals who are born male and adopt a female identity and social role; many are castrated. The hijras traditionally occupy a special role in Indian society and perform at weddings and births. But they also suffer from social discrimination. A majority work as prostitutes and HIV rates are very high in this population.[5] I was also surprised at the number of heroin users in Bombay who came from poor villages, including young girls.

At the time of my visit, the global AIDS debate was still fixed on the effectiveness of generic versus patented drugs. Around the world, many HIV doctors and NGOs were hoping to access low-cost generics, but wanted reassurance about their quality and efficacy. The big pharma companies claimed generics were of poor quality compared with their patented drugs. At the time, WHO officials had approved products from the pioneer, Cipla, but were avoiding any actions or statements that appeared to favor generics over brand-name drugs. I wanted to look at technical documents and tests related to their efficacy. I also wanted to find out how generic companies viewed their role, and which governments were visiting their factories to secure deals.

Before embarking, I spoke to experts at the Food and Drug Administration, the Centers for Disease Control and Prevention, the WHO, and watchdog groups like the Dutch-based International Dispensary Association, IDA, a wholesale distributor of essential medicines for non-profit organizations. These groups independently conduct quality control inspections of drug manufacturing plants and products, including generic producers. I wanted to know what to expect from a plant visit, and what to look for. These groups provided me with a long list of questions that focused on very technical details of chemical manufacturing, and highlighted such factors as drug purity, stability, absorption and other matters that they use to measure drug quality.

I visited three companies and toured their plants. Officials at Cipla, Hetero and Ranbaxy were generous with their time, and made available their chemists, managers, account ledgers and – most important to me – the log books of results of bioequivalence tests done on their new HIV pills. I was able to verify that these products had passed stringent quality control tests, and in many cases had been independently approved by outside laboratories and regulatory agencies in other countries that are equivalent to the US Food and Drug Administration.

At the same time, I wasn't naive about the motives behind generic drug manufacture: it's about money and business, the same interests driving the multinationals. Today's generic producers might be tomorrow's captains of industry, and in India some already are. Ultimately, what matters is how quickly needy individuals in poor countries get access to high-quality, low-cost, lifesaving anhtiretrovirals for HIV. The sad fact is that while generic anti-HIV drugs were saving lives in countries like Brazil, they had done little for local citizens who were desperate to survive. The government was claiming it couldn't afford generics, though activists from the Lawyers Collective pointed out that although India is poor, the government finds plenty of money to maintain troops in a state of alert along the Pakistan border.

Cipla Enters the Fray

Seen from the air, the sprawling port city of Mumbai (formerly Bombay) looks like a rough gray-and-brown patchwork. There are shiny, well-scrubbed areas like Malabar Hill with sleek high-rise hotels and designer boutiques, favored by Bollywood stars. Lying cheek-by-jowl with such extravagant wealth is a network of vast, dusty slums that spill into the surrounding countryside. Like New York City, Mumbai is a diverse, culturally dynamic Mecca that attracts many with the promise of money and fame.[6]

Since the early 1990s, Mumbai has also earned the unfortunate moniker, "AIDS capital of India." HIV infection itself has been dubbed "the Bombay plague" or "Mumbai disease." Over 250,000 city residents have HIV, including many of the city's 100,000 sex workers in its famed red light district, a dusty twelve-block area with 10,000 brothels.

It seems particularly fitting to find the corporate headquarters of Cipla Ltd, the now-famous Indian generic HIV drug manufacturer, located a stone's throw from the city's red light district. Cipla burst onto the world stage in February 2001 when its maverick president, a chemist named

Yusuf Hamied, offered a copycat three-drug anti-HIV regimen to poor African countries and aid groups like MSF at $360 a year, a thirtieth of the standard price.

The move tipped the scales in a high-pitched battle for global drug access being waged by AIDS activists and groups like MSF against the multinational pharmaceutical companies controlling drug patents. These companies denounced Cipla's act as a threat to the international patent system that makes pharmaceutical research possible. They also warned that Indian knockoffs were likely to be of poor quality, and would contribute to drug resistance across Africa and Asia.

Undeterred, Hamied defended his company's reputation and his action as perfectly legal under a 1970 Indian Patent Act, which protects the patents on drug-making processes but not on the final product. Indian companies can create alternative manufacturing steps to copy patented drugs, and then legally sell those drugs in India. They can also export their products to countries or markets where no patents exist for them. Where compulsory licensing laws apply, the Indian manufacturers can apply to sell their generic versions of patented drugs, and pay a licensing fee to the patent holder. That market, it turns out, covers much of Africa, Asia, Latin America and Eastern Europe, but not the US and Western Europe. The drugs involved include medicines for life-threatening opportunistic infections as well as for HIV.

"What Cipla did was show everyone that the emperor had no clothes," stated Mumbai lawyer Anand Grover of the Lawyers Collective, an advocacy group working on AIDS drug access issues, in March 2002. "For years, the multinationals claimed it cost so much to make their AIDS drugs, and they were so hard to make. Now we know it's simply not true. The generics make these drugs for pennies, and they make other drugs too. So the secret is finally out. The truth is, the profits in this industry have been just staggering."

As Grover points out, the patent battle has revealed the real stakes involved. It is not really the African HIV market, which in fact represents only 1 percent of global HIV sales, but "their [the multinational brand-name companies'] hegemony in the multibillion-dollar global pharmaceutical industry." The international corporations worry that AIDS provides a wedge for foreign generic producers to gain legitimacy and a foothold in other markets.

It is a valid concern: Cipla, the third-largest generic drug maker in India at the moment, is an 87-year-old company with 1,023 generic products in 130 markets; its US marketing partner is Andrx. Cipla's eight HIV drugs are making money, but it sees bigger profits in the blockbuster drugs of the 1990s, like antidepressants, which are going off-patent soon. While HIV drugs have caught the world's attention, the Indian generic companies have made steady gains in major drug markets including the US, Germany, Britain, Brazil, China and Japan.[7]

As of early 2002, the HIV market for developing countries was roughly $2.2 billion in sales, at a low estimate. This number was based on a generic industry estimate of the number of people living with HIV outside the US and Western Europe – some 38 million – and the percentage who probably need antiretroviral treatment – around 15 percent, or 5.7 million. That number was then multiplied by the current generic HIV drug price of around $400 per person per year. If universal access is extended to people who want to begin therapy in order to stay healthy and avoid getting sick, the pie becomes much bigger.

Familiar Bedfellows

One of the richest ironies of the HIV drug war – and there are many – is that large multinationals generally accept the quality of products made by their Indian competitors. Outside of HIV, foreign generic companies, including those in India, have been supplying raw materials for drugs to brand-name producers for years. So what is labeled a brand-name, FDA-approved and patented pill in the US may begin life as a cheap generic.

Dehli-based Ranbaxy, for example, is the largest generic maker in India, and has moved into the HIV market. It has sold raw materials (called Active Pharmaceutical Ingredients or APIs) to Bristol-Myers Squibb for doxycycline, cefalexone and amoxycillin. The FDA has approved four Ranbaxy raw material plants in India. The company also has a manufacturing facility in New Jersey. As of 2002, it had concluded marketing pacts with GlaxoSmithKline for cefuroxime axetil, with Eli Lilly for a half-dozen generic pain products, and with smaller US companies like Penwest Pharmaceuticals and Wockhardt.

The closer one looks, the more the lines blur. The public fights over HIV patents and profits are certainly real, but "a lot of that is also for a consumer audience," explained Amar Lulla, Cipla's outspoken joint managing director, in 2002. "What we do among ourselves in the industry is another matter. If [the multinationals] have a problem, they can come to us and we will try to address it." Behind closed doors, Lulla said, the rivals work out disagreements. "They aren't interested in this [HIV] market. It is not commercially viable for them. They're not idiots to sell drugs at low prices like us," he quipped. Or as Hetero's Reddy put it frankly, "It's just business. That's what we all have in common."

And profits. Since the generic producers don't have to invest a lot of up-front money to develop the drugs, compared with brand-name makers, they spend less. They don't have to submit their products to years of costly testing in clinical trials. They also spend less on advertising than brand-name companies. The cost of labor in India is a lot less than in richer countries. That includes managers and chemists and the women from local villages near the drug company plants who are hired to pack generic drugs. All of these spell savings that are passed on to consumers in the form of cheaper drugs, but allow generic companies to make a decent profit by marking their products a bit higher than the base cost of production.

Given the potential profits in the world HIV market, there are plenty of reasons to anticipate "new strategic alliances," as Lulla calls current and future deals between the brand-name multinationals and generic competitors. Sir Richard Sykes, chairman of GlaxoSmithKline, recently admitted that the company was considering an alliance with a quality Indian producer in order to do low-cost clinical trials of its HIV products. He mentioned Ranbaxy and Dr. Reddy's Laboratories, another large Indian generic producer, as possible partners. Never mind that Sykes has lambasted the Indian biotechs in the media. Meanwhile, a daily rivalry exists between the Indian companies. "It's cutthroat competition," said Hetero's Reddy, smiling. "I can talk to you, but not with Cipla."

Seizing a Trade Window of Opportunity

In the past, developing countries traditionally excluded food and medicine from intellectual property laws to ensure they would be accessible and affordable by keeping them out of monopoly control. But the lure of globalization and profits has caused a change in global policy. Many middle-income countries like India, as well as poorer ones, now belong to the World Trade Organization, a global body that was set up in 1994 in a meeting called the Uruguay Round. The WTO has been given final authority to rule on patent, copyright and other laws related to global imports and exports of commercial products, including pharmaceuticals.

The WTO established the Agreement on Trade Related Aspects of Intellectual Property (TRIPs), which seeks to reconcile disparate national laws governing each WTO member country, and bring their patent, trademark and copyright protections up to a uniform global standard that reflects a higher US standard. The process is called "harmonization", and in theory, it should benefit consumers by providing a guarantee of food and drug safety. Under TRIPs, pharmaceutical companies will enjoy a minimum twenty-year monopoly for patents on their brand-name drugs, allowing them to block the entry of generic competitors.

And corporations have found clever loopholes to extend their patent protection on products. When patents are about to expire, they tweak formulations, or seek "second-medical-use" patents, or file patent infringement lawsuits against potential generic rivals which, in the past, has bought an automatic extension of twenty to twenty-four months in the US and Canada to delay generic competition.[8] Generic competitors can also be complicit by colluding with big pharma to keep generic products off the market.

It wasn't always so. India's parliament refused to implement TRIPs in the 1994 Uruguay Round. Later that year, India's prime minister issued an Executive Decree that enacted TRIPs rules on pharmaceutical and agricultural chemical patents, but both houses of parliament fought it. India's Patent Act stayed firmly in place. It bans patents for substances "intended for use, or capable of being used, as food or as medicine or a drug." Its laws mandated that India's Patent Office refuse any applications for patents on non-patentable substances.

The US challenged India, taking its complaint to the WTO, which ruled in September 1997 that India had to establish some statutory procedures for receiving applications on patents so that, come 2005, when the new TRIPs law goes into effect, patents can be backdated to the day of filing. India balked at that. In March 1999 the Indian parliament finally reached an agreement with the WTO. Drug companies can file for patents before 2005, but that does not guarantee that patent applications they submit while it is still illegal to do so will be reviewed or accepted after 2005, when patent laws go into effect.

Clearly, the big drug companies have India's huge consumer market in mind as they prepare for the day the lid comes off. Big pharma companies have been hiring Indian lawyers specialized in intellectual property to scour India's patent laws, looking for opportunities and new markets that will break open in 2005. As have their generic rivals, who are rushing to manufacture, introduce – and prepare to register for patent – as many generic drugs as possible by the 2005 WTO deadline. When I remarked to Cipla's Lulla that the upstarts were becoming the establishment, he smiled.[9] Suddenly, patent protection is all the rage in India. For Indian consumers, the news is less positive. The move to a universal standard under the WTO is likely to spell increased prices of drugs (and food and other products) as generic competition ends and the patent holders enter the market with a monopoly on their higher-priced products.

WTO member countries must change their intellectual property laws to conform to TRIPs by 2005 – India included. But "Least Developed Countries" (LDCs) have a ten-year extension – till 2016 – instead of 2006, to implement patent protection in conformity with WTO rules.

The Doha Declaration

The conflict over HIV generics reached a peak at the November 2002 WTO meeting in Doha, Qatar, when the then 142-member body issued the Doha Declaration on Public Health. The agreement allowed countries to override drug patents under certain circumstances through compulsory licensing. By issuing a compulsory license, governments can suspend a pharmaceutical company's exclusive marketing rights so that others can also produce the drug by paying a royalty to the patent holder. This opens the door to public and private generic manufacturing, and ultimately lower prices. But compulsory licensing can only be used to manufacture drugs for "predominantly" domestic consumption, and not for export markets.

Furthermore, the Doha Declaration requires developing countries to establish a local manufacturing base if they wish to import or make generic drugs; it has no provision allowing export of these drugs. Since most countries lack an infrastructure for producing drugs, they can't easily take advantage of the generics option. Paragraph 6 of the Doha Declaration rec-ognized this contradiction, and called for resolution of the issue by the end of 2002 – a deadline long passed, despite several attempts at negotiation. Doha's failure to cover exports, declared Lulla, "is a complete eyewash and there is no gain. Not allowing exports is a major deterrent."[10]

The Doha Declaration created a catch-22 situation: if producer coun-tries like India, Brazil, and Thailand cannot export generics, poorer and smaller countries without domestic generic industries have no source for drug imports. Like India, these countries must also bring their intellectual property laws into alignment with TRIPs by 2005 or face potential trade sanctions.

"For Africa and Latin America, there is hardly anybody with capability to produce finished product," explained Ranbaxy senior vice-president Bimal K. Raizada, who oversees global marketing for the company, in March 2002.[11]

Even when allowed to export, generic companies must register their products in each country and market, something that can take many months and a lot of bureaucratic red tape. "The country-by-country appli-cation process is very time consuming," explained Hetero Drugs' director of global and domestic marketing, M. Srinivas Reddy. As he noted, many governments are not on top of their own patent applications and may not have enough experts trained in intellectual property or trade law to approve generic drug applications.[12]

Local Rivals

While Cipla highlighted needs in Africa, several other rival Indian drug companies quietly entered the race, focusing their attention on South America and Southeast Asia. As of early 2002, Cipla had an edge as the leading exporter of finished products (FP) for HIV to forty countries, including much of Africa, the Caribbean and Southeast Asia. But other companies, like Hetero, were making a lot of money selling the active phar-maceutical ingredients, or APIs, for antiretrovirals.

Domestically, Ranbaxy captured one sixth of domestic generic HIV pre-scription sales in 2002; the rest mostly went to Cipla. But Ranbaxy was also competing well globally. It was the first to export APIs to Brazil, and claimed $12 million in sales of bulk indinavir to that country in 2002. The company was spliting a tender with Cipla to supply anti-HIV drugs to 10,000 Nigerian patients. Ranbaxy also has partners in China, a huge exporter of raw materials, and had begun marketing a generic hepatitis-B drug there.

Hetero Drugs is an aggressive Hyderabad-based company that makes heart and antidepressant medicines, and had eight HIV products as of March 2002. With $12 million in sales of raw materials used to make AIDS drugs in Brazil and $26 million to Argentina in 2002, it was the leader in the overall market. By comparison, Cipla's total antiretroviral sales that year were no more than 20 percent of Hetero's, according to figures compiled by Hetero.

Another newcomer, Aurobindo Pharma, has several finished drugs being marketed in India. Aurobindo is chasing Hetero for a share of the "bulk actives" market, as APIs are also called, by offering low prices. In 2002 its manufacturing plants and products were being reviewed by the WHO for global export, as were Hetero's. Sun Pharma was recently rated the fastest-growing pharmaceutical company in India; it also manufactures bulk APIs. Others in the game in 2002 included well-reputed Zydus-Cadila, along with Torrent Pharma, RPF Life, Micro Labs, Sol Pharma, FDC, Pure Health Products, East India and Kopran.[13] Dr. Reddy's Laboratories, a large, established company, was rumored to be considering entry into the HIV market.

Other Products

In addition to manufacturing HIV drugs, the companies are making forays into HIV diagnostics and herbal drugs, and are moving into R&D for new HIV drugs. Ranbaxy initially sold low-cost T-cell and viral load tests through a partnership with Specialty Labs that proved difficult; it then began producing its own kits.

Beyond the Indian companies, generic rivals have been emerging in a dozen other countries, including Brazil, Egypt, China and Thailand. They are poised to keep competition healthy, although only a few companies now produce high-quality APIs. The Brazilian and Thai governments pioneered the use of Indian generics in national treatment programs involving thousands of patients, and imported Indian technical knowhow. Brazil now makes its own HIV pills using Indian source material, as does Argentina. Elsewhere in the region, manufacturers in Mexico, Cuba, Costa Rica and Peru are planning to make pills from Indian raw goods. The regulatory agencies in several countries have independently reviewed Indian factories and products, providing outside proof of their laboratory quality and efficacy. The Asian countries of Cambodia, China, Indonesia and South Korea are importing and gearing up to produce their own drugs with Indian help.

In Africa, the governments of Uganda, Zimbabwe, Ivory Coast, Cameroon, Nigeria, Botswana, Kenya and Congo are moving fast to import pills and technical help from Indian producers, as are Ghana, Tanzania, Ethiopia and Sudan. Other African countries are also looking around for good deals. Several intend to manufacture the drugs using bulk-source APIs from India – or a cheaper competitor.

The situation is finally changing in AIDS-stricken South Africa, where President Thabo Mbeki has long been publicly opposed to the importation and use of HIV drugs – brand-name or generic.[14] Ironically, Mbeki signed a cooperative agreement with Fidel Castro in March 2001 to jointly develop generic drugs. That occurred during the time when thirty-nine big pharma companies had filed a lawsuit against South Africa to prevent it from either making or licensing generic antiretrovirals. Cuba makes its own and has long-standing ties to South Africa (see Chapter 5).

GlaxoSmithKline, which was one of the plaintiffs in the later-withdrawn lawsuit against South Africa, recently assigned a compulsory license to a local generic manufacturer, Aspen Pharmacare, to sell versions of AZT and 3TC. This will effectively block Indian competition – except that Hetero will supply the ingredients. In a counter-move, Brazil's state-owned Far Manguinhos, which makes HIV drugs from Hetero's raw materials, recently shipped anti-HIV medicines for fifty patients in MSF's South African clinics.

Quality is the Sticking Point

The brand-name drug companies have argued that manufacturing standards are lower in India and other developing countries, and that corruption is a huge problem. Product quality is not an idle concern, since generic manufacturers make money by cutting corners to keep costs low. Although

Cipla, Hetero and Ranbaxy all have excellent industry reputations, the fact remains that a thriving, unregulated gray market exists in India for many products, including medicines.

"Quality is an issue all of us are and must be concerned about," admitted Hetero Drugs' Reddy. "There are different standards in this industry, as with all industries. We realize there are many people who are unfamiliar with our products and need to be reassured."

The key data set used to evaluate the quality and efficacy of a generic drug is something called a biological equivalence (BE) study, which is typically done in twenty-four to thirty-six healthy volunteers, according to WHO guidelines. The BE test must show that the generic compound is equivalent to the FDA-approved brand-name or innovator drug, meaning that it affects the body in the same way. To be considered bioequivalent, a generic product must yield maximum and average blood levels that lie between 80 percent and 125 percent of the brand-name drug.

Bioequivalence studies typically cost several thousand dollars in India, and take from several weeks to months to complete. But this is nothing compared with the testing a new drug goes through before US marketing approval.[15]

In mid March 2002 the Indian companies celebrated another victory when the WHO issued its long-awaited list of approved drugs for HIV, and included Cipla's HIV products for the first time. Since none of the other Indian companies had yet been inspected by the agency, Cipla was able to extend its edge over rivals for a little while.

For Cipla, the WHO endorsement was bittersweet. Just days before the WHO announcement, Cipla officials in Mumbai were openly complaining that the agency was deliberately delaying public approval of their HIV drugs. "Do you think the WHO is exempt from the influence of the multinationals? Not at all. It's all political," declared Lulla hotly. "They keep saying they want proof. But we've given it. They analyzed our products. Our plants have been inspected." Frustrated, he added that the brand-name multinationals had "tried every trick in the book to say, 'Hey, Cipla isn't quite, you know, up to snuff.'"

In Lulla's view, WHO officials went the extra mile to review Cipla products and found no problems, but refused to say so publicly for a long time. "In their talks with us, they keep saying there is so much politics and please do not push us to make a statement," Lulla said. Now that the agency has given its thumbs-up, Lulla is mollified, but his views about the deeply political nature of the battle have not changed.

Soon the Indian companies hope to offer clinical proof of the efficacy of their drugs in patients, something Brazil has publicly documented.[16]

Developing New Manufacturing Processes

In India, HIV medicines are made in a process called reverse engineering, to avoid the patents that cover how a brand-name drug is manufactured. Chemists trace back the complex steps, or chemical reactions, used to make a given molecule, and substitute these to produce the same final product. Each alternative reaction can introduce impurities or be hazardous. It takes trial and error and very experienced technicians to get the process right. "In terms of reverse engineering, the only advantage is that the drug has been clinically tried and evaluated in trials by the multinationals. But everything else we have to start from scratch," said Reddy of Hetero Drugs.

Compared with antibiotics, which require five to six chemical reactions and a production cycle of around fifteen days, HIV antiretrovirals may involve up to twenty stages and a production cycle of thirty-five to seventy-five days. "Our own experience is that each molecule is hard because it has a different chemistry," said Reddy. "The larger the time cycle, the more the problems involved in that manufacturing process." Over time, Indian companies have become more adept at using fewer steps to make the drugs. That has led to reduced costs for consumers.

According to Reddy, the Hetero team found that nucleoside analog drugs like 3TC, d4T and AZT are "relatively quick and easier to make than protease inhibitors, which have long time cycles." Some aspects of manufacturing are more dangerous for certain drugs, namely nevirapine and 3TC. "We have to do it proficiently with so much caution," he said about 3TC. "In other products like ritonavir, the time is long, but there aren't the same hazards as with lamivudine [3TC] and nevirapine."

A surprise was efavirenz (Sustiva). "It is a most difficult process," Reddy explained, getting technical. "We use butyl lithium [a catalyst]. If things are fine, only the good reaction will come. If there is some small variation due to some mistake . . . the explosion will be venomous." So far, so good, he remarked there haven't been any explosions in Hyderabad.

Once the BE studies are ready, the Indian companies contract outside laboratories to review them and submit the results to regulatory agencies, including the WHO and the US Food and Drug Administration. If an inspection turns up a shortcoming, the companies are given a period of time to correct the problem.

Since the global HIV market calls for companies to market the cheapest drugs possible, they are all making and testing nucleoside analogs first, then putting them into double- and triple-combination tablets. Up to now, the third drug has been nevirapine, which has turned out to be especially inexpensive. Indinavir is the cheapest protease inhibitor to copy, so it has been the most popular generic protease inhibitor.

The result of this strategy is a number of generic non-protease drugs and new "fixed-dose" combination pills that are effective as alternatives for first-line therapy in treatment-naive patients, following the WHO guidelines. The companies are planning to make more fixed-dose pills that are easier for patients to adhere to, since they spell fewer pills and an easier daily regimen. These combinations have not been tested in clinical trials, though – something the WHO is hoping to do in the future.

"Strategic Alliances" with the Brand-Name Multinationals

Quality control is a continual process after the equivalence studies are complete and manufacturing begins. Indian generic drugs come under the purview of several regulatory agencies, notably the Drug Controller General of India (DCGI), which approves new drugs for the domestic market, and the CDIR, an Indian authority over bulk drugs. Foreign regulatory bodies such as the FDA also inspect plants that export to their countries. The main seal of approval for the companies is an inspection certificate of Good Manufacturing Practice (GMP), which shows their plants and other operations are up to industry standards. The drug companies then do regular testing of the individual products as they are manufactured, and randomly test samples taken from warehouses and pharmacy shelves.

The competitive need for companies to keep their inventions secret from rivals makes it harder for outsiders to analyze the Indian industry accurately, or to compare the various products to one another. All the companies – the brand-name multinationals included – regularly test their products against their competitors', yet the press and consumers never hear about it, or only selectively. "I can tell you that if some big company has a problem with one of our HIV products, they make sure the right people know," said Ranbaxy's Bimal Raizada, adding, "No one has. We are confident of their quality."

Nonetheless, independent auditing of the manufacturing process remains an important concern for consumers. The International Dispensary Association (IDA) is a non-profit organization based in the Netherlands that procures generic and essential drugs and provides an independent review of their quality for international agencies, including UN agencies. They are now developing a plan to procure and distribute HIV drugs to non-profit groups. According to IDA spokesperson Guido Bakker, "It's not that hard for a plant to get a GMP. They have their own people and labs. So you have to have outside laboratories that you can trust to review quality."[17] The IDA is initiating an independent inspection of the Indian companies, and has plans to distribute their generic products to non-profit and donor groups if the results are acceptable.

Extending Treatment Access around the Globe

Despite all this movement, not a lot of drugs are actually getting into bodies. According to a 2002 estimate by MSF, only 25,000 to 30,000 out of the 2.5 to 3 million Africans with HIV/AIDS had access to low-cost anti-HIV drugs from the brand-name companies through a much-touted Accelerating Access Initiative. The number receiving generic drugs is growing, but remains difficult to estimate. In 2002, it was still only in the tens of thousands, according to various company reports. Nearly every African and Asian government had sent a representative to visit Cipla or the other companies to shop for a good deal; but few have come through with the cash. Many were hoping that the United Nations' new Global Fund for AIDS, Tuberculosis and Malaria would help them buy the drugs. In late April 2002, the Fund announced it was granting $378 million to thirty-one poor countries, with nearly half the money going to drugs for HIV and AIDS. That opened the door for the purchase of generics, but the money is taking time to flow.

Of course, getting the money for generic purchases is only a small part of the battle. There is still a huge gap in terms of infrastructure to distribute anti-HIV medicines and use them properly in settings of poverty. Money is also urgently needed to educate doctors and community health workers about HIV disease, employ trained technicians in clinics and laboratories, buy HIV diagnostic tests and monitoring equipment, educate the general public about HIV, and counsel those who are affected.

While the multinationals invest big bucks to market their drugs and back clinical trials of their products, the generic companies have smaller budgets. In India, as in the US and elsewhere, drug company representatives lobby physicians and pharmacists to prescribe their drugs.[18] But they do little advertising direct to consumers compared with what is done in the US. "The drug companies deal with doctors, not HIV patients," explained Shashank Joshi, MD, an Indian doctor and HIV specialist who practises in Mumbai.

There are other reasons for delays in access. It takes years and millions of dollars for a developing country or even a private company to build a manufacturing capacity to make generic HIV drugs. Few countries are in a position to do that today, though several are considering it.

Brazil's experience shows how quickly the treatment train can move when a track has been laid. As a large country with a functioning economy, it had a decent public health-care infrastructure, as well as a large number of agencies ready to support a national AIDS treatment program. The government has committed major resources to educating a core of physicians and health technicians on the finer points of HIV management and monitoring. It initiated pilot treatment programs to see what worked and to pinpoint problem areas. Similarly, private companies took the lead in manufacturing generic medicines. Only then did the state-owned company, Far-Manguinhos, get involved. "We used to supply to small manufacturers in Brazil and Argentina," said Srinivas Reddy at Hetero Drugs. "They started with 50 to 100 kilogram batches in the initial lots. Now it's up to 200 to 500 kilogram lots."

Back in 1997, when Hetero began making generic 3TC, GlaxoSmithKline was selling the drug at $80,000 per kilogram, said Reddy. "We gave the Brazilian government the drug at $5,100 per kilogram. Now we sell it to them at $700, and we have been able to reduce costs further." The result has been huge savings for Brazil, something that has inspired other governments hoping to do the same.

Today, the transfer of technology and hands-on training is part of the package that all the Indian generic producers are selling to interested governments. These new business relationships will also help the companies market other drugs in these countries.

Waiting for the Global Fund

The Global Fund grants are likely to alter current consumption radically. Aside from India, Brazil and Argentina have been the largest users of generic drug ingredients and pills until now. In Africa, Uganda, Kenya, Nigeria and Cameroon have imported finished generic medicines for small national pilot programs. Up to now, MSF and Oxfam have been the main users among nongovernmental organizations, but here, too, the scale is small. Other private groups have started to use generics along with discounted brand-name drugs in small pilot projects in several countries. In Latin America, the Pan American Health Organization has traditionally been the main agency involved in helping countries to access essential medicines, and it is beginning to play a middle-man role in the HIV arena.

African private-sector use of generic drugs is scattered, but growing, though corporate use has been almost nonexistent. Anglo-American and Debswana, two mining giants in South Africa and Botswana, respectively, have announced plans to buy generic drugs and give them to some employees, as has Coca-Cola, the largest employer in Africa.

In Asia, private hospitals and AIDS centers have been the main users of generics, and it's not uncommon for private doctors with their own pharmacies to fly to India to fill their suitcases with bulk purchases of generic pills bought directly from the companies. The exception is Thailand, where a state-owned company produces generic antitretrovirals.

In India, anti-HIV drugs are readily available in major cities, but less so in rural areas. Around 100 Indian physicians were pioneering the use of the generic versions in 2002, and more are being trained to do so through educational seminars sponsored by the generic producers. Several drug companies have HIV clinics and centers where their products are distributed free. Around twenty-five NGOs distribute generic drugs, some for free. These agencies are also beginning treatment education for people with AIDS. "A year ago, only 1 percent of people [with HIV] were getting access to anti-HIV drugs; in private settings, it is now 6 to 7 percent," said Reddy in 2002.

At the time of my visit, the Indian government had no plan to buy or provide homemade generic HIV drugs to its citizens, despite pressure by activist groups like the Lawyers Collective. The government had announced a plan to use anti-HIV drugs to treat pregnant women in twenty-two infectious disease centers with designated AIDS wards – a first step. It also decided – after pressure by the generic drug companies and activists in India – to drop the excise tax on domestic HIV generics. That reduced retail HIV drug prices by 10 percent.

Still, AIDS activists in India are not impressed, and they spread the blame. "These companies like Cipla began making HIV drugs without providing educational materials for the public," complained attorney-cum-activist Vivek Diwan of the Lawyers Collective.[19] "Now there is a gap in terms of who's going to do the education, and we are left holding the bag. The government isn't going to do it. Don't the companies have some responsibility?" To its credit, Cipla launched a major HIV public education campaign that was hailed by activists, but Diwan says, "It's a drop in the bucket."

Globally, there are other complaints. Smaller donor agencies and community networks hoping to acquire Indian drugs report limited success. "We've tried for months to order them from Cipla and couldn't get anyone to answer our e-mails," said Richard Stern of Agua Buena, a Costa Rican AIDS advocacy group, in March 2002. His network wants to donate generic drugs to needy patients, which is technically legal, not to sell them. "The generic companies say they'll provide the drugs, but no one has been able to get them. People are dying as we wait for an answer," said Stern.[20]

The companies acknowledge that few organizations outside MSF have received drugs. One reason, contended Cipla's Lulla, is that "we are ignorant of who these agencies and patient groups are. We know MSF. We can't afford to just give the drugs away carelessly. And we can't break patents." For the record, officials at several companies said they were willing to sell drugs to licensed physicians and legitimate donor groups, as long as they received assurances the drugs would not be resold.

How quickly such words will be followed by action is anyone's guess. In April 2002 the physician-run Honduran AIDS Network happily reported that it had received its first batch of Cipla drugs. Bought directly from the company, the drugs took a few weeks to arrive.[21] They were then given free

of charge to very ill patients, and physicians in the network strictly monitored their use. With the United Nations agencies and groups like IDA
poised to act as middle-men, access could readily expand. "There is a learning curve because we are new to this whole area," Lulla admitted. "It's all
moved so quickly none of us can even keep up."

Many do not know that there is any progress to keep up with. Outside
Cipla's well-guarded entrance, the district sex workers pay no heed as they
pass by on their way to the brothels. For them, universal access to cheap
AIDS drugs remains somebody's dream, not – yet – their reality.

From India to the World: 2002–03

On August 19, 2003, southern Africa's largest generic drug manufacturer,
Aspen Pharmacare, announced a plan to produce a generic combination of
three HIV drugs that will sell for under $1 a day per person.[22] Aspen
launched the first generic antiretroviral drug manufactured in Africa earlier
in the month. Aspen-Stavudine is produced under an exclusive voluntary
license from Bristol-Myers Squibb, which markets stavudine (d4T) as
Zerit. With similar licenses from GSK and Boehringer Ingelheim, Aspen
submitted registration applications to the country's Medicines Control
Council for its generic versions of AZT, 3TC and Combivir (AZT/3TC), as
well as ddI and nevirapine.

The news comes on the heels of an historic August 8, 2003 decision by
President Thabo Mbeki's administration – which had long opposed the use
of antiretrovirals – to develop a national HIV treatment plan by October,
in the country with the worst AIDS epidemic in the world. The government recently applied for a grant from the Global Fund that would help
pay for treatment for some of South Africa's 5 million HIV-positive citizens, 600,000 of whom need antiretrovirals immediately.

This pivotal event reflects a major victory for AIDS activists from South
Africa's Treatment Action Campaign (TAC), who have long advocated the use
of generics in their campaign for HIV treatment. In one of the opening salvoes
of the drug access battle, TAC members illegally imported generic fluconazole from Thailand in 2000 to treat opportunistic infections. TAC recently
upped the ante by allying itself with frontline physicians to create the Generic
Antiretroviral Procurement Project (GARPP), a private company that will

act as a wholesale procurer of high-quality generics. GARPP's launch is a symbol of pent-up frustration over the continued delays in access to anti-retrovirals.

Generics at Last?

Spying a new market, Aspen said it hoped the government, UNAIDS and the Global Fund would be big customers for its new products. After months of stalemate and bitter disputes over the WTO block on exports, Aspen is now following leading Indian generic rivals like Cipla. So are about forty other companies around the world.

Meanwhile, states like Brazil, Cuba and Thailand have continued to import raw materials from Indian companies and manufacture their own generic antiretrovirals within the public sector. Brazil provides universal access to HIV therapy through a combination of state production of generics and aggressive negotiation with patent holders for steep discounts on brand-name drugs (see Chapter 4). Officials there recently warned Abbott, Roche and Merck that Brazil would override their patents on lopinavir, nelfinavir and efavirenz if it could not obtain lower prices. They gave the drug companies an August 30, 2003 deadline to offer a good deal on their brand-name drugs, and promised to issue a compulsory license to produce generic versions if the negotiations failed.

For big pharma, then, the pressure has steadily increased. In a historic first, generic antiretroviral producers recently beat brand-name companies in open bidding by nine Andean countries and Mexico, which established a maximum price for HIV drugs. The Pan American Health Organization helped broker what's called the Andean Agreement, in which a model of pooled procurement was used to achieve record-low regional prices of the drugs. Centralized procurement allows countries to pool their resources and be stronger at the bargaining table. Negotiators estimate that savings will allow them to treat another 150,000 people.

The deal was also hailed as a global breakthrough by generic manufacturers. "The Andean agreement is a breakthrough because it sets a worldwide reference price for antiretrovirals that is based on a generic price," explained Bill Haddad, who has represented Cipla and Ranbaxy at international meetings.

As more countries in Africa and Asia have also begun using generic anti-retrovirals, central procurement looks like the wave of the future. Using this model, Cameroon was able to import a generic combination costing under $300 a year per patient and now treats 7,000 people. Thailand treats 10,000 people with similar low-cost state-produced generics.

Looking ahead, generics are very much a part of the WHO 3×5 scale-up plan to reach 3 million people by 2005. As they move forward, the WHO, the IDA, Unicef, PAHO and other groups are actively setting up centralized procurement systems that allow fair, transparent purchasing of essential drugs – be they brand-name or generic – with price being the critical factor determining purchases.[23]

More Patent Wars

Why, after the Cipla miracle, have so few generic drugs reached people with AIDS in Africa and elsewhere? Three years after its groundbreaking offer, company officials complained in early 2003 that some of their cheap, high-quality AIDS drugs were sitting inside warehouses in India, while across Asia, Africa and other poor regions, 8,000 people a day were dying due to a lack to affordable medicine. Instead of a revolution, there was a stalemate.

What's preventing governments from acquiring or making generics? Funding is still an obstacle; even current generic prices vastly exceed what most countries can afford without the assistance of international donors. But with multiple funding sources emerging, it's clear that money is only half the story. As Lulla predicted, the Doha Declaration has remained an effective stumbling block. Only Namibia and Guyana had taken steps by mid 2003 to manufacture their own drugs. Others had sought to do so, and been threatened by US trade sanctions, according to insiders.[24]

Drug manufacturing is a complex business that calls for purchasing materials, processing, production, packaging, quality control, release of drugs, storage and related controls. Generics are also a tough business, especially when the local market for a product like AIDS drugs is not well established. Even when companies succeed, generic drugs may not be cheaper than imported drugs because big companies have more resources with which to compete in the market. In a recent review of the prospects for establishing local generic production of drugs in developing countries,

Warren Kaplan and colleagues at the Boston University School of Public Health found that African economies could not support generic industries efficient enough to compete with multinationals on price.[25] Other developing countries, like the Philippines, have the necessary manufacturing capacity in place, but their HIV rates are too low to justify producing generic drugs solely for the domestic market. These countries will only have affordable HIV treatment if allowed to import generics.

From Doha to Cancún

The next chance to resolve the WTO block on generic exports for AIDS drugs came in September 2003 at the WTO Ministerial Conference in Cancún, Mexico. Weeks before the highly anticipated meeting, the Bush administration hinted at a willingness to compromise on draft language in the Motta Text – an accord that attempts to clarify the Paragraph 6 contradiction in the 2001 WTO agreement. By then, the US had dropped its demand to limit the scope of diseases that constitute a national health emergency, a major sticking point in previous talks. In August, US trade officials tentatively laid out four conditions for a revision of the Motta Text. The first demanded that generic suppliers could provide drugs designed for "not for profit" or "humanitarian" purposes. The second required a clause enabling countries to "opt out" of exercising their right to import generics. According to Asia Russell of Health Gap, the opt-out provision could then allow the US to pressure countries into accepting more restrictive conditions for use of generics through other bilateral and multilateral trade agreements. The third US condition was a review mechanism or "audit" of how the WTO solution would be used. The language did not spell out who the ruling arbiter or auditor might be, whether a trade committee of the WTO or a health body like the WHO. The fourth was a request for an "explicit statement" that would distinguish generically produced medicine through special packaging. This would help prevent re-importation of cheap generics into wealthy countries, where they might be resold and undercut sales of their brand-name equivalents.

As Cancún approached, the WTO debate was pitched, with little consensus – and few could predict the outcome. Health Gap's Russell remained pessimistic on the prospects of a breakthrough. There were two potential scenarios being anticipated: if the WTO agreed to a pro-generics revision, countries could issue a compulsory license to import generic AIDS drugs regardless of their ability to make the drugs or the status of drug patents. Even then, activists felt, there would be many hoops to jump through. But if no solution was reached, then countries could still legally use compulsory licensing or parallel importing to get or make generic drugs, as long as they had the political will and muscle to confront the US. But as activists pointed out, the opposite has been true.

The US has aggressively defended the interests of big pharma, and activists say that many countries have held back from introducing generic anti-retrovirals, fearing US reprisals.[26] Both the US and big pharma have tried to block countries from taking measures legal under TRIPs that would facilitate access to generic HIV drugs. Beginning in 1998, South Africa faced a protracted lawsuit by forty major pharmaceutical companies seeking to block the new Medicines Act governing pricing and promoting access to drugs.

There was also the US WTO complaint against Brazil that was viewed as the Bush administration's attempt to limit generic access; it too was dropped partly in response to activist pressure. Also in 2000, GlaxoSmithKline issued legal threats over the use of Cipla's generic version of Combivir in Ghana. A 2001 United Nations Development Programme Human Development Report concluded that "pressure from Europe and the United States makes many developing countries fear that they will lose foreign direct investment if they legislate for or use compulsory licenses." Poor governments cannot afford long, expensive legal battles with the multinationals. In the meantime, the unresolved WTO Paragraph 6 paradox had made it difficult for countries to plan for any long-term access to generic drugs.

There's also the looming 2005 WTO deadline, when member countries must adhere to TRIPs rules upholding patents. As things stand today, Brazil, India and Thailand will no longer be able to make new generic drugs after that, because they will have to respect patent laws as WTO members. They will only be able use the generic versions they already make, and will have to pay market prices for imported drugs. Finally, there's the proposed Free Trade for the Americas Agreement (FTAA) – a successor to the North American Free Trade Agreement. If passed, it will also take effect in 2005. FTAA talks will take place in November 2003 in Miami.

"The US wants to export US-style patent protection which exceeds levels of protection guaranteed under TRIPs," said Russell, worried. "If the US gets its way, there would be an extension of patent terms past twenty years. There would be a five-year block on any country doing a compulsory license once a patent gets filed. So it has the potential to dramatically limit access to medicines in the future." Her take on the FTAA: "It's one more bit of evidence that the US is giving with one hand and taking with the other."[27]

Does the WHO Want Generics?

Regardless of the outcome of trade talks in Cancún and Miami, the momentum is still squarely behind scaling up antiretroviral therapy. With the Global Fund money, more and more governments and non-profit organizations have drafted HIV treatment plans that call for use of the lowest-cost drugs – generics. The WHO is developing several strategies to support scale-up. High on the WHO's list is a pooled procurement system for antiretrovirals, intended to streamline purchasing and distribution, reduce drug costs, and ensure quality. The WHO is also offering technical expertise and other "best practice" resources to developing countries to build up their ability to buy, deliver and make drugs – including generic drugs. The agency aims "to ensure that access to drugs is not an obstacle in reaching the target of 3 million in treatment by 2005," says WHO advisor Jim Yong Kim.[28]

The WHO has also played an important role in vouching for the quality of generic drugs after intensive assessment. National regulatory bodies like South Africa's Medicines Control Council oversee generic products for domestic use, but local standards vary and many countries lack the resources for quality assurance. Although only four generic producers have made the WHO list of prequalified suppliers of anti-HIV drugs, more products and companies will be added. Much will depend on how quickly the WHO moves. Officials there hope to vouch for the quality of new "fixed-dose" pills and combinations that have been introduced.

For now, generic manufacturing of anti-HIV drugs is growing more rapidly in the private than the public sector. That's because the private companies have merely shifted their focus onto HIV, while governments and state producers are blocked by the WTO quagmire. Private Indian and Latin American companies lead the industry for pills, while Chinese and Korean manufacturers are well poised to supply raw materials for HIV drugs. Although state production is stalled, there are signs of movement. Brazil has given $100,000 in technology transfer grants to ten countries – five in Africa, five in Latin America – to help develop local industries for generic AIDS drugs. The Thai state producer, GPO, is giving technical help to Ghana, Zimbabwe and Zambia to set up pilot manufacturing plants. Zambia hopes eventually to supply antiretrovirals to thirteen neighboring countries. Nigeria, with its large manufacturing base and skilled population, is also moving forward.

Experts now predict that most countries will rely on a mix of brand-name and quality generic drugs to scale up treatment, based on availability and price. Even the US displays a new pragmatism towards generic antiretrovirals, with administration spokespersons indicating that global AIDS funds for treatment will not be restricted to brand-name HIV drugs. The guidelines of the Global Fund – now chaired by Tommy Thompson, US Secretary of Health and Human Services – do not directly endorse generic antiretrovirals, but encourage procurement of quality drugs at the lowest prices. With more competition, prices will fall, while pooled procurement plans could lower costs more. Some predict combination therapies in the near future for $0.50 a day, or less – half the price of today's dollar-a-day regimens.

"It's clear that generics have completely changed the equation," says Joep Lange, head of the International AIDS Society and a key force behind the WHO's 3×5 plan. "If it weren't for Cipla and other Indian companies, we wouldn't be talking today about the possibility of treating millions of people. In the end it doesn't matter whether the drug is a generic or brand name; what matters is that the drug works and is affordable."

5

CUBA FIGHTS AIDS ITS OWN WAY

In the early 1980s, Cuba was internationally criticized for its controversial policy of keeping HIV-positive individuals quarantined in a system of sanitariums. To outsiders, the image of the sanitarium is a throwback to a draconian 1950s institution where uncaring doctors keep patients with contagious diseases apart from the rest of society. Although HIV is transmitted via a blood-borne virus, not in airborne particles like tuberculosis, Cubans with HIV are still initially required to stay in the sanitarium for a short period. But a lot has changed there.

Cuba's socialist model of universal health-care is impressive, especially considering it is a poor country, one that has greatly suffered due to the US trade embargo. The blockade affects not only food and other goods, but essential medicines, which are lacking on the island. Since these drugs are used to treat HIV illnesses, the embargo has directly and negatively affected Cuba's AIDS effort. The Castro government has always invested in public health, and had a long-standing policy of sending Cuban doctors (as well as teachers and other workers) abroad to train and work in other developing countries, especially in the countryside. Today, Cuban physicians are helping to fight HIV in Haiti and other neighboring Caribbean countries, as well as in some of the poorest African countries. They are known for their skills in treating tropical diseases like malaria, and now in managing HIV and TB in co-infected patients.

Amid this glowing praise for Cuba's AIDS effort, particularly in the arena of prevention, there are reportedly brutal conditions inside Cuba's overcrowded prisons, with heavy censorship of the press and new threats made against pro-democracy activists. This makes it difficult for outsiders to evaluate the current status of AIDS programs in the country.

Two decades after the first HIV case was diagnosed in Cuba in 1986, the AIDS picture there has changed dramatically, however. Statistically, Cuba is a poster-child for HIV prevention, having succeeded in the Holy Grail of public health: reducing the spread of HIV and gaining control over the epidemic.

Compared with nearby Haiti, which has a 6.1 percent national prevalence rate – the highest in the western hemisphere and just behind sub-Saharan Africa – Cuba has a very low 0.03 percent adult HIV rate – ten to sixty-fold below that of its Caribbean neighbors. That is one of the lowest incidences in the world. Cuba registered 3,200 cases of HIV in early 2003, almost entirely in gay and bisexual men.[1] Its integration of HIV and AIDS control into a community- and family-based model of care has also been praised by public health officials outside Cuba. Unfortunately, the government's reliance on quarantine and other heavy-handed disease-control strategies that discriminate against individuals with HIV overshadow this progress.

Even if Cuba's AIDS program is flawed, it offers lessons for other developing countries. In planning my visit there, I was particularly interested in talking to HIV-positive individuals about treatment, to find out the degree and quality of care they received from the state system. I knew that Cuba manufactured several generic HIV medicines, but not all, and not enough to meet the current need on the island. Before leaving for Havana, I visited the offices of Global Exchange in San Francisco, one of a number of progressive US organizations that educate Americans about Cuba. They send essential medicines to the island, and gave me a box of antibiotics, basic medical equipment and, most importantly, a few boxes of recycled antiretroviral drugs, to donate to the main AIDS research clinic there.

As any American who's gone to Cuba recently will tell you, the biggest barrier is the misinformation that persists about the island in the United States. But I wasn't sure what to expect from contact with ordinary Cubans. Would they feel open about talking to a foreign journalist about AIDS? What was their aware-ness of the disease? Of the government's program and policies? What about Cuban health officials? Would they speak openly to me? Would I be allowed to interview residents openly at the sanitarium? What about HIV-positive and gay activists outside the sanitariums? How open would they feel about talking to a Western journalist?

These were my thoughts as I flew directly from Miami to Havana in late December 2002, with a State Department-approved visa tucked into my passport. It was a short trip that has now become difficult to make. In March 2003 the Castro government took a serious step back – toward repression. It carried out the worst crackdown on the political opposition in decades, arresting seventy-five pro-democracy and human rights advocates who were given prison terms of up to twenty-eight years.[2] A month later, Castro executed three people attempting to flee the island – the same week that a major international AIDS conference took place highlighting Cuba's progress against the epidemic.[3]

These actions have caused Bush and hard-line members of his administration to shut several US doors to Cuba. The administration has enforced travel restrictions to Cuba that were relaxed by the Clinton administration. Although a majority in Congress are pushing to end the embargo, Castro's actions – and Bush's reactions – have caused a political standstill. All of this bodes badly for AIDS activists, physicians, researchers, and particularly HIV-positive Cubans who are already suffering from the embargo on food, aid, medicine, communication and travel.

To an outside visitor, the sanatorium at Santiago de las Vegas in Cuba feels like an army base, set apart from civilian life in a self-sufficient world. It is located half an hour's drive from Havana and is the biggest and oldest AIDS center of the seventeen in Cuba. The main facility is hidden behind a walled entrance and presents an odd sight: an architectural hybrid of heavy, almost Soviet-style institution and Alpine ski resort – but set in the tropics. Across the highway, smatterings of low Florida-style bungalows serve as laboratories and medical wards and house some 450 patients. Residents walk through an underpass from the main facility to their homes, passing a basketball court and a garden.

From the highway the bungalows are visible. In the evening, when the daytime heat and humidity have subsided a bit, sanatorium residents often hang out by the long-running fence, chatting with locals and friends on the other side. Many of them are gay men in their twenties and thirties. But some residents, including a heterosexual married couple, have been there for two decades now. In fact, Santiago de las Vegas has become a home for many and, for different reasons, some prefer it to life outside.

That may strike some as surprising, considering the controversy that the sanatorium model has generated in and outside the country.[4] From 1986 to 1993, Santiago de las Vegas epitomized the country's much-criticized quarantine policy that kept people with HIV apart from the general public. Forced quarantine ended in 1993, but the government retains an aggressive public-health approach to controlling HIV.[5] The sanatorium model reflects an emphasis on preventive care over acute care, and on early diagnosis and quick treatment of infectious diseases like tuberculosis.

Like TB, HIV is viewed by the state as a medical condition for which an individual bears social responsibility. Individuals who test positive for HIV are required to spend at least three months in an AIDS sanatorium, where they take a training course in living with HIV and protecting others from exposure. They now have the option of attending the training on an outpatient basis. Today, half of Cuba's HIV population live in the sanatoriums, can come and go freely, and receive daily visits from relatives and friends. The rest live outside and receive care at a few specialist centers.

Of the 1,000-plus people who have passed through the Santiago de las Vegas sanatorium since it opened, 380 live there. An extended medical and social support staff of over 300 attends to them. The facility includes a hospital ward and laboratory, as well as specialized clinics to provide surgical, dental, gynecological, hematological and psychological services. It also offers legal and social aid, including peer support groups. Between 1998 and 2000 there were twenty-two outpatient groups. Some members of the outpatient groups have become community educators who go into people's homes to talk about AIDS. They are part of the "Cara a Cara" or "Face to Face" national HIV initiative.

Life Inside

Although residents have more freedom to come and go, outside visitors to the sanatorium are escorted. My visit was arranged by Dr. Jorge Perez Avila, medical director of the Pedro Kouri Tropical Medicine Institute in Havana, known here as IPK, an infectious disease hospital and the main center for AIDS research. The institute serves as the central clearing-house for all

Cubans receiving anti-HIV drugs, which it distributes to their clinics. Perez ran the sanatorium here for several years, and now runs the national HIV treatment program. Affable and intelligent, he is credited by many people with single-handedly opening up the sanatorium system, reforming many of the more abusive policies. He's also been instrumental in getting Cuba to move forward on the treatment front.

Over the years, sanatorium rules at Santiago de las Vegas have relaxed further, said Perez, though officials stress that it remains a medical facility, one where patients have to agree to some rules. "They have very good living conditions there," he explained, adding that many residents inside are poor, previously unemployed, or lack family support to live so well outside. "They have a house, air conditioner, color TV, 100 percent of their salary and a diet very high in calories and rich in protein. No one else has so much." Some residents have told journalists that they live better than they would outside, given the economic uncertainty in Cuba.[6] Perez echoed that view.

Still, he was shocked back in 1993, when only 10 percent of residents opted to leave the sanatorium when offered the chance. "It was not discrimination, it was fear," he explained. "Those were the years of the really bad 'Special Period' when people were hungry."[7]

The situation today is greatly changed, he added. "We have made a lot of progress, despite not having all the resources we need," said Perez. "You'll see for yourself."

Upon his referral, sanatorium officials welcomed me for a visit and a tour of the facility. Like Perez, they were eager to dispel any notions of the forced confinement or repression that, they admitted, were features of the earlier era. That said, they also stayed close by while I interviewed residents.[8]

Four gay men were gathered on a porch of a small two-bedroom house, sparsely furnished but clean and comfortable, and offering a luxury item: an air conditioner. Residents live as couples or four to a house at the sanatorium. Compared with apartments I'd seen in Havana, it was better than average housing. These men had been at the sanatorium for relatively short periods of time, not years. They said they received superior medical care compared with outside hospitals, and they ate well. Friends and family could visit. They also received a special stipend for working on the premises. Sanatorium residents are entitled to receive 100 percent of their former salary. Persons with HIV outside the system get 50 percent. Given the difficult economic situation in Cuba, this financial support is impressive, especially since those who are ill may not be able to work. (And, as I learned later, some people lose their jobs when they have to go into the sanitorium, though this is not supposed to happen.[9])

They confirmed that many sanatorium residents require treatment for their HIV, something that isn't accessible outside the system. Two of the men were managing their antiretroviral drugs without much difficulty. One had experienced some initial side-effects. The fourth, a younger man, was preparing to begin treatment. He was unsure of what medicine he would take or how it worked. Although he had been taught the basics about HIV and treatment at the sanatorium, he was unfamiliar with some of the drugs available outside Cuba. Nor did he have access to information from abroad. His knowledge of HIV came primarily from his housemates. All four residents expressed a desire to know more about new developments in AIDS, and to have more contact with HIV-positive persons outside Cuba.

In an earlier private interview, the staff psychiatrist informed me that residents were free to leave the sanatorium if they were healthy, had completed the HIV training course, and were enrolled for social services. "If they have health problems and they want to go, they can, but we don't recommend it," he added. "Or if they've started triple therapy, we suggest they stay a while to see if there are any adverse reactions."

Like other health officials, he disagreed that the sanatoriums were velvet prisons, though he agreed that they were de facto gay ghettos. In his view, the sanatoriums also offer gay men a refuge from a socially intolerant society. "There is a sense of community here," he explained:

> Here, gay men can be together in their houses; they have that freedom and they also have privacy. There are support groups and people are confronting similar problems. I think that's one reason why people stay: they like it and they find things they wouldn't if they were just living by themselves in an apartment somewhere or with their families.

Positive Prevention

Quarantine is a classic public health approach to controlling the emergency threat of contagion, and in this sense the sanatorium reflects an early step in epidemic control. In Africa, quarantine was critical to stopping the outbreaks of Ebola, a lethal virus that has no cure and spreads rapidly, causing people to internally bleed to death. It is a critical part of managing active tuberculosis, which is spread via airborne particles, just like the SARS virus. Whenever a fast-moving, lethal infectious organism crops up, a key task of public health officials and epidemiologists is to track the origin of the illness and its pattern. That often involves putting all the potentially exposed individuals under surveillance – and keeping them apart from others until the threat of contagion is understood and a cure or vaccine is found. The focus is on rapid assistance for those exposed, and protection for those unexposed.

Unfortunately, by its very nature, quarantine spells an automatic – usually temporary – loss of rights. It can also be used punitively – as is the case with SARS. After initially covering up the outbreak of SARS, Chinese health officials enacted a strict quarantine of people who had been, or were suspected of being, exposed to the virus, and moved people who defied the policy to jail. SARS had struck 5,000 people when the regime went further: in May 2003, China passed laws that allowed authorities to imprison for life or execute anyone who violates SARS quarantine and spreads the disease. Globally, this move was denounced.[10]

Whenever there is public panic and fear, public health officials are given support for taking drastic emergency steps that, by their nature, infringe the civil rights of citizens. When that threat diminishes, so does the justification for quarantine.

Cuba's HIV quarantine policy is of a different stripe, but it, too, limits the rights of HIV-positive citizens. It sends a message to an already frightened public that those who harbor the HIV virus are dangerous to others. That is the opposite of the goal of educational campaigns to destigmatize HIV and reduce discrimination against those affected. From a purely public health point of view, the question is different: once you have identified the source, methods of contagion, and treatment of an epidemic, is quarantine an appropriate solution? Most health experts say no, because other strategies become available, and the longer the quarantine, the more punitive it becomes for those inside and their families on the outside. I would argue that, as a public health measure, long-term quarantine interferes with educational and prevention efforts because it makes those who don't know their status fear HIV, possibly reducing their interest in getting an HIV test and any necessary care.

HIV is also arguably different from TB, SARS and Ebola. It is not casually transmitted: you don't get it by sitting next to someone, or even if they cough or spit on you. There are two routes of exposure: blood and sexual fluids. Exposure to blood is commonly through accidental needle sticks or surgery for health professionals, or via injection drug use for drug users; exposure otherwise occurs most commonly through unprotected sex. In 1983, one of Cuba's first steps was to institute screening in blood banks,[11] and they quickly made sure the national blood supply was free from HIV.

As there are very few intravenous drug users in Cuba, quarantine is a method designed to stop the sexual transmission chain of HIV. A second step is education and counseling, through mandatory classes at the sanatorium. If these steps succeed, the ultimate goal is achieved: sexual responsibility – namely safer sex, including the use of condoms.

Instead of putting the onus of HIV prevention on all citizens, then, Cuba implicitly puts the responsibility for containing the AIDS epidemic on those with HIV. A key criterion for residents wishing to live outside the sanatoriums is disclosure of their sexual partners, and provision to the health authorities of "confidence" that they are sexually responsible.

"Here we view the idea of a person being responsible for the health of another as a very relative term," explained a staff psychiatrist at the sanatorium.

> We say that person has a right to a higher quality of life and social rights. But they must modify their behavior to care for themselves and others. If you meet someone who has psychological issues, who has no family to support them, or if they are a person who has infected several people because they have no conscience, then we have to make a plan for that person. For them, it can take longer.

The program works, he argued. "Out of the 1,000-odd people who have stayed here, or as outpatients, very few have infected others."

The health authorities also actively pursue the contact tracing and HIV testing of sexual partners – other common epidemiological strategies borrowed from TB and STD control. There is mandatory HIV testing of pregnant women, soldiers and blood donors, while anonymous testing is available for the general public. In 2001 over a million HIV tests were carried out in Cuba, out of a population of 11 million. The use of condoms has doubled, and they are distributed in bars, clubs and pharmacies, though they are in limited supply.[12]

Rights and Responsibilities

The government's heavy-handed approach to disease control continues to give ammunition to critics. Though forced quarantine is no longer official policy, it continues to be a threat if one doesn't play the game by the government's rules. Away from the eyes and ears of health officials, Cubans living outside the sanatoriums offer a different picture of life for those with HIV, both inside and outside the sanatoriums. "I have always disagreed with this decision by the state," remarked Cheo [a pseudonym], a leading HIV activist, about the sanatorium system. We met at an HIV support group at the Monserrate Church in Havana, but conducted our interview in a park.[13]

In Cheo's view, life at the sanatoriums "is not a normal life, because it is very controlled. It is all about illness. People may get quality medical care, but they remain socially isolated." Though he knows that some who have lived there for long periods have adjusted, Cheo felt that "[i]f they could afford to, most would live outside. How can you call something a choice if you don't have another option?"

He is very critical of policies like contact tracing. "It's supposed to be a decision of the person to disclose, to take charge of their situation and inform the people they've had relationships with," Cheo explained. "But the thing is, the authorities need to know and there is a lot of pressure to tell them. If you don't say, and if they take you to the sanatorium, they won't release you because they won't have confidence in you."

Cheo isn't alone in complaining about the lack of privacy or consent for Cubans living with HIV. Several activists I spoke to referred to the paternalistic nature of the AIDS program, and to the prevailing stigma and isolation they suffer. "There is a lack of freedom here in Cuba, and when you have HIV it's that much harder," he explained. "You are seen as a threat to society by the authorities. These views are changing, but people still think that way."

Critics contend that there is a gap between official AIDS policy and discriminatory routine practices. Manuel,[14] who is a gay, HIV-positive, and in his forties, said gay people who test positive are asked to name their sexual partners of the previous five years. "Some people are afraid to name more than five persons because they will be labeled promiscuous," he noted, "but if you name too few, they'll say you are not disclosing." "There is no privacy," he added. "The minute you are diagnosed, everyone seems to know. The state can't protect you."

Although a new labor law forbids the firing of HIV-positive individuals, both men have friends who lost their jobs after being diagnosed. They know people who have had unsafe sex with positive partners but won't get tested, out of fear of being sent to a sanatorium and losing their jobs. "A lot of people are in hiding or denial," added Cheo, who feels official HIV statistics are too low.

Past Scars

Cheo's criticism stems from personal experience. Forty-one years old and bisexual, he was diagnosed with HIV in 1993, just as Perez was reforming the sanatorium system. An HIV test was done without his knowledge after he went to a hospital for what doctor's thought was glandular cancer. "For me, it was obligatory to be in the sanatorium; there was no other option. But I didn't want to go," he related. "For two years they tried to pressure me, saying I had to go and learn to live with HIV, that there was good food, etc. But I said my parents supported me very well. I didn't want to be separated from them."

Cheo said he received regular visits from health officials and was threatened with arrest, as were his parents. He pleaded his case with higher officials and was allowed to take a training course in a Havana center. He then obtained treatment at the Pedro Kouri institute. But for years, he says, "I had no support because I had no friends with HIV, and my family was ignorant about it. I thought I would die right away."

Despite such complaints, critics don't hold AIDS officials responsible for the problems of the system today. They sympathize with physicians, who also contend with Cuba's strict laws and bureaucracy. "Dr. Perez doesn't make the rules. Nor do the people who work at the sanatorium," said Manuel. "They can't speak out any more than we can. If they did, they'd be risking their jobs. A lot of people are doing what they can to help us. We appreciate that."

The Early Years

It's useful to look back at the origins of Cuba's policies to judge the progress it has made. The first AIDS case turned up there in the early 1980s, when HIV was still a mystery virus. There was no cure, no effective treatments, and a high degree of public fear. Cuba had clear policies for the control of infectious diseases like TB, which included quarantine. The sanatorium model derived from already existing strategies.

Under the National Commission to Face AIDS, founded in 1983, Cuban doctors aggressively traced Cubans who had studied abroad, served in the military, or worked in Africa. The first of twenty-three AIDS patients admitted to the newly created sanatorium system in 1995 was Reynaldo Morales, a man who had volunteered to do his military service in Angola in 1984. Morales was also one of the first Cubans admitted to the island's Naval Hospital, where HIV patients were first treated.[15] His wife, Maria Julia, seroconverted shortly after his return from Angola. They later set up a home in the sanatorium, and coped with the challenge of family life in these circumstances. When their diagnosis was known, their teenage son was given a scholarship to sports school by the government.

Maria Julia is among the oldest survivors of HIV, and has been a leader in advocating for the rights of people with HIV. She also helped start the HIV Prevention Center in Havana, where she works. Morales died of AIDS in 1995. During the first years at the sanatorium, patients and doctors agree today that life was difficult for all, and especially so for some. The first patients essentially lived in a medical ward where they wore hospital pajamas and were closely supervised. Later they were housed in the small apartments and houses that now make up the sanatorium. There was care, but AIDS treatment was limited until Cuba was able to manufacture its own drugs. Patients relied on a limited supply of imported drugs, or on those donated by humanitarian groups. "When there was no treatment, it was hard for the patients and for the persons caring for them to confront [the absence of medical options]," said the staff psychologist at Santiago de las Vegas. "This was a very difficult situation."

Some adapted better than others, including Reynaldo and Maria Julia, who were given their own home within the sanatorium. But most patients reported too little privacy and freedom.

From the start, Morales and other patients organized to begin pressing for more rights, including the right to wear normal clothing, receive more visitors, and for outside passes to visit family and friends. Life got much better when Perez took over. He began by tearing down a wall that made the sanatorium feel like a prison, and built housing for residents. He also gained the trust of patients and instituted other changes that improved their quality of life.

Perez backed support groups for patients, helped establish work programs, and extended a pass to leave the premises for a day to residents who were not ill. Initially, patients leaving the premises were accompanied by a doctor or sanatorium workers, to make sure they would not expose others to HIV, and to safeguard their medical treatment. That too was relaxed with some patients, as they proved to authorities that they would not engage in unsafe sexual practices. Those who could not leave the premises were granted supervised visits by family members.

A key reform was the establishment of the HIV education and training program that allowed residents to leave and receive outpatient care at other centers. To carry out these changes, Cuban officials had to build other provincial facilities, train staff to provide HIV care, and extend this training to local family doctors who would follow patients once they returned home. The government also worked with social workers and other educators to prepare local communities and try to reduce stigma as a step prior to releasing residents from the sanatoriums. Here, residents played a key role, helping Perez to shape what some other Cuban officials viewed as policies that were too lenient.

Sanatorium residents continued to be active as advocates and educators, forming political councils within the sanatorium to lobby officials for changes, and forming Grupo Prevencion SIDA (GPSIDA), a patients' HIV prevention and education group that helped spawn the HIV Prevention Center, where a number of HIV-positive ex-residents found work.

The Unofficial Picture

According to some AIDS activists on the outside, it's not as easy to get out of the sanatorium as officials claim. It's not by accident, critics feel, that mostly gay men are kept apart from general society in these sanatoriums.

The other way that happens is through incarceration. Although the Castro government doesn't lock up gays or expel them as "undesirables," as it has in the past,[16] homophobia is still strong in Cuba. Despite changing social attitudes on the island, AIDS is still equated with *maricones*, or "faggots," even though some early AIDS cases were among heterosexual men and women. There is an obvious current of homophobia that underlies the sanatorium policy on "sexual responsibility," in which authorities view gay men and their sexuality as promiscuous, irresponsible, and a potential threat to the rest of society.

"They may not come out and say something like that, but we encounter it all the time," said Manuel.[17] There are no gay or lesbian bars or public social clubs in Cuba, and the government doesn't openly support such organizations, he said. There's no gay or lesbian center. Instead, gay social life tends to take place inside people's homes and, to a growing extent, in the streets. It's also different for those living in big cities, as opposed to small towns, as it is everywhere.

"The official attitude toward gays has changed – that's true," Manuel added. "There has been some evolution. But people can't be that open about it. And every night you'll still find the police coming along late at night to harass us and threaten to arrest us. Though I am Cuban and I love my country, the Cuban revolution has never been open to gays," he concluded. Instead, Cuba remains a very macho society. Many Cubans are also practicing Catholics and oppose homosexuality on religious grounds. In Castro's Cuba, religious groups were repressed for years, but religion plays an important role in the private lives of citizens.

Here again one finds an inherent contradiction in Cuban policies as they relate to AIDS: on one hand, health officials want gay men to be sexually responsible and use condoms when they have sex; on the other, the authorities police public gay activity, and there is a social intolerance of homosexuality. How can gay men in Cuba feel comfortable and open about their sexuality if it is being repressed and criminalized? The same can be said for Cubans with HIV.

As a sign of changing attitudes, Cuban health officials are funding an HIV prevention program aimed at gay men, called HSH – "Hombres que tienen sexo con hombres" (Men who have sex with men). It is one of many interventions, including programs targeting youths and teachers. Still, the law makes it hard for people with HIV to organize or get support outside of state-run organizations. Though independent self-help groups have been permitted to form since 1997, they can't legally raise funds or apply for government money. Nor can informal gay groups.

Safe Havens

Around sixty people attend a support group at the Montserrate church in Havana, the largest of its kind. It meets once a week and visitors from abroad often drop in, bringing donations of medicine and information. The church provides a haven, Cheo said, because the police cannot enter it. But people are careful about being overly critical of the government in this still-public forum, he said.

The church program was started by Father Fernando de la Vega, and has over 100 members. On the evening I visited, the church's meeting room was packed, and included several American students. A number of US organizations are helping Cubans with HIV, including the Cuba AIDS Project,[18] the Disarm Education Fund, Global Exchange, and drug recycling projects like the River Fund in Florida and AID for AIDS in New York.

At the meeting, participants were mostly concerned with issues related to daily life with HIV, disclosure, and discrimination from family, friends or co-workers. As a group, they discussed their need to increase access to HIV information, materials and magazines, which are in short supply. Few support group members had regular access to the internet; in Havana, for example, there is a handful of public internet cafes, but they are not advertised. By and large, Cubans depend on other media for regular news coverage.

At Monserrate, support group members have formed close ties with activists in Spain, Latin America and the US, who provide Spanish-language HIV information that is shared with group members. The Cuba AIDS Project regularly sent twenty-person groups to travel within Cuba and do educational work, especially in rural areas. Most of the support group members had passed through the sanatorium. When asked, they expressed support for those inside, who are given passes and transportation to attend the evening meetings.

Economic Pressures

After forty years of the US embargo against Fidel Castro, Cuba has lifted itself out of economic dependence on foreign aid, but it continues to struggle with poverty and economic problems. People aren't starving as they are in nearby Haiti, but there are shortages of all kinds – food, adequate housing, work, electricity – especially in the countryside. There isn't enough money in the national coffers to maintain roads and buildings, to the point where entire sections of cities like Havana have simply collapsed.[19]

By comparison, Cubans are generally well educated and in good health – major achievements of the Cuban revolution. Despite the embargo, Cuba has developed extensive ties with other countries and become not only self-sufficient, but also a major exporter of goods. And although Americans can't travel easily to Cuba, the rest of the world can – and has. Today, tourism is a major industry, even if it's nothing on the scale of what you'd find in the Bahamas or other popular island vacation destinations. And plenty of Americans have found their way around the US travel embargo, traveling via Mexico or Canada. So have companies doing business with America.

These include, notably, one of the big multinational HIV drug makers. Not long ago, Cuba licensed the meningitis-B drug it manufactures to Britain's GlaxoSmithKline. GSK planned to sell the drug in the US under an exemption to the trade embargo granted by the Clinton administration.[20] That was in keeping with Clinton's actions to ease the ban against Cuba, including "people-to-people ties." As a result, more Americans than ever have traveled to Cuba in recent years, many through groups like Global Exchange, which sponsors politico-cultural tours on the island.

But not many tourists visit the sanatoriums, and nor do ordinary Cubans. I asked a half-dozen Cubans in Havana about the sanatorium, including several living nearby; they knew about the facility, but had never been inside. After two decades, these institutions remain a life apart.

"Free and Easy Access"

"One of the characteristics of the health system is that it is free and has easy access. Everyone is entitled to the same level of care," explained Dr. Perez.

"Even though I am a specialist and in charge here, a patient from anywhere can decide to come and see me." Like other health officials, Dr. Perez cites the US trade blockade of Cuba as a critical factor that has affected the AIDS program, and contributes to the chronic shortage of medicine, food and other necessities. But he's also proud of what has been done with limited resources. "It's true we are hurt by economic problems and our patients have suffered from a lack of medicine," said Perez. "The lack of money is a constant problem for everybody. But now that we are producing our own drugs, things have started to change."

The Pedro Kouri Institute (IPK) is located outside the capital and is comparable with the National Institutes of Health in the US because it combines frontline clinical research with treatment. Its physical appearance betrays Cuba's lack of resources: it is a relatively small facility, and the walls badly need a paint job. But the care is first rate. HIV patients praise the free medical services they get, which include both medicine and diagnostic tests. HIV patients have their CD4 counts tested every three months, and those on treatment also receive viral load tests. They return to the institute for monthly follow-up visits and are monitored at home by a family doctor.

Before 2001 some patients were getting dual therapy through foreign donors, and drug availability was problematic. As of December 2002, around 900 people were receiving a triple generic cocktail of two nucleoside analogs and the protease inhibitor indinavir. Two new medicines in other classes were being readied. The government was also training the specialists who treat AIDS patients and other health professionals as well, but budget restrictions had hampered this effort.

Of the 900 people on therapy in late 2002, 72 percent were men and 28 percent women. One hundred and thirty had received drugs since 1996, and required salvage therapy regimens. They relied mostly on donated drugs. Perez will not start a patient on a salvage regimen unless he has a guaranteed six months' supply of the drugs, and there were still gaps in the supply.

Cheo's is a case in point. At the time of our interview in 2002, he had survived two opportunistic infections. His health was better now, but he had become resistant to two previous HIV regimens, and was now off therapy, waiting for a salvage regimen. The doctors at the IPK didn't have enough medicine yet. Without the drugs, he worried his HIV viral load level would shoot back up – a sign that the virus was taking over again –

and that he would get sick again. Without an effective salvage regimen, he felt vulnerable to a recurring opportunistic infection.

His case was not unique. In his experience, new HIV patients have no problem accessing generic Cuban HIV medicines, but some people, like him, are struggling due to their long treatment histories. His physicians were sympathetic, and had urged him to start his own mutual-aid group to seek foreign donations of the needed drugs. He'd done that, but in the spring of 2003, when I got an update on his health, he was again struggling with illnesses, still lacking medicine, and his pleas to outside visitors for recycled salvage drugs had intensified.

For the majority, anti-HIV drugs are seen as a godsend. After eighteen months, Dr. Perez reported, in December 2002, "Most of the people on therapy are doing very well." His one-year follow-up data showed that almost all had undetectable viral levels, higher CD4 counts and improved weight. After three months of therapy, 74 percent who began with CD4 counts below 200 jumped to over 200, then climbed progressively to over 350 after a year. Those who began with CD4 counts around 350 went up to 500 within three months – "and very easily," the doctor added. Around fifty people were waiting to get their first anti-HIV medications – but not because first-line drugs were lacking, Perez explained. It takes four to eight weeks to meet with referring doctors and complete the paperwork.

A Decentralized Model

One reason for Cuba's success is its uniquely decentralized, family-centered health-care structure. It relies on a local team of a family doctor, nurse, and social worker assigned to care for 120 people in a given community. In 2002 there were over 60,000 practising doctors – approximately one for every 185 residents – and over 70,000 nurses in Cuba.[21] Local health officials report up the ladder to regional and national authorities. "At each level, there are people invested in how the patient is doing," explained Dr. Perez. That includes the pharmacists at the IPK, who track every pill given out, and the psychiatrist who evaluates how patients are coping.

One area in which Cuba has made progress is against tuberculosis, which is a common co-infection with HIV around the world. TB expert Juan Carlos Millan works with Perez at the IPK and oversees the use of Directly

Observed Therapy for TB patients (see Chapter 6). This also relies on care provided by a small team. "With tuberculosis you have an incidence of .0017, so really there are very few people with TB here, and you can monitor those people very well," explained Perez.[22] Not so with HIV. "The treatment at the sanatorium and the institute is supervised, but the [HIV] treatment at home is not," he explained. "You give them medicine for thirty days." Many people hide their HIV status from their families – a factor that impacts on their adherence to drug regimens.

Adherence to dosing schedules remains a daily challenge. "The difference between TB and HIV – it's completely different," said Perez. The stigma around HIV prevents health professionals from monitoring HIV drug adherence as they do for TB. The family doctor or social worker is supposed to follow up each patient, but in reality, "many people don't like their families to know they have HIV. It's difficult to send a nurse in – it's an ethical issue," Perez said. He's had patients who stopped taking their medicine without telling anyone, and even died. How does he know when patients stop taking this medicine? "They have to come here or to the sanatorium every month to get treatment. So if they do not come, you know they have run out."

The biggest challenge is caring for patients with advanced AIDS. Treating their HIV does not help them much, Perez observed. In 2000, 141 people with AIDS died. In 2001, when triple therapy commenced, the number dropped to 116. The mortality rate is now 7 percent. Most new HIV cases are diagnosed early, within six months to a year of exposure, so AIDS itself should now be avoidable.

Reliance on Generics

Cuba boasts one of the most advanced premier biotech and engineering programs in Latin America. In west Havana, over 1,000 people work at the Genetic Engineering and Biotechnology Center, one of thirty-eight institutes that make up Cuba's version of the US National Institutes of Health. The CIGB's high-quality biotech products and technology are sold in over forty countries, totaling over $100 million annually.[23] The center is famous for making cancer drugs, and is the sole producer of a meningitis-B vaccine, sold globally. It also pioneered the use of interferon to treat dengue fever and several other tropical infections. AIDS physicians now use interferon to boost the immune system in HIV patients taking antitretroviral therapy. It makes many drugs and vaccines, such as hepatitis-B, dengue, cholera and tuberculosis.

As in India, Cuba's national drug laws allow it to make generic versions of patented drugs. As of mid 2002, it made five drugs: AZT, ddI, d4T, 3TC and indinavir, the last being the only protease inhibitor. It was also testing two new AIDS vaccines. As a member of the WTO, Cuba can sell its generic drugs to countries where drug patents don't exist without breaking intellectual property laws, and that includes markets in much of the developing world. In March 2001, when South Africa was battling thirty-nine big pharma companies over the right to make or license generic AIDS drugs, Castro signed an agreement with Thabo Mbeki that involved cooperation in making generic anti-AIDS drugs. The ties between the two countries are well established. Over 400 Cuban doctors now work in South Africa, and around 200 Cubans study in schools there. South Africa already receives several Cuban-made vaccines, including one for hepatitis-B. Following Mbeki's tour of the CIGB plant, Castro told reporters in a press conference that he welcomed the US's response to the agreement. "I would like to hear a protest so that I can grin from ear to ear," said Castro.[24]

Castro made a similar offer of technology transfer to Brazil, and has since extended a drugs-plus-technology transfer offer to neighboring countries in the Caribbean, and other poor nations. By early 2003, several Caribbean leaders were considering the use of generic antiretrovirals from Cuba. Unfortunately, the CIGB plant and its generic AIDS drugs have not been evaluated by the WHO, in order to provide consumers with an independent verification of their quality and – more importantly – to be listed in the WHO formulary. Nevertheless, experts say that state-produced Cuban medicines must have the highest standards to achieve regulatory approval for export, which they do. They also produce HIV and other diagnostic test kits for local use.

Outside the area of AIDS, Cuba created a marketing subsidiary, Heber Biotec SA, in 1991, which reported sales of $45 million in 1999.[25] It set up joint ventures to make drugs for Iran, Egypt and India, and was eyeing the huge Chinese market. Cuba and Iran have also worked together since 1996 to build drug research and production facilities outside Teheran, in one of a variety of joint technical transfer projects in fourteen developing countries. New agreements were in the works in 1999 with Brazil and nine other countries: Malaysia, the Netherlands, Spain, Mexico, Venezuela, Vietnam, Ukraine, Germany, and the United States. Cuba also works with Canadian companies like YM Biosciences to develop cancer drugs. On the vaccine front, Heber Biotec formed a joint venture with the Indian giant Panacea Biotec to mass-produce vaccines. Should its AIDS vaccine succeed, India would be well placed to help distribute it globally.

On September 19, 2002, Cuba also received a $26 million grant from the Global Fund for AIDS, Tuberculosis and Malaria, strengthening its multisector AIDS effort being channeled through the United Nations Development Program. Goals include an improved quality of life for those with HIV, greater education and outreach to workers in different sectors, and a reduction of high-risk behavior among vulnerable groups, including commercial sex workers, men who have sex with men, and young people. At that time, the government estimated that there were 454,500 men who have sex with men in Cuba. It also estimated that there were 3,168 individuals with HIV, and 1,500 who needed antiretrovirals. At the time, 693 people were receiving therapy, and 822 were on waiting lists. As the national program expanded, officials estimated that the number of people with HIV could double, due to the proliferation of testing services.

Looking Ahead

In May 2003 Cuban officials hosted Foro 2003, a biannual Latin American AIDS conference, which attracted over 3,000 participants, including activists, physicians, scientists and a good number of Cubans with HIV. For three days, participants openly met in workshops, and many told US activists in attendance that they were generally satisfied with their country's AIDS program.[26] But that was in a public setting. According to Richard Stern, an American treatment activist based in Costa Rica who attended, other activists offered different stories when he left the conference site and met them at the Monserrate support group.[27]

Stern also heard from two men on therapy that, while HIV care was good, they had developed resistance to the first-line regimens they were given. Like Cheo, they needed salvage drugs such as Agenerase and Amprenavir, which were not available. They also lacked access to updated treatment information. Access to the internet in Cuba requires owning a business or government permission, he was told. Even if the support group had a computer, they couldn't legally use it because they are not an official government group.

A Political Step Back

Fidel Castro opened Foro 2003, which chose human rights as its theme. It proved a bitterly ironic choice, given that, less than a mile away from where he spoke, the government executed three Cubans. They were caught hijacking a ferry on April 2 to escape the island. After what human rights monitors called a sham trial, a judge found them guilty and they were shot. News of the impending trial had caused some US AIDS activists to boycott the conference.

Even within Cuba the executions were a shock, coming on the heels of a crackdown on the opposition a month earlier.[28] In March, without warning, the Cuban government arrested seventy-five democratic "dissidents" – opposition leaders, human rights advocates, and others pushing for increased trade with the US – and jailed them for up to twenty-eight years. Some had been meeting with US Congressional officials in the weeks prior to their arrest, pressing them to drop the embargo. In 2002 the House of Representatives voted to end the enforcement of travel restrictions to Cuba, and, prior to the crackdown, the Senate was moving to do the same.

Since the executions, Cuba and its record on human rights have again become the subject of headlines in the US and global press. The attacks on pro-democracy groups reflect the most punitive aspects of a regime that continues to take extreme measures to police its citizens. The executions also stole global media attention that should have gone to Foro 2003 and the progress that Cuban health officials, doctors, drug manufacturers and activists are making against AIDS, despite economic and political difficulties.

In the US the Bush administration reacted to developments in Cuba by seriously tightening restrictions on travel or any trade with the island by US residents. It will again enforce the travel restrictions that were eased under Clinton, and ordinary Americans who try to travel to or do business with Cuba face stiff penalities. In 2002, 160,000 Americans visited the island, half of them Cuban-Americans.[29] The rules now technically allow

US citizens to visit Cuba, but unless they are journalists, academics, or government officials, or receive a special license, they can't spend money on the island. Those caught violating the rules face ten years in prison, a $250,000 criminal fine and a $50,000 civil penalty.

Needless to say, my special visa and direct flight from Miami to Havana are not options for most American travelers. And the Bush administration has made it clear that it is going to make it harder for pro-Cuba groups to support Cuba. Recently, Global Exchange, the progressive organization that has operated "reality tours" to the island for a decade, was informed that its special license would not be renewed.

Human rights groups have responded by demanding that Bush reconsider his policy. These groups have also condemned Castro's political crackdown, and are allied with a number of key congressional leaders who favor easing the travel rules and increasing US contact with Cuba – including business relations. With the Cuba debate raging, the US Senate passed an amendment in November 2002 to end the embargo that mirrors last year's House bill. Both will go to Bush for approval, or more likely a veto.

The new block on US relations with the island will cause more economic shortages and shut down avenues of communication and support for democratic activists and others in Cuba, including AIDS groups. It will make it harder to bring or send medicine, medical journals or other donations like cash to Cuba. It will also limit the important exchange of information between AIDS physicians and researchers in Cuba and the US. That's especially unfortunate, given that Cuba has important experience in battling AIDS – quarantine aside.

Cuban activists hope that there is a global audience to hear what they so urgently have to say. By speaking out, critics like Cheo and Manuel are seeking international support from HIV-positive and human rights groups as they lobby the Castro regime to increase access to treatment information and drugs, and to do more for prisoners with HIV and those in less well-furnished sanatoriums. As of mid 2003, Cubans with HIV urgently needed more medicines, including non-nucleoside and protease drugs, as well as food and other basic necessities that remained scarce. With the crackdown on dissent, they also need more support from the global community than ever.

AIDS is currently more under control in Cuba than it is almost anywhere else. That success is based on a mix of controversial strategies, including early quarantine – globally condemned – and generic innovation – globally hailed. The benefits of its aggressive program of testing, prevention and now treatment remain remarkable – a success story that reflects Cuba's focus on bettering the lot of its citizens as a group over individual rights. One can easily appreciate this success by looking at Haiti, just next door, where 30 million have died in two decades. On a global level, Cuban trade and health officials have also shown that they are ready to provide leadership and resources to countries seeking access to low-cost, high-quality medicines and vaccines. Cuba has continued to ally itself with Brazil and South Africa in a developing-bloc challenge to the US positions at the WTO.[30] Whether the international community will allow poor countries to buy Cuba's generic drugs with donor funds from multilateral sources like the Global Fund is another question. It seems doubtful given the influence the US has on that organization.

The downside of Cuba's AIDS program can also be measured in human terms: decreased quality of life and a loss of freedom and sense of identity for those with HIV and AIDS. On that scale, the rights of those who are uninfected in Cuba continue to outweigh those HIV-positive people, and that spells inequality and, often, discrimination.

In the wake of the crackdown on free speech, as US hawks call for more punitive measures against Castro and progressives push for actions to help the Cuban people, it's hard to imagine a major change in US policy toward Cuba. For now, activists on both sides, including AIDS activists, will continue to push a political agenda that emphasizes greater human and civil rights for Cubans, including those with HIV.

6

HIV MEDICINES COME TO RURAL HAITI

Haiti, once the nineteenth-century pride of the Antilles, remains the poorest country in the western hemisphere, a small island the size of Maryland that shares a 360-kilometer border with its wealthier neighbor, the Dominican Republic. It also has the biggest AIDS epidemic in the region. For that reason, it's surprising to see that Haiti has taken a global lead in confronting AIDS in several arenas: prevention, vaccine development, and most recently treatment.

A stone's throw from glittering Miami, rural Haiti more closely resembles southern Africa – the other global AIDS hotspot. For that reason, Haiti offers the ideal comparative test case of how well or quickly treatment can be scaled up in a setting of dire poverty and limited resources, one where the epidemic is already entrenched and exists alongside other endemic co-diseases like malaria and tuberculosis. The majority of its 9 million citizens live in small towns and villages where jobs and food are scarce. Half of all rural residents are illiterate and work as subsistence farmers, scraping a living out of eroded soil. An ongoing three-year US economic blockade of international loans for clean water and other basic resources has contributed to declining health conditions, especially in the countryside.

The aid embargo was enacted in protest against alleged improprieties during the May 2000 election, under the government of Rene Preval, one of President Aristide's closest associates and his successor.[1] Despite being out of office, critics say Aristide still called the shots. The marred elections marked a blatant grab for power by the Lavalas ("The flood") camp, a coalition of populist, grassroots organizations that first swept Aristide into office.

In 1990, Jean-Bertrand Aristide, a former Salesian priest who embraces liberation theology, won the presidency by a landslide in what is seen as Haiti's first democratic election, ending decades of military rule. After seven months he was overthrown in a military coup, and served most of his term in exile in Washington, D.C., until his return in September 1994, courtesy of a UN-sanctioned US military operation called Operation Uphold Democracy. He helped Preval win in 1996, then in 2000 won a second term by another landslide.[2]

During the rocky period since he resumed power, many NGOs and donors have followed the Bush administration's lead and curtailed their activities in Haiti, contributing to a sharp decline in services to Haiti's rural poor, including healthcare. Without money to run the country, Haiti has fallen into further chaos: hunger and unemployment remain at desperate levels, and there's been a rise in drug trafficking, crime and fresh waves of "boat people" seeking Miami's shores.[3] Although Haiti's poverty and political crisis have deep roots, activists like Paul Farmer, a Harvard physician who works in Haiti's interior, draw a direct connection between the suffering of AIDS patients and the embargo. Illness and poverty are like the marassas, the twins of voudon, Haiti's animist religion of spirits – inseparable.[4]

The harshness of Haitian rural life only underscores the dramatic success of an ongoing AIDS program in Haiti's central plateau. There, a group of Harvard physicans led by Paul Farmer – who heads Partners In Health, a Boston-based non-profit organization – have successfully treated TB and now HIV patients who are poor villagers. The PIH team has argued that poverty is not an impediment to successful treatment if other ingredients are in place. PIH's innovative approach to curing resistant TB, and now HIV, has highlighted a strategy called Directly Observed Therapy, or DOT.[5] Theirs is a community-based DOT model that stresses empowerment and emotional support to boost patient adherence to treatment. The key to management of AIDS in Haiti, Farmer argues, involves political will and a basic commitment to health for the poor, as well as an investment in local community development. This approach views patients as potential peers and allies in the fight.

While that sounds good on paper, I wanted to know how well the PIH program really functioned on the ground, and under what conditions their DOT model can be applied in other settings, health infrastructures and countries. I wanted to know who was being left out of treatment, and why. I was interested in comparing a *rural program in Cange with a larger AIDS project in the capital, called Gheskio, headed by Bill Pape, a pioneering Haitian physician. How well would DOT work in Port-au-Prince, a bustling, overcrowded port city? I also knew Farmer and Pape wanted to scale up their pilot treatment programs. How were these plans coming along? How easily could the results of their pilot efforts be reproduced at the national level? Was Aristide supportive? What about the political opposition? Was the Bush administration helping or hindering the plan? I was especially curious to see how they viewed Haiti's volatile political situation, and what steps could be taken to overcome the foreign aid impasse.*

I wanted to know whether the stigma surrounding AIDS and homosexuality was changing there. In the 1980s and 1990s, I'd reported on AIDS and gay issues in Haiti and encountered a deep, entrenched vein of homophobia, partly linked to Catholicism.[6] I had met a few gay Haitians who were openly HIV-positive, but they had all died. Others remained closeted and hid their status from their families.

Globally, Paul Farmer, who is a white doctor, was speaking on behalf of Haitians with HIV. I went to visit the PIH program there in the fall of 2001. Through my work and family relations, I know many of the frontline players in AIDS, including Paul, who I regard as a friend, President Aristide and his dynamic wife Mildred, herself a leader in the AIDS fight, Bill Pape and the team at Gheskio, and a number of physicians. I also know the activists and journalists who once lionized Aristide and now bitterly denounce him.[7] Before my visit, I re-read a barrage of e-mail updates from colleagues, Haitian and foreign, who work as journalists and human rights activists there. They lamented the country's intensified poverty and economic woes, the negative impact of the aid embargo on daily life, the civil insecurity and rise of drug gangs, the pitched battles between pro- and anti-Aristide groups. Life had become even more impossible, they agreed. The situation would only get worse unless Haiti could improve its economy – and here the US was calling the shots. The situation would continue to negatively affect AIDS and health-care for Haitians. But to what degree? What would I really find up in the mountains at Cange?

Over the years, the dun-colored mountains of central Haiti have come to resemble a giant ridge-backed dinosaur frozen in time. The stark peaks are often void of a single tree, and further below, all that is left of Haiti's once-lush forest and valleys is semi-arable land dotted with cactus and spiky acacia bushes. Long-gone are the slopes of coffee trees, and fields of bananas and mangoes.

From the air, the paved highway that leads from the capital, Port-au-Prince, into Haiti's high, forested interior becomes a broken line, disappearing altogether in places. Thirty years ago this road was a winding feat of engineering, a proud sign of rural Haiti's continuing development. Today it would be generous to call what remains of it a road, especially after midday summer rains. Better to view the steep, gutted dirt track as an ideal test for the most powerful, rugged four-wheel-drive jeep, one that requires a driver to continually monitor the vertical angle of ascent and wonder at the sight of rusting overturned trucks that litter the mountain pass.

For the majority of people heading for the village of Cange, where the Zanmi Lasante (Creole for "Partners In Health") medical clinic is located, there is little choice in making the journey. They and their family members are sick, desperate and penniless. Many live in tiny mud shacks clinging to the mountain, without electricity, eking out a living as subsistence farmers. Their faces and bodies bear the signs of chronic hunger and toil; children have distended bellies, their hair rust-colored from malnutrition. Many have tuberculosis, parasitic diseases, and now HIV. They leave their shacks in the mountains to arrive at all hours of the day and night, some shouldering dying relatives on hard-wood pallets like an awkward religious cortege. By dawn, dozens are camped out, waiting to be seen by the clinic's small staff.

The sight of the large Cange complex suddenly looming above the trees in this otherwise barren landscape seems nothing short of a miracle, a kind of Oz. How, one thinks, did this get here? And who in their right mind would build it?

Championing Human Rights

The answer is a group of idealists led by Dr. Paul Farmer, an American doctor and anthropologist from Harvard who has become world famous as a champion of the poor who views health as a fundamental human-rights issue. Farmer came to the region in 1983 and quickly found his calling in Cange, a small hamlet not far from the border with the Dominican

Republic. Many of the district's sharecropping families had recently been displaced by a huge hydroelectric dam built on the nearby Artibonite River. The dam now provides most of the electricity for Port-au-Prince, but none to the surrounding villages. The whole area lacked health services, and regional clinics had little to offer in the way of medicine.

Farmer had a vision of a medical center that could provide care to rival a rich place like Harvard, but one that was developed on the basis of community ownership and investment. He benefited from the commitment of Père Fritz Lafontant, a well-respected Episcopal priest who mobilized community support for the project. With several friends, Farmer launched Partners in Health (PIH), a small non-profit organization that sponsors the Cange center and similar projects in Peru, Mexico, Cambodia and Roxbury, Massachusetts, a poor Boston neighborhood.

Today, PIH's modest staff at Cange provides care for well over a million people, including 100,000 in its primary catchment area. Word of mouth attracts residents from across Haiti who have heard about their AIDS program. Fees for health services are nominal or nonexistent. In addition to primary care and a focus on endemic illnesses like typhoid, malaria and dengue fever, the project has a maternal health and pediatric program, a state-of-the-art STD clinic, a recently built tuberculosis and infectious disease center, and it provides comprehensive HIV care. PIH has also built schools, homes and communal water systems, and provides work for residents of the area. Many have become health workers and counselors, trained midwives and nurses. No wonder locals regard Dokte Paul, or Blan (Whitey) Paul, as the closest thing to a saint or God they're likely to encounter.

Battling Stigma

The country has a per capita gross domestic product of less than $400, and an unemployment rate that rose from 70 percent to almost 80 percent between 2000 and 2003. For decades, the country has relied heavily on foreign and humanitarian aid. Health services are poor and only 40 percent of the population have access to clean water. For every 1,000 babies born, five mothers die – a situation a hundred times worse than in the most developed countries.[8] Malaria and tuberculosis are endemic, along with waterborne illnesses. There's also meningitis and polio – diseases eradicated elsewhere in the western hemisphere.

In the countryside, there are few doctors or nurses, and nationally only 1.2 doctors for every 10,000 citizens.[9] Many rural residents travel two hours or more to reach the nearest clinic, and so often don't bother unless they're near death; instead, they rely on traditional healers who use herbs and roots to treat illnesses. Around 400 to 500 Cuban doctors work in Haiti for one- to three-year stints as part of the Castro government's mission to help support development in other poor countries. Many work in the countryside, where they have made a difference in treating AIDS patients. But the need is extreme. Now, in the new millennium, hunger has sharply risen in Haiti, due in large part to the three-year blockade of $500 million in promised foreign-aid development money by the Bush administration and European allies from January 1999 through to Aristide's second inauguration in February 2001.[10] They also froze $146 million in Inter-American Development Bank (IDB) loans, including $22.5 million for medical supplies, $54 million for clean water programs, and money for education programs.[11] The blockade left Haiti economically paralyzed and effectively prevented Aristide's fledgling administration from running the country. What's worse, Haiti has had to pay millions of dollars in interest and "commission" fees to the IDB for loans it can't access. Farmer is among those who have called the payment of such fees "illegal."[12]

Japan is among the countries that broke the embargo by providing a small amount of emergency aid – $2.8 million – to boost food production in April 2001.[13] But many NGOs and other agencies, themselves dependent on the goodwill of governments and major donors, observed the embargo, sharply curtailing their activities in Haiti. Across Haiti, community projects that depend on the support of outside organizations were hit hard: services to Haiti's rural poor, including health-care, were sharply affected.

"The [$46 million] in IDB loans that are blocked by the US administration is urgently needed," wrote Farmer in an angry *Lancet* article of February 1, 2003, blaming the declining health conditions in rural Haiti on the embargo. "During the past two years, we have seen further deterioration in regional public health infrastructure," he said, adding that "[h]umanitarian assistance is being withheld while the country's health profile is deteriorating."

The Bush administration, Farmer charged, "is playing politics with the lives of Haitians in order to punish a democratically-elected leader who they no longer like." Calling the present embargo "immoral," Farmer wrote that "[s]uch policies are both unjust and a cause of great harm to the Haitian population, especially for those living in poverty." Critics point out that the US gave foreign aid to the former Duvalier dictatorship and successive military regimes for decades.[14] They turned a blind eye to the abuses of the notorious "Papa Doc" and his son "Baby Doc." The US also stands accused of failing to enforce a trade and oil embargo against the Duvalierist coup-makers who ousted Aristide on September 29, 1991 – seven months after he was elected by a landslide.[15]

Exposing US Interests

The US embargo of Haiti has everything to do with US economic interests and Aristide's – really Haiti's – inability to follow the rules of an agenda set by US economists and their allies at the World Bank and other bilateral donors.[16] That agenda is for economic reform and privatization, and is being pushed onto many poor countries by free-market economists who contend that unfettered capitalism leads to development.[17] Since Aristide resumed power, Haiti's economy and state-run institutions have been increasingly opened up to free-trade competition, and private and foreign development.[18]

Unfortunately, structural adjustment hasn't worked. Haiti signed on to this program in the late 1980s, but the result has been greater poverty, particularly in rural areas.[19] For example in 1991, before Aristide's overthrow, there were 60,000 jobs in the light manufacturing sector; in 2000 there were 25,000.[20]

As Farmer has remarked, there is a bitter irony here, since Aristide's government stands accused by leftist groups and even supporters of totally caving in to the World Bank and IDB over its acceptance of $1.2 million in foreign aid in January 1995. Aristide, long viewed as a radical critic of capitalism, was excoriated for paying the interest and commission fees on these loans.[21]

Throughout 2001, world leaders, humanitarian agencies and lending institutions were pressured to end the embargo. Harvard's Jeffrey Sachs and

Congressman Joe Kennedy were among those who penned editorials arguing that America's treatment of Haiti was unfair.[22] Eventually, donors agreed. In November 2001, the IDB approved a $1 million grant to the Pan American Health Organization for technical assistance to Haiti in the area of HIV/AIDS. But in reality the money was intended to support PAHO consultations with Aristide's government. Many groups noted the irony, since the IDB was still blocking release of $76 million in health-related grants and loans that would help the administration fight AIDS.[23]

They finally offered Haiti new World Bank and IDB loans in late 2001. But the aid had political strings attached to it. To begin with, the money would be channeled through NGOs, not Aristide's government. As critics like Farmer noted, that allowed NGOs to avoid recording that they had helped Haiti in their institutional ledgers – lest they be accused of taking sides against the Bush administration.[24] In addition, the loans given to NGOs would not directly strengthen Haiti's public institutions or public health system. In May 2003 Haiti was promised access to between $100 million and $150 million in IMF funds for poverty reduction and growth, after agreeing to further economic reforms that are especially harsh for a country reeling from AIDS and dealing with a staggering poverty level. Haiti then had a year to cut deficit spending in half, from 5.2 percent to 2.7 percent, to reduce inflation from 13 percent to 10 percent, and to monitor spending in public sector enterprises. If it fulfills these obligations after twelve months, it will be given the funds; if it fails, it might lose the money. At the time of the new loan agreement, Haiti had accrued debts of $60 million to the World Bank and IDB.[25] But the banking institutions were continuing to use the carrot-and-stick approach of foreign aid to bring Haiti in line with US economic and political thinking.

A Hidden Epidemic

After two decades the HIV epidemic has killed 260,000 Haitians – 30,000 in 2002. Nearly the same number of new cases crops up each year. Already, between 150,000 and 200,000 children have become orphans, having lost one or both parents. The latest figures show 6 percent of adults are HIV-positive – approximately 276,000 people. That's the higher estimate. The lower estimate is half that: closer to 132,000, based on epidemiological surveys. The numbers are hard to pin down because they derive from those who voluntarily seek an HIV test, and only 4.5 percent of Haitians have opted to do so. There are only sixty private and public testing centers that offer HIV tests. Most offer only a rapid test for diagnosis, with limited counseling. But among new cases, half are in women – often young women. Another 36,000 babies and children are estimated to have HIV or AIDS – again, as a generous estimate.

The prevailing attitude of many Haitians toward AIDS and HIV is characterised by fear and ignorance. Those who believe in voudon often say AIDS is the product of a curse by a neighbor, something requiring divine intervention. To this day, few people have openly declared their HIV status, fearing discrimination. Instead, those with AIDS remain isolated, afraid of telling the truth to their families. In much of rural Haiti, AIDS patients who can't afford hospital care typically return home to their villages to die, and lie for weeks inside darkened huts without even basic medicines to alleviate their pain.

The Roots of Stigma

The issue of stigma has special resonance for Haitians, due to an early 1980s policy by US health authorities that branded Haitians a high-risk group for AIDS – one of the four H's, along with homosexuals, heroin users and hemophiliacs. There was a backlash against Haitian-Americans and a fall in tourism. An unknown number of HIV cases were the result of exposure to dirty blood, before the national blood supply was cleaned; some were paid donors who regularly sold their blood to commercial plasma companies – a largely unregulated practice in Port-au-Prince, which was stopped.

Today the majority of cases are heterosexual. But the early association with male homosexuality – officially outlawed in Haiti – led to a backlash of homophobia. Today, Haiti remains a traditional society, one where the Catholic Church plays an important role, as do Protestant and other religious groups. Homosexuality is not openly discussed and is viewed as taboo by many. There is no openly gay movement, and few openly gay activists. Instead, gays in Haiti live private, semi-closeted lives. As in much of Latin America, many gays and bisexuals marry to conform to social and parental

expectations. Social attitudes toward gays and lesbians are steadily changing, but not quickly enough.

Most Haitians with HIV also choose to hide it, fearing rejection by
their families or other repercussions. Discrimination is a serious problem.
In the early years, the few wealthy Haitians who could afford to travel
went to Canada, Europe or the US to seek care and medicine for HIV.
They died away from home, virtually exiled. Even today, it's not uncommon to hear of people abandoned by their families when their HIV status
is known, according to doctors treating these patients. For years, few
people died of AIDS in Haiti – at least officially. Death certificates listed
tuberculosis as the cause of death in many young people. TB is a common
co-infection in Haiti linked to poverty, not necessarily to a suspect
sexuality.

Today, people with HIV are still turned away by many institutions.
Businesses fire employees, who have no protection against discrimination.
Some churches require testing before marrying couples, and refuse if one
partner is HIV-positive. Communities routinely isolate members who fall
sick and are suspected of being HIV positive. Orphanages refuse to accept
HIV-positive infants. Even hospitals turn away people who are referred to
these institutions for care by HIV testing facilities.

This level of stigma makes it very hard for Haitian health officials to
combat the epidemic on the island. The number of openly HIV-positive
activists is small. One of them, Esther Beaucicault, was recently honored
by the American embassy for her leadership as an HIV-positive woman who
set up a foundation in her hometown of St. Marc and began doing outreach
work with other HIV-positive women. Well educated and well spoken,
she's a role model for others with HIV, and is linking Haitians with HIV
to the global networks of HIV-positive people. For years she worked on her
own, investing her own funds to set up her small program, until recently
securing international support. Much of the growing, but still limited
AIDS advocacy comes from women's groups in Haiti.[26]

There are also advocates like Danielle and Robert Pennette, a
French–Canadian couple, who began the first orphanage for HIV-positive
children in Haiti and are providing treatment to a growing caseload of children.

Due to the high degree of poverty in Haiti and the absence of medicine
and doctors, there has been a strong focus on home-based and palliative

care for the very ill and dying. Here, as in other countries, there is an acute shortage of pain medicine for those with advanced AIDS. Several larger NGOs, like CARE and Promotion Objectif Zéro SIDA, are active in a few districts. They provide food aid and other forms of material assistance, as well as emotional support for families. Other NGOs, like World Relief and Catholic Relief Services, provide food supplements. Haiti has a lot of smaller NGOs who are now belatedly beginning to address the AIDS problem. But the blocking of donor aid due to the embargo has left these grassroots groups with only limited resources to address the huge demand for care.

Bringing Medicine to the Country

Between 2000 and 2003, Farmer and his team generated a slew of headlines and more visitors to Haiti for their boldest project ever. It is one that put Cange at the center of the international AIDS map and fueled a passionate debate among public health policy-makers. His team is determined to prove that it is possible to treat the poorest Haitians with HIV and AIDS using an expensive drug combination (called HAART, or highly active antiretroviral therapy), and to offer a community-based model of HIV care that can be applied in other poor countries. The key to their success is community mobilization, an empowerment model that views patients as equal allies in this effort. It also situates HIV care at home, not only at the clinic.

PIH began battling AIDS in Cange in 1986 (the same year Baby Doc and his Duvalierist cronies were sent into exile in France with US help, with the millions they stole from the national coffers safe inside Swiss bank accounts). At first, all they could do was to treat TB and HIV-related illnesses with traditional antibiotics, and offer palliative care. In 1995 they began administering AZT to pregnant women to prevent maternal transmission of HIV, with great success. In 1997 a prophylactic regimen (typically AZT, 3TC, and a protease inhibitor) was first offered to exposed health workers and victims of rape. A year later, ongoing antiretroviral therapy was added to the mix.

For PIH, the chief HIV treatment lesson has come from resistant tuberculosis, a chronic infectious illness. Although TB is clearly different from

AIDS, it shares certain features that pose a tremendous challenge to daily and long-term management. Both diseases require patients to take several powerful drugs daily and to substitute "second-line" or less effective drugs to overcome cases of drug failure and resistance, including multi-drug resistance. The medicines often trigger noxious drug-related side effects, and are hard to take without food. MDR-TB patients often have severe lung damage after failing for years on previous regimens. They must brave an additional two years of daily combination therapy, including injectable antibiotics. A key difference with HIV is that resistant TB can be cured, whereas antiretroviral drugs can only keep an active HIV infection in check. HIV persists as a latent infection that may rebound if a patient goes off therapy.

The PIH teams are strong advocates of Directly Observed Therapy (DOT), which they first used against MDR-TB.[27] The DOT approach calls for a nurse or third party to observe a patient swallowing their medicine. The primary goal is to help patients comply with difficult regimens in order to reduce the risk of drug resistance and subsequent drug failure. Those taking antiretroviral drugs for HIV must take a combination of potent, often noxious pills every day on a strict schedule, for life, to avoid resistance, which can occur quickly with some regimens. The longer one must take drugs, the greater the risk of developing drug resistance. In recent years, simplified, three-in-one "fixed-dose" pills have been introduced that greatly reduce the complexity of HIV treatment.

The issue of resistance and concerns about consistent drug supplies are often cited by critics as good reasons for avoiding the introduction of anti-HIV therapy in poor countries. Skeptics argue that, aside from the cost, it's just too hard to treat patients like those in Haiti without an adequate health infrastructure and trained professionals to ensure adherence. They point to TB and warn that the universal use of HIV drugs will give rise to novel MDR-HIV strains that will make it harder to treat and control AIDS in the future throughout the world.

Although he admits that drug resistance is a challenge, Farmer says he does not believe that it should "serve as an excuse to let the destitute die of AIDS." The PIH initiative is called HIV Equity, for good reason. The fight for access to HIV drugs is fundamentally one for justice. "The people who say you can't treat the poor with these drugs are just looking for a reason not to do it," said Farmer, taking square aim at what he calls the heart of the problem: greed and indifference.

It's amazing how many excuses people can come up with when they don't want to do something. The bottom line is that rich countries and governments don't want to pay for medical care for poor people. Not here, not there. I'm not saying HIV disease isn't a complex medical disease – it is – but it can be managed with existing medicine and closer supervision.[28]

If it can be done in Haiti, he maintains, it can be done anywhere.

TB is the Model

When Farmer starts talking about how his team approached the HIV problem, his anger is quickly replaced with enthusiasm.

I wish everyone could see what we are doing here. I really think MDR-TB is a great model for HIV because it's even harder to treat resistant TB in my opinion. Of course, it's true that people don't have to take the TB drugs for as long, but the TB drugs are tougher to tolerate and they don't always work as well. The problem is that not many people really know how to treat resistant TB.

Farmer's group had had several cases in Cange in the early 1990s. "Most had been cured, as were all of our regular TB patients."

An estimated 2 million people a year die of TB, a contagious disease caused by a bacterium that thrives in settings of poverty and overcrowding. Around the world, many governments have adopted a standard aggressive treatment for active TB called DOTS – the S stands for "short-course" – a regimen using first-line drugs that was created by the WHO for global TB management. In Haiti, as in many poor countries, TB is often the first marker of HIV infection, and remains the primary cause of death among HIV-positive individuals when people literally stop being able to breathe.

Very few strategies exist to combat MDR-TB strains, which are spreading throughout the world. It is considered a chronic illness that is very expensive and almost impossible to treat, even when second-line drugs are available.

In 1995, Farmer and a PIH colleague named Jim Kim, also an MD and anthropologist, learned that a priest and friend of theirs from Moscow had died of drug-resistant TB. The man, Father Jack, had previously worked in

Carabayllo, a shantytown outside Lima, Peru. There the PIH duo discovered a fast-growing epidemic of MDR-TB, with most patients resistant to all five "first-line" TB drugs. Since Peru had a strong national DOTS-TB program in place, with high cure rates, the news was especially alarming.

"They were not happy," said Farmer of Peru's Fujimori government. "And neither were we. They did not want to hear about flaws in their model program. And we'd lost a friend. We know he must've acquired this strain in the slum in which he served."[29]

He paused, sighing. "The problem is, people with MDR-TB can infect other people with resistant strains. So it becomes necessary to treat. What's the point of treating active cases of drug-susceptible disease and allowing the spread of more resistant strains? That's a recipe for a public health disaster."

Bucking conventional wisdom, he and Kim started using second-line TB drugs in individually tailored regimens. They called their strategy DOTS-Plus. In Lima, and soon in Haiti (where Cange had become the national reference center for drug-resistant TB), they set up support groups for MDR-TB patients, and trained community residents to become drug buddies who would provide emotional support and administer the medicine. Soon, the once-incurable regained their health.

Overall, the results have been quick and impressive. In both Carabayllo and Cange, MDR-TB cure rates were higher than those registered in US hospitals. In 2002, 90 percent of all registered TB cases were considered cured in Zanmi Lasante's facility, compared with only 26 percent in other regions of Haiti. Now the challenge is how to extend such TB success to the rest of the country.

Dr. Joia Mukherjee is Farmer's right-hand woman at the Peru project. She is also an AIDS specialist active in Haiti who recently replaced Farmer as PIH's medical director. Another outspoken activist-physician, Mukherjee did stints in Uganda before tackling MDR-TB and HIV. "Our programs in Haiti, Peru and Russia are focused on treatment equity – we treat with the best drugs, if it's here or there," she said. "That would not seem to be controversial, but of course it vaulted us onto the international TB stage because it was expensive – nothing more – and complicated." She paused, adding a mantra that Farmer is apt to repeat to visitors: "We've been successful because we remove the barriers to compliance. The doctor may be noncompliant, but not the patient."

The PIH team has since applied its community-based DOTS-Plus

model to HIV and in other challenging settings, notably Russian prisons –
with equally promising results (see Chapter 12). For these reasons,
Mukherjee believes that MDR-TB provides a critical new paradigm for
public health and global HIV control:

> What has succeeded before in public health are answers that are fairly
> straightforward and one-shot, like vaccination and the eradication of guinea
> worm. MDR-TB is the first example that looks at treatment of a compli-
> cated medical disease with a complicated treatment regimen on a public
> health scale, rather than a doctor–patient individual scale. I think the treat-
> ment of HIV will fall under that category. We're talking about the public
> health treatment of a chronic condition.

The Ethics of DOT

As a strategy to boost drug adherence DOT works very well, but its use is
hardly new. It's been a standard public health practice in institutional settings for decades, including hospitals, prisons, and mental institutions.
Historically, DOT has been directed at patients with highly communicable
diseases like TB, or at patients who were viewed as somehow deviant, noncompliant in their behavior, or otherwise unable to cope with therapy and
required supervision. While DOT does help patients manage their medicines, it began as a disease control strategy aimed at protecting the wider
society from contagion. Ethically, then, there are power dynamics that
underlie the DOT model and have led some critics to question why it is
often directed at poor or marginalized groups.[30]

Today DOT is not only popular in prison health settings, but in methadone and TB clinics and, increasingly, in HIV care settings.

As an anthropologist and activist, Farmer is keenly aware of the past and
potential abuses of the DOT approach. He defends the efficacy of PIH's
DOT model – but with a twist. In Cange, the ones giving out pills and
supervising patient behavior in a clinic are not doctors, but peers and community members who go to patients' homes. This introduces social equality and the concept of trust and emotional support into the formula, which
sustain adherence over the long haul. In Cange, community health workers
are called "accompagnateurs" – those who accompany. They don't just hand

over pills; they listen, they talk, they help individuals and their families cope with a range of daily, personal needs.

This home-based approach puts the onus of success on providers, not patients, and closely monitors the obstacles to patient access to care. In Cange, accompagnateurs crisscross the mountains daily on donkeys or on foot to see patients. At the first visit, they provide medication for a second daily dose. But often they return at other times in the day. Even by Haitian standards, this is a Herculean endeavor, for which they receive a modest salary and some food. Since the medicines are hard to take without food, patients are also given a small stipend for food (US$10) and some clean water.

"I can talk to the accompagnateurs about what I need and they try to help," explained Ti Ofa, 34, né Bernardin Garcia, one of Farmer's patients on therapy in Cange. "The biggest challenge for me at first was fear and isolation. People are so afraid of AIDS here. But the accompagnateurs are here to support me and my family. I like knowing that they care about my health and survival."[31]

"Until we arrived, people viewed AIDS as a death sentence," explains Dr. Leandre, an easy-going Haitian doctor who directs AIDS and TB programs at the Cange clinic. "Now they aren't so sure," he adds smiling.

In defense of DOT, Farmer points out that many of the best educated HIV and TB patients in the US and other rich countries fail to adhere to their complex, lifelong regimens. If DOT programs are administered by uncaring doctors or institutional providers with little relationship to the communities and patients they serve, they will fail to achieve PIH's larger goal: patient self-sufficiency.

For his part, Farmer has grown impatient of what he calls the "DOT debates" over the effectiveness and viability of this approach in various settings. "Frankly, I think a lot of it is a smokescreen," he says.

We never argued that DOT was the most important ingredient. After all, most of our patients have twice-a-day regimens. And we never asked the accompagnateurs to go to the patients' houses twice a day, although many of them do. What we ask is for them to care for their neighbors. That's why we call them accompagnateurs, not DOT workers. Solidarity and compassion, not supervision, is the key to program success.[32]

A Pilot HIV Program

The HIV Equity initiative technically began in 1998, when antiretroviral drugs were offered to several patients with severe AIDS who no longer responded to treatment of their opportunistic infections (OIs). In Cange, pulmonary TB is the biggest OI, followed by wasting (chronic digestive disease) and neurological complications of HIV. Like most PIH projects, the program began on a shoestring, using recycled drugs donated from Boston doctor friends and hospitals. In 2001, sixty-five people with advanced HIV disease received what Haitians call "tritherapie," a three-drug antiretroviral regimen. At the time, there was a very long waiting list for drugs.[33]

Patients are selected for HIV treatment according to clinical criteria that include advanced HIV disease, wasting, severe neurological complications of HIV, anemia or thrombocytopenia (low platelets), and recurrent OIs that don't respond to antibacterial or antifungal treatment. Initially, Farmer's team avoided splashing out on expensive CD4 cell and viral-load tests. They relied on basic laboratory data available in most rural health clinics to monitor patients, using clinical parameters such as weight gain and body mass index, renewed energy, and resolution of opportunistic infections. Within a short period, their data showed, most patients on triple therapy feel better and begin to gain weight and strength.

To counter their critics and test the thesis, PIH sent some patient blood samples to Boston for viral-load analysis. The first results were indisputable: 83 percent of patients in the HIV Equity initiative had undetectable viral-load counts. In some patients, the drop occurred within days of initiating therapy. CD4 cell counts rose quickly in some, more slowly in others. With few exceptions, the patients tolerated the regimens well and adhered to their medication. Initial drug-related side-effects like vomiting were minimal and easily managed. Prior to 2001, forty-eight patients had gone back to working and caring for their children.

"We were so stunned to see that some patients fell to undetectable within two weeks," remarks Dr. Leandre. As to drug-related toxicities, he notes that "[n]othing significant has emerged yet, nothing like metabolic problems. But we know such reactions can occur and so we are really paying attention to any signs of that."[34]

Drug resistance is a factor PIH anticipates. If and when a patient appears to be failing therapy, based on clinical markers, resistance testing will be used prior to switching their regimens – that is, if there's money for those expensive tests.

Publicizing the Personal Experience

In August 2002, a forum was held at Zanmi Lasante on "Health and Human Rights." Over 1,000 local residents crammed inside a church there, along with a number of outside Haitian doctors, politicians, and Farmer's colleagues from Carabayllo and Chiapas. Several of the treated HIV patients testified about their experience to date. All were converts to tritherapie, with nothing but good things to say about the HIV Equity initiative. As they testified to the Lazarus-like effect of HAART, amazed voices at the back of the church whispered in Creole, "Gade gwo moun la!" – "Look at that fat guy!" For Cange residents, the clinical details of combination treatment are hard to grasp, but not the sight of a neighbor given up for dead who now looks healthy.

Ti Ofa laughs, nodding, when he hears this. At thirty-five, he looks more like a teenager. But he was frail and unable to work when Farmer first placed him on therapy. Like his neighbors, he had heard about AIDS and knew about condoms, but he regarded the epidemic as a distant threat. He was married, with three children, and sexually faithful to his common-law wife. He had no idea HIV was the cause of the illness. His wife, it turns out, is also HIV positive and ill; she also started antiretroviral therapy. Their children are all HIV-negative.

"I was doing so badly; I hadn't prepared my funeral yet, but others were talking about it," explains Ti Ofa. "The minute Dokte Paul put me under treatment I became normal. There are a lot of people who say that you people in such a small poor country, you can't get access to those drugs, you can't manage them," he continues. "But for me, it's not true." That includes managing drug resistance, since he was among 7 percent of patients who have had to switch to a new drug combination. "We are the evidence of the success," he adds defiantly. "There is poverty, and we are poor, but that's not a reason to say we can't manage a big thing like this. And if we succeed, it shows all of us can manage this."[35]

The drugs are tough to take day-in and day-out, but Ti Ofa has never missed a dose. Food makes all the difference: "I took my medicines without food this morning because I didn't have any," he says. "The problem is that then it makes me feel bad. I have nausea; I have to lie down. If I eat, it doesn't do that."

Could there be a link between lack of food, poor drug absorption, lowered adherence and HIV resistance? There are no studies to document such a link, but some doctors wonder. At Cange, PIH staffers stress that adequate nutrition plays an essential, overlooked role in HIV care, particularly in poorer settings. "We talk about that in the support groups, where we focus on unexpected reactions, side-effects, what you must do, what the ideal behavior is to manage," says Dr. Leandre.[36] Many experts argue that food programs must be integrated into HIV programs.

The highlight of the 2002 forum was a declaration by the HAART patients to the world, a passionate defense of their right to HIV therapy: "We have a message for all people here and anyone who will listen. We are seeking solidarity. The fight we wage to get care for people with AIDS, with tuberculosis and other diseases, is the same fight we've been waging for a long time – for the right of all people to be able to live as humans."

The New Challenge: Scaling Up

The success of the Cange treatment project led to a new challenge: how to replicate this success at the national level. In July 2002, the PIH team presented their latest data at the Fourteenth AIDS Conference in Barcelona.[37] By then over 3,000 HIV patients were being followed, and 250 were on antiretroviral treatment – about 10 percent of the total number of HIV-positive clinic patients.

Those with advanced HIV illnesses that failed to respond to standard OI treatment showed dramatic improvements in their health within weeks. In late 2002, the Bon Sauveur clinic received a flow cytometer machine to measure CD4 T-cells on site. That now allows patients to be screened for therapy before the onset of advanced symptoms. In late 2002, the Haitian government adopted new antiretroviral treatment guidelines modeled on WHO guidelines for resource-poor settings. The guidelines call for a primary first-line regimen of d4T-3TC-NVP. AZT is used as a second-line regimen because it causes anemia, and many chronically malnourished patients with AIDS and TB suffer from anemia.

In a recent update, their group reported that the initial 300 patients who began therapy in 1999 were doing well. The dropout rate for the program was under 2 percent since 1999. Side-effects continued to be rare, and only a few patients had to switch regimens. That doesn't mean it was a perfect picture. For a subset of the first 300 patients on therapy who appeared well, "death will occur in the first two years, and is likely due to sub-clinical immune suppression leading to aggressive opportunistic infections," PIH predicts. Late diagnoses also played a part in this outcome.

Many of the Cange patients have active TB. Since TB and HIV drugs shouldn't be taken together, those who are not in advanced stages of AIDS are treated first for TB – an arduous regimen in itself. But Farmer still loses these patients – though rarely – and each death remains a personally felt tragedy. "It's never something one should get used to," he said in 2001, after a young girl in his care died of advanced pulmonary TB. The girl had arrived at the clinic too late for the drugs to work quickly enough. "I thought we'd be able to save her," he said. "We just needed a little more time." These days, the word has spread throughout Haiti that help is available at Cange, prompting ill patients to seek care earlier.

Impact on Prevention

The combining of treatment with prevention and epidemiological efforts is another success story. According to PIH, "Decreased stigma is reflected in an increased willingness of patients to discuss their diagnosis openly, an increased demand for HIV testing, and a reduced number of patients' complaints regarding abusive behavior of family members of neighbors."

Within two years of the launch of the HIV Equity program, there has been a 300 percent increase in use of the clinic's free HIV counseling and testing services. In 2002, over 4,000 HIV-positive people were being followed on the program, whose services and facilities have duly expanded. In two years, outpatient visits have increased from 30,000 to 200,000 annually. Today the clinic includes general medicine, women's health, pediatric and infectious disease clinics, adult and pediatric inpatient wards, two operating rooms and a village school. Visiting surgeons from Harvard have offered surgery and eye care; and medical teams from Cuba and Mexico have been welcomed for years.

Another victory has come from PIH's shrewd negotiations with drug suppliers. In the late 1990s, PIH helped found the Green Light Committee to stop TB, which pioneered a pooled procurement plan of first- and second-line TB drugs from multiple sources. They've done the same with anti-retrovirals, securing discounts on brand-name drugs, buying generics from WHO-approved pre-qualified manufacturers, and teaming up with the International Dispensary Association, or IDA, a Dutch non-profit whole-sale distributor of essential drugs. The IDA and UNICEF are among groups developing pooled procurement and distribution systems that will be available to UN agencies and NGOs. In Haiti, these actions have led to a steep drop in drug prices, from $10,000 per patient per year in 1999 to $300 for a standard three-drug combination by 2003.

But none of this was easy. For years, the story goes, Farmer and Jim Kim would regularly raid the drug stockrooms of Harvard hospitals in Cambridge and Boston, promising to replace them later.[38] PIH also relied on donations by recycling groups and physicians at Harvard who would send regular donations. And Farmer, a prolific author of books on medical anthropology and public health, has donated a sizeable percentage of his earnings as a lecturer and global AIDS superstar to his Cange program.

Farmer's group has concluded that DOT-HAART can work in rural Haiti if there is an uninterrupted supply of high-quality drugs, and they have urged international authorities to develop mechanisms to deliver medicines and funding quickly to Haiti and other poor nations. In a keynote speech to a world audience at the Barcelona conference, Farmer delivered that message, and received a standing ovation.

The Race to Scale Up

"What Paul has done so well is mobilize the community," said Jean (Bill) Pape, MD, another treatment pioneer who heads Gheskio, the biggest AIDS care center in Haiti and a premier HIV vaccine and research facility. "That's a lesson for all of us." But as Pape remarked to me in 2001, "There is a difference between a private initiative with private resources and a public health program. The key difference is money. Haiti doesn't have much. Well, Haiti doesn't have any."

But as the saying goes: that was then, this is now.

Almost overnight, Pape has had to radically amend his views to reflect rapid changes in Haiti's landscape. In fact, he's been a key figure behind much of this change. Following Barcelona, he and Farmer pled Haiti's case with President Bush and top US health advisors like Dr. Tony Fauci, head of the US federal AIDS research effort. He's also had the support of Aristide and his government. First Lady Mildred Aristide has taken a direct role in pushing the plan forward and making access to care a priority for the administration. Aside from money, then, political will is the new ingredient behind a sudden flow of money, new partners and opportunities into Haiti. With the dam broken, everyone's now scrambling to keep pace.

In December 2002, Haiti was among the first countries outside Africa to receive a $24.7 million grant from the Global Fund for AIDS, TB and Malaria, to carry out a comprehensive national AIDS program that includes treatment.[39] Pape helped draft the plan, along with officials in Haiti's health ministry and, of course, Paul Farmer. In all, Haiti has an open pipeline to $67 million in grants over five years. Over in Cange, PIH received $2.5 million from the Global Fund to expand treatment in the central plateau region. The Haitian health ministry will receive about $1 million to develop its capacity to coordinate the national rollout.[40]

Before the beginning of the scale-up, only 3 percent of an estimated 41,000 Haitians who needed treatment were getting it – around 1,200 people. The first Global Fund installment arrived in Cange in March, and as of June 2003, 5,000 patients were on treatment there. PIH's goal was to reach 8,000 people in a year.[41]

The national plan reflects a public–private effort spearheaded by the Haitian health ministry and Gheskio, with strong support from the Aristide government. There are many partners, including seventeen local civic groups, the private sector, multilateral organizations, and bilateral donors. Four US medical centers are also onboard: Cornell, Harvard, and Vanderbilt – reflecting Pape's and Farmer's existing ties to these institutions; and medical teams from the University of Miami are also working in rural Haiti and will be involved. Nationally, AIDS centers will be set up in twenty-five existing hospitals and health centers – one public and one private in each of Haiti's departments.

If all goes well, at least 2004 Haitians will be on treatment by January 1, 2004 – to coincide with the 200th anniversary of Haiti in 2004. Half the patients (actually 1004) will be treated by Gheskio in the capital, and the remainder by PIH in the central plateau. Farmer notes that, if at all possible, he'd like to have "2004 by 2004" in his region, "because faster rollout is how we'd celebrate Haiti's bicentennial."[42] In both programs, generic drugs will be used, and the first-line regimen for most new patients will be AZT, 3TC and nevirapine or efavirenz. (This last drug, made by Merck, was not yet available generically in Haiti in mid 2003.)

To meet the urgent scale-up need, a large infectious disease center is being built for Gheskio on six acres of land by the airport in the capital, with funding from two of Haiti's biggest banks. And in a sign of the shifting political winds, the US and French ambassadors in Haiti have held fundraising events for the new center. French money is paying salaries for Gheskio mobile teams to train staff at these new sites, while USAID funds will help renovate the sites and pay staff salaries there. Global Fund money will pay for drugs and test reagents.[43] More funding has come from the Bush administration, which is backing the rollout of seventy maternal HIV prevention programs (MTCT) across Haiti.[44] But since the Bush money is being disbursed by USAID and directed at NGOs, not the government, that move has generated considerable criticism from activists.

Finally, the William Jefferson Clinton Foundation, through its new global HIV/AIDS initiative, helped the government develop its detailed scale-up plan, one that relies on a partnership between the government and private groups.[45] The Clinton plan for Haiti focuses on repairing weaknesses in the public health infrastructure and integrating HIV treatment with beefed-up TB and STD programs, as well as OB/GYN services for pregnant women.[46]

Under the plan, Haiti hopes to identify and monitor an additional 142,000 individuals, and provide drugs for 26,000, by 2008. By then, other programs are slated to provide care for another 40,000 individuals and drugs for 6,500 more. If all goes smoothly, 32,000-plus people will be on therapy by 2008, and another 181,000-plus will be getting comprehensive care – between 60 percent to 70 percent of Haitians with HIV, based on current figures.

As the program rolls out, there is expected to be an increase in the demand for voluntary counseling and testing (VCT) and care services. Haiti hopes to test 2,600,000 people by 2008, and provide services for 260,000 HIV-positive pregnant women. It will launch four mobile VCT centers to reach groups in remote areas. Special groups at risk include women, sex workers and their clients, and young people, including some 15,000 street children and 30,000 "*restaveks*" (literally "to stay with") – domestic servants. In Haiti, 70 percent of *restaveks* are girls who are literally sold into forced life-time labor with families in exchange for room and board. Rape and sexual abuse of these children is common.[47]

Aside from clinical and medical services, the national plan focuses on supporting community-based organizations that will be critical in delivering services at the local level. Building upon Farmer's success, the program will adopt the accompagnateur model in selected areas, to support use of DOT. The plan notes the urgent need to support the empowerment of HIV-positive groups. Of course, these groups are few in Haiti now. Here the Clinton plan offers fewer details about how communities can overcome the prevailing stigma that discourages so many from seeking HIV testing and care.

Finally, there's a pressing need for a focus on Haiti's larger socioeconomic problems: hunger, widespread poverty and underemployment, lack of clean water and infant formula, lack of roads to Cange. Partnerships are envisaged with NGOs and private groups to provide basic services that are directly related to health. Farmer is among those pressuring US authorities to drop the aid embargo, which would release badly needed funds for clean water, food and agricultural programs.

On paper, the Clinton plan is impressive in its scope and long-term ambition. If it succeeds, it will not only save the lives of tens of thousands of Haitians who will otherwise die of AIDS, but will help build up other aspects of Haiti's infrastructure besides health.

"I'm all for public–private partnerships and Haiti's success story is of that stripe," says Farmer. "But we need to make sure that the public health infrastructure of these vulnerable countries gets the lion's share of the resources, however they are to be managed. Because it's the public sector that has the formal obligation to care for the poor, who happen to be the global risk group for HIV."

Other Positive Steps

Other projects are underway that focus on the treatment needs of particular groups, including orphans with HIV. In Port-au-Prince, over 150 children at Rainbow House, an orphanage run for HIV-positive children by the Pennettes, are getting help and care from Pape's team. By mid 2003, the orphanage had secured food and other support from UNICEF, smaller NGOs and private church-based donors in the US and elsewhere. In 2001 the Rainbow House had enough drugs for around forty children, with fifty more on a waiting list. "That's the hardest part – accompanying the children and supporting them as they get sick, knowing they are going to die and it can be prevented. It's heartbreaking," said Danielle Pennette in August of that year.[48]

Armed with new funds and drugs, she's started to focus on the future of these children – not just their immediate survival. They need love, families, financial and social support, schooling, and talented health providers to help them stay healthy and manage a life on antiretroviral therapy. In the US, pediatric HIV requires a team approach, and usually involves social workers to address the additional emotional needs of children and adolescents with HIV. Adherence is much harder for children; they require extra support. In Haiti there are no centers or resources dedicated to their multiple needs. More than anything, these children seek to live normal lives. But in a country where HIV is so stigmatized, this won't be easy. As HIV testing increases, there are also likely to be more HIV-positive children identified, increasing the demand for pediatric HIV services.

"We have to build the infrastructure, to make sure we succeed," said Pape, while admitting a tendency toward caution. He's especially worried about adherence and drug resistance. "We can't afford to fail, because the consequences would be too enormous," he explained. Still, he champions HIV treatment as an opportunity to rebuild Haiti's shattered health system, which will greatly benefit its society as a whole.

The Model: Integration

Haiti's national scale-up plan reflects an integrated model that links HIV services to a range of other care programs, including STD and TB control, family planning and prenatal care – all offered free at a single site. This model was developed in the early 1980s by Gheskio in Port-au-Prince, and has expanded to include other activities such as research, including clinical and vaccine trials for several diseases.[49]

The Gheskio center was started by a group of Haitian physicians in the mid 1980s, led by Pape. He has collaborated closely with US partners like Cornell and officials from Haiti's Ministry of Health to put in place a strong national HIV prevention program, which reduced the rate of infection to 4 percent by 2003. Gheskio also treated a small number of wealthy private patients who could afford access to US-priced drugs, and offered post-expo-sure prophylaxis to health professionals and rape victims when possible, and AZT to pregnant women, with good results.

In the future, Gheskio expects to offer VCT services for HIV to over 20,000 new people in 2003. They now offer rapid testing and MTCT ser-vices for pregnant women, including teenage girls – a rising caseload. Although overall seroprevalence rates in Haiti have declined in recent years, the percentage has increased in women and young people. By June 2003, eight Gheskio sites were up, and two had started working. All will be ready by Haiti's 200th anniversary.

Focusing on Research

Pape has kept the fires burning high on other fronts too. The Gheskio team has built up a first-rate vaccine and clinical research facility. Their center has provided an epidemiological picture of the spread of the virus since the early days.[50] They have also published important studies on sexually trans-mitted diseases and HIV in Haiti. Gheskio researchers have had impressive results using standard antibiotics to treat severe diarrhea, and relying on less expensive drug combinations to treat AIDS.[51]

In 2001 Gheskio successfully launched one of the first human phase II HIV vaccine trials, which also took place in Brazil and Trinidad and Tobago.[52] Each of these steps has called for the engagement of civil groups in targeted communities, including local leaders, Catholic and voudon priests, and HIV-positive patients who make up a community advisory board, or CAB, which approves Gheskio's various projects. These community actors have also had a say in the national plan and, along with nascent NGOs, now have a key role to play in educating and mobilizing civil society, and especially HIV-positive individuals, to con-front AIDS.

In the central plateau, PIH has been working overtime too. In 2002 they had 200,000 patients in Cange alone, more than Gheskio. By July a new clinic was up in Lascahobas, and CD4 tests were already available there. Next there were plans to rebuild the hospitals in Boucan Carre, Thomonde, and Hinche. According to Dr. Farmer, "[w]ithin a couple of years, the Département du Centre will have HIV prevention and care that is as good as the States. Better – since we have community-based care with accompagnateurs."

The Urban Challenge

Cange is a world apart from overcrowded Port-au-Prince. Many residents of the capital are displaced peasants who live in the slums with no ties to the local community or officialdom. Will HIV patients encounter doctors and health workers as dedicated as Pape and Farmer and their teams in public health centers? Will DOT work as well in other sites, where solidarity and compassion for neighbors is in shorter supply?

Farmer points out that Lima is an urban setting similar to Port-au-Prince, and that the PIH DOTS-Plus model works well there. In Lima, a sense of community ownership grew out of an investment of compassion, as well as money and resources. "It can be done," insisted Farmer. "Whether people want to do it is another matter."

While PIH has tackled the challenges of rural health delivery, Gheskio's team has dealt with the explosion of an urban pandemic in an overcrowded, deteriorating city of over 2 million people. It is located a stone's throw from a sprawling shantytown where some 20,000 people live in tightly-packed cardboard and aluminum-siding houses. There, living conditions are hazardous to health: there is no potable water, people bathe in open sewers, pigs forage for food in the alleyways, and a layer of smog from city traffic mixes with the smell of charcoal from cooking fires.

As Haiti's poverty has increased, so have crime, violence, prostitution and the illegal drug industry. Haiti today has become a major trans-shipment point for cocaine destined for the US, and drug gangs rule the streets. Drug money has created a climate of civil violence and daily insecurity throughout Haiti, especially in the poorest shantytowns. With its economy at a standstill, due in part to the international embargo, the Aristide government has been able to do little to stop gang or drug activity. It's not surprising that many returning exiles have launched private security businesses – the rare growth industry on the island. Meanwhile, tourism – long Haiti's top industry – is dead.

Future Threats

In the volatile brew that constitutes Haitian political life, things have become more tense recently, and the violence threatens to derail the well-funded national AIDS plan.[53] A recent example comes from Cange. On May 7, 2003 a group of armed men in army fatigues who claimed to be anti-Aristide attacked a jeep ferrying a PIH doctor and four nurses, and also packed with medicine. The nurses had come up to Cange to interview for jobs at the refurbished hospital in Lascahobas, and at a site in Belladares. Earlier that night the commandos had shot and killed two security guards at the hydroelectric power plant and tried to shut it down. They set the plant on fire, and took the medical team hostage before releasing them – and after much pleading – their precious cargo.

The attack was the second against PIH's team; in December 2002, a similar paramilitary group had harassed them. The violence, says Farmer, is linked to the government's efforts to root out a band of former military men on the Haitian border. In April 2003 PIH staffers had cared for some of those wounded in the border conflicts.[54]

Farmer is an outspoken activist, one who supports the democratically elected Aristide government and denounces efforts to topple it. Though he supports the AIDS effort of the Bush administration and its allies, he's critical of their anti-Aristide position and of outside efforts to undermine his presidency. Others who view Aristide differently, and may even oppose him, also worry that if political fighting prevails in Haiti, the ray of hope represented by the AIDS plan may be dimmed.

As veterans of Haiti's internecine politics, Farmer and Pape try to stay above the fray, keeping their eyes on the prize: saving lives and rebuilding Haiti. Now that funds are arriving, maybe someone will rebuild the road up to Cange. That would allow outsiders to evaluate the merits of

PIH's community HIV program for themselves. "If they can get here, we'll give them lunch," Farmer joked. "If they stay too long, we'll put them to work."

7

TWO MEXICOS:
ONE URBAN, ONE RURAL

For the better part of two decades, most AIDS experts have ignored America's southern neighbor, Mexico. Yet the epidemic there is serious and steadily growing, a problem that is fueled by poverty and Mexico's economic crises. In the mid 1980s, desperate American activists with HIV were crossing the border to bring back cheaper drugs they bought in Mexican pharmacies. In the mid 1990s, the reverse began to happen: US groups began sending recycled medicines across the border. The scale of these projects has remained very small, while the need for access to medicines has increased.

Given its large size and diversity, Mexico is a society that is modern, yet which retains many aspects of traditional culture. The Catholic Church continues to have a strong influence on social policies, including those that affect attitudes toward sexuality, including homosexuality. At the same time, Mexico boasts a revolutionary history, strong feminist and labor movements, and a nascent gay and lesbian movement. Sprawling Mexico City has the biggest population of any metropolis, reflecting the very rapid growth of a city that can't keep pace with the demands of so many new residents for housing, work, clean water, education and health services. Meanwhile, life for Mexico's poorest rural residents, including some indigenous Indian groups, remains at the subsistence level.

I decided to focus on the issue of access to AIDS care in Mexico because I think it provides a good test case to examine the issue of infrastructure as it relates to access for different groups in a given country. In recent years, critics of global AIDS treatment have cited lack of infrastructure as a legitimate reason to delay providing antiretroviral therapy to individuals in poor countries. What do critics really mean when they talk about infrastructure? How much of a barrier is it? Is lack of infrastructure just a code phrase for lack of development?

Over the years, I'd visited Mexico a number of times and worked as a newspaper journalist in Mexico City in 1985. I'd reported on the student strikes at the national university, on labor and land struggles, on drug trafficking and the struggles of new residents of the capital who were often from rural areas. I was familiar with Oaxaca, and decided to compare the HIV situation there with that in Mexico City. In the southern states of Chiapas and Oaxaca, indigenous Indian groups have been locked in a sometimes violent struggle with the government over civil rights, land and political power. How much do politics contribute to the issue of access to health-care? Does the government provide access to HIV care to these communities? How much do indigenous women benefit – or not – from these services?

In the post-9/11 period, as the US has tightened control of its border to Mexico, poverty has increased, tourist dollars have become scarce, and unemployment high. Sex work and drug trafficking are increasing – two factors fueling HIV's continued spread. I know from colleagues that these activities are increasing along both the northern and southern border regions of Mexico, particularly among women.[1] HIV among migrants is another factor contributing to the spread of the epidemic, particularly in poor, rural regions.

Before heading to Mexico City, I did an internet search and was surprised to find comparatively few articles about the treatment of HIV in Mexico compared with many other countries I'd researched. When I got there, I found it just as hard to get information about individuals and groups working in remote regions. The internet was not a good means of communication with local groups in Oaxaca. Nor was the telephone that useful. Instead I learned to rely on names and addresses written on scraps of paper to track down activists and groups. It required a car and traveling long distances. Along the Pacific coast and in Oaxaca City, AIDS groups said they felt cut off from events and news in Mexico City, and lacked access to information and resources that were plentiful in the capital. On a global level, this communication gap leaves the rest of us without much information about life for people with HIV in el otro

Mexico, *as residents of the mountains of Oaxaca joked to me – the rest of the country outside of Mexico City.*

"There are two worlds, two completely different realities when it comes to AIDS in Mexico," reported Dr. Gustavo Reyes-Teran, a native of Oaxaca who is an HIV specialist at Mexico City's leading respiratory hospital. "You cannot compare what you find in Oaxaca to Mexico City. Unfortunately, what exists up in the mountains is the truer picture. There you find a lack of infrastructure and medical attention, lack of training of doctors, and totally inadequate combinations of drugs prescribed for HIV. This is what we see in a huge percentage of cases. Patients are not only dying of AIDS, but are dying without any medical attention at all."[2]

Mexico's urban–rural disparity isn't limited to AIDS, of course, but applies to many aspects of life in this large nation. Life in the capital might resemble life in Switzerland for the richest citizens, but living conditions in the interior of the southern states of Oaxaca and Chiapas more closely resemble impoverished Africa. Health officials say rural Mexicans now have three times the risk of dying that urban citizens have. The situation is most critical for indigenous communities. For example, 40 percent of indigenous women in Mexico have anemia – a direct result of inadequate nutrition.[3] Among Indian groups who live in the Sierra Madre zone, hunger is constant, government services limited, and health-care fragmentary at best.

Many live in remote villages lost in the dense fog that settles over the peaks of this mountain range, located between the Pacific beach towns of Puerto Escondido and Puerto Angel and the state capital, Oaxaca City. To seek care, they spend hours walking down the mountain to one of two worn, curving highways to flag down a rare public bus or truck picking up passengers. In the rainy season when I visted, the daily torrential downpours made visibility almost zero, and completely washed away several sections of the highway. Locals waiting at the edge of the highway for rides appeared like blurry ghosts, suddenly looming up, chasing down trucks to no avail.

Imagine now having HIV and being very ill, suffering as many do from serious diarrheal diseases, high fevers, tuberculosis or lung infections. Little medical treatment is available in the mountains, and only basic care in coastal towns. Patients suspected of having HIV are automatically referred to Oaxaca City for testing and treatment. Many arrive in late stages of AIDS and tuberculosis, unaware of having HIV – that is, if they make it down the mountain. The length and cost of the trip alone rule out seeking medical treatment for some, say activists. For others, the cost of shelter and food in the city is a major obstacle.

"We are in a bad situation because it's a huge coast and everything along it is totally unprotected in terms of health services," explained Alfredo Ramos Garcia, an Oaxacan member of Frenpavih (National Front of People with HIV), a national PWA network, in 2002.[4] "It's impossible for a patient in a terminal stage to come to the city of Oaxaca for medicine. If they must cross one road, then the other, it can take up to fifteen hours." It's no surprise, say local activists, that rural residents die uncommonly fast, progressing from diagnosis to death in two years. In 2002, Frenpavih and other groups were lobbying the state Secretary of Health to set up emergency plans to help persons with AIDS in Oaxaca's most affected zones. But little was happening.

Lack of Government Response

Throughout Mexico, the distance between coast, mountain and city is as great as the various estimates of its AIDS problem. In mid 2002, the government put the official figure at 46,000 AIDS cases, based partly on death and disability certificates. Registered HIV cases numbered 150,000–200,000. But others say those figures are way off, and that HIV rates may be ten times higher. "I say there are no fewer than 450,000 people with HIV and most of them don't know it," said Dr. Reyes-Teran at that time. "They are poor and what is going to happen to them? We'll see them here in five or six years when they are dying of HIV wasting."

Activists agree the official numbers are underestimated. "The problem is that the government intentionally doesn't gather statistics," added Armando Belmares-Sarabia, a former state legislator from Puerto Escondido and a leader in local AIDS efforts. "As they see it, if we don't have statistics then we don't have a problem and we don't have to put our money into that," he said. "There is money in the state, but it is far from adequate. They are denying the problem and it just becomes harder to manage." Early on, the epidemic affected mostly gay and bisexual men in the capital and bigger cities. Now it has moved to rural parts and affects mainly heterosexuals, though activists believe that closeted bisexual cases constitute a portion. A growing percentage of women make up the newly exposed.

Like other countries, Mexico has begun to tackle the enormous challenge of providing life-saving HIV medicine to this growing rural population. The government says that an estimated 60 percent of eligible Mexicans with AIDS are getting free drugs through the social security system. Of course, that leaves out 40 percent who don't qualify. And then there are those who are not part of the social security system, including farmers, fishers and others who work for themselves.

The lucky ones getting treatment are mostly in the national capital. Many states have waiting lists for HIV medicines, and even for drugs to manage opportunistic infections. In 2002 there were only two state-run treatment programs outside of Mexico City distributing HIV drugs for free – one in Oaxaca city, the other in Guadalajara.

Infrastructure and Politics

"The problem with access to medicines in Mexico is only one part of the larger problem that relates to services provided by the social security system, which are deficient," said Anuar Luna, director of La Red Mexicana, a national network of people with AIDS that is at the forefront of the access battle. "The problem can't be appreciated in such an isolated way. There is some money to buy drugs, okay, but not to manage the needs of people with HIV. It's just that we have more politics than money."[5]

Like many Mexican institutions, the health sector lacks money and is plagued by bureaucracy, corruption and local turf wars. "We do have a serious problem in that there are few people in positions of leadership to really discuss policy regarding treatment and use of HIV drugs," Luna added.

"The public health system is universal, but limited. And that's due to political reasons really," said Dr. Reyes-Teran.

In the D.F. [Federal District], where most of the AIDS cases are, there are no waiting lists and all do get free treatment – if they are registered. They have to confirm residency in the D.F.; if they can't, they have to get it [treatment] in another state, or from the state of Mexico. But in the other states, there are waiting lists; there is not total coverage and this is significant. There are people needing treatment and there is no support for giving it to them.

In 2002, the progressive newspaper *La Jornada* chastised President Vicente Fox's administration for dedicating less than 1 percent of the 2002 national health budget to people with AIDS.[6] Fox also took an ax to the social security budget. "If the budget is less than 1 percent, what does that say?" asked Reyes-Teran at the time. "If AIDS and TB are priorities, they should assign a lot more money. Yet this issue is one of the most important to public health."

A year later little had changed in the government's attitude, said Reyes-Teran, but the death rate had climbed. By his count, closer to half a million Mexicans may have had HIV. He also noted that in 2002, by the official count, AIDS cases – again extrapolated from death rates – jumped from 46,000 to 64,000. How, then, could HIV cases have plateaued? "I'm telling you, we have a serious problem. It's due to late diagnosis of AIDS cases, and lack of early detection of HIV." He cited the two immediate obstacles that prevented care from reaching beyond big cities: lack of widespread testing and sites to detect new HIV cases, and lack of training for doctors, especially at the level of provinces, though not in the capital.

Reyes-Teran said that AIDS was the leading cause of mortality in young people aged between eighteen and forty years at his institute and in many general hospitals in Mexico. It is also the third-highest cause of death of young people in the country. "If there is no infrastructure, no financial support, then it's hard for our fight to succeed," he noted in 2002.[7] How can Mexico get money to fight AIDS if the government is denying the extent of the problem? "They are not dealing with it. Really, there aren't many cases in their view," he added.

"What is happening now in Mexico in relation to health-care assistance is worrisome," said Dr. Patricia Volkow-Fernandez, an outspoken, popular physician who treats women with cancer and HIV at a top facility in the capital.[8]

Mexico is facing a transition and medical care is passing from the public sector to the private – health-care and illness are becoming a good business. The socialized health-care system that was built in the last decades of post-revolutionary governments, led by the PRI (Institutional Revolutionary

Party) which became the establishment party in Mexico, is being destroyed by the present government.

Turning to AIDS, she added,

The access to drugs is a fight won by the NGOs and affected patients and relatives. But what is the use of drugs if you don't have a health-care system to maintain good standards of care, follow-up of patients, laboratory exams, adverse event management, and prevention of complications related to HIV infection and therapy?

She pointed to TB as a proven example of the need for a comprehensive approach to disease control. "If you don't integrate a complete program, that means diagnosis, access to treatment and follow-up simply doesn't work."

For her, the AIDS fight is inseparable from the fight to strengthen the public health system and avoid privatizing it; the latter, she feels, will not benefit the majority of Mexicans. "AIDS in this country is an illness of the poorest, as it is in Africa and the rest of Latin America. If you don't socialize health-care, just giving pills makes no sense." The other problem was the lack of trained workers in public hospitals. "As wages are low, many are leaving the public hospitals, and leaving them with less trained and experienced staff," she explained. "That can impact on treatment results. So to talk about treatment access is not enough. If we want to have really good results and impact on life expectancy and quality of life, we need a strong health-care infrastructure and access of patients to it. But at a fundamental level, what is happening to the public system is not optimistic."[9]

"The problem is with the political parties," said Reyes-Teran. "They have lost all credibility in Mexico and I think this is the primary problem related to AIDS." In the most recent elections, he noted, there was 70 percent popular abstention. "That's as never before," he said. "But it's because no one has improved the situation here and the poverty is increasing."

Up in the Mountains

Oaxaca State has 2 million inhabitants, many living in the 7,000 rural localities covering its six regions. These largely poor indigenous communities produce coffee for export and are struggling to survive the current worldwide slump in coffee prices. Nearly half of the rural population is illiterate, and 15 percent speak no Spanish at all. Surveys show that few are aware of AIDS.[10] Some Indian groups consider talking publicly about sexuality taboo, and this makes it hard to educate women in particular about health-care. "In general there is a great absence of government campaigns to combat HIV," said Armando Belmares-Sarabia. "There is a complete ignorance in places that are more remote."[11]

A 2002 survey by Coesida, Oaxaca's state AIDS council, found that half the state's 1,637 officially reported HIV cases were in Oaxaca City and the surrounding Central Valley. They regarded this as an underestimate since HIV testing is either unavailable or not generally offered outside the state capital.

Those who do receive care from village *casas de salud*, or community clinics are often referred to one of fourteen regional social security hospitals, each of which has two infectious disease doctors. In 2002 these physicians had yet to receive specialized HIV training. If they suspect someone of having HIV, they automatically refer them to Coesida. Unfortunately, HIV can be hard to spot based on symptoms alone, since weight loss, diarrhea and pulmonary problems commonly affect non-HIV patients.

"Basically they become infected and have opportunistic infections and many just die," said Belmares-Sarabia. "If you see the statistics, they have a short second stage. Between infection and death, it can be two years, maybe three or four. It is far from the famous ten years that is the average in the US." Others like Reyes-Teran report a similar short period between primary infection and the onset of AIDS in poor Mexican patients, often because they fail to get medical attention until they are very sick. By late 2003, that trend had not changed.[12]

Tapping Local Resources

That is the grim picture, seen from below the mountain. From up above, remote indigenous communities have always had to fend for themselves. Their customs and healing practices represent elements of local and community-based infrastructures that could be built up to deliver better HIV care. Along with the *casas de salud*, there are trained midwives, lay birth attendants and traditional healers who could be trained to provide HIV education and promote wellness. They could help identify and refer individuals for HIV testing and care before they become too sick. Community caregivers could provide long-term support to patients on therapy, while providing critical information about the epidemic. In Juchitan, where a majority of Zapotecan Indians live, the community has been active in HIV prevention. A substantial number of transgendered individuals live in Juchitan, where the community openly accepts them, though there is still homophobia. They have led the AIDS fight in Juchitan and raised awareness about the disease among other Indian groups.

Such a community-based approach demands a shift in the official mentality away from federal and state control of resources. For years, Mexico's Indian communities in Oaxaca and Chiapas have violently fought the federal government and local officials over land disputes, demanding more attention and resources from the government to address the needs and rights of indigenous communities. The current national administration is not likely to embrace Indian community leadership of the rural AIDS effort. The nation's health infrastructure may be weak, but historical political structures are firmly intact.[13]

Although Indian political groups such as the Zapatistas in Chiapas, and others in Oaxaca, are fighting for health rights within a larger civil rights platform, Reyes-Teran is not hopeful: "[T]here they are trying, but they are completely isolated. This is partly due to bad press, and partly due to errors they made. But they didn't get the support in Congress they should have gotten, to give them their rights and their dignity."

A Pilot Clinic for Oaxaca's Central Valley

The woman everyone comes to see for HIV care in Oaxaca City tends to be more optimistic about the pace of change. "Oaxaca is one of the lucky states because the political will has existed here since 1996," explained Dr. Gabriela Velásquez-Rosas, an infectious disease specialist who heads Coesida.[14] Coesida was set up in 1994, and provides a range of services including HIV testing, support groups, legal advocacy, medical care and, increasingly, HIV therapy. From 1996 to 1999, a small number of Coesida patients were given two-drug therapy. In 2000, triple-drug combinations without protease inhibitors became available. The figure was up to 120 by June 2002, and another eighty people with HIV were slated to begin therapy.[15] The federal government provided money to cover eighty-nine patients in May 2003.

In a mid-2003 update, Reyes-Teran, who does lab work for the Oaxaca clinic, said that around forty people had been added to the roster in the past year. "We're going up to 200 there, but that's not the number of people with AIDS in the state. . . . There is not total coverage and this is significant. There are people who need treatment and there is no support for giving it to them."

Coesida spent 75 percent of its small budget on treatment in 2002. It provides services to patients with or without social security benefits. Referred patients are given an HIV rapid test and basic blood work.[16] Blood samples are sent to Reyes-Teran in Mexico City for CD4 count and viral load testing. "But not in all cases," he admitted, acknowledging that more T-cell tests are being done than viral load tests.

In Oaxaca, a CD4 count test cost 350 pesos (US $35) in 2002, and a viral load test 1,250 pesos (US $100). The patients pay for these tests. Today, although generic drugs are becoming available in Mexico, low-cost diagnostics – indeed any diagnostics – are hard to access in rural areas. "The issue of the lab is the hardest part," said Velásquez-Rosas, who noted that patient follow-up is hard without diagnostics, especially for those outside the city. She confirmed that many rural patients arrive at the Coesida clinic in declining health. Aside from weight loss and diarrhea, TB and PCP pneumonia are common first symptoms. Later on patients have cytomegalovirus.[17]

"Only infectious disease specialists and internists should manage these patients," she added, since few community doctors have had HIV training. "The only thing they can do is make sure [patients] are taking their medicine. If they show up with an OI, they will send them back here or attend to them. But they aren't trained to follow them on treatment." Velásquez-Rosas was focusing on training the twenty-eight local infectious disease doctors in social security hospitals, where HIV therapy will be extended as capacity is developed. That training began in 2002 and is ongoing.

To date, those who have received therapy at the Coesida clinic generally do well, but diet remains a problem. "The overall nutrition of patients is an issue because they are poor," explained Velásques-Rosas in 2002. Many Indians survive on a tortilla diet with too little protein. They also have limited access to clean water, which increases their exposure to pathogens.

Back in Puerto Escondido, Belmares-Sarabia said in 2002 that the state

Coesida program has a good reputation, but he had heard criticism: "Everyone who is referred there is treated with a limited number of antiretrovirals." The other complaint is that there is not a continuous supply, and that necessary lab work is not done there, like viral load [testing]." Reyes-Teran confirmed that neither T-cell nor viral load testing was available, though access to generic AZT or d4T had improved.

"Access to antiretrovirals is not the only issue," stressed Reyes-Teran. "Who is going to train the doctors to give medicine correctly? Who's going to intervene with a sociocultural strategy so that patients really understand the disease, and how it is to be treated, how these complex drugs are taken, so that we can control this illness? This has to be in the whole system."

In an effort to help their colleagues in the provinces, frontline HIV experts recently drafted Mexican treatment guidelines for HIV. The guidelines emphasize a clinical "low-tech" approach to managing patients when testing is limited. This approach is similar to HIV treatment guidelines issued in 2002 by the WHO in 2002. The Mexican guide has been widely distributed throughout the country and welcomed by doctors and health providers, said Reyes-Teran.

Concerns about Low-Quality Drugs

For now, the lack of affordable, high-quality drugs and diagnostics for HIV remains a key obstacle to increased access in rural areas. As of mid 2003, the public health system has provided discounted brand-name and generic antiretroviral drugs. Mexico has had mixed success in securing steep discounts on antiretrovirals from some large manufacturers, but not all. "Prices have dropped in the overall health system," said Reyes-Teran. The biggest cut in prices has come from Merck, with lesser discounts from GlaxoSmithKline and Abbott. "Merck makes and sells efavirenz and indinavir for Mexico, and sells it at a 70 percent to 80 percent discount," he added. As a result Merck's drugs are more widely used than other anti-HIV drugs.

Access to generic antiretroviral drugs has steadily grown, and is expected to increase further as the result of a new deal. In Spring 2003, Latin American countries collectively succeeded in negotiating lower prices for generic antiretrovirals, and brand-name drugs and will get them under a pooled procurement plan called the Andean agreement. The agreement means Mexico will use the cheapest drugs available, be they generic or brand-name.

Like many developing countries, Mexico has a domestic pharmaceutical industry that produces high-quality drugs – as well as low- and no-quality ones. There is an overall lack of adequate quality control by Mexican drug regulation agencies, say Mexican doctors like Reyes-Teran, and widespread corruption. He is particularly concerned about the growing use of locally produced drugs known as Similares.

"In Mexico there is an industry called Similares that wants to sell drugs as if they were generics when they aren't," explained Reyes-Teran. "Similares is a brand. There are no controls on their drugs." These local drugs are gaining wider use due to the influence and marketing dollars of Similares' owner Victor Gonzales Torres, who "has tried and succeeded in putting his products into the health system," said Reyes-Teran. "He has a lot of pharmacies and he gives the drugs free or cheaply to pharmacists. Torres has done a lot of publicity to get a law changed in [Mexico's] Congress to allow Similares products to be put on the list of patented drugs," he added, "which would be really dangerous for a patient infected with HIV, because there is no regulation. We don't know if they are pure."

Actually, he's convinced Similares are not comparable to approved patented drugs or generics. "I'll take you to get some fluconazole that is sold by Similares and the normal generic fluconazole; you'll see the difference – you can taste it on your tongue, you understand?" he said. "It has such poor quality. It's far from pure." Under the new Andean agreement, only drugs approved by the WHO, an arbiter of drug quality, will be purchased for governments. But this still leaves a growing private market that is less regulated.

The Need for Grassroots Activism

The key problem in all these areas is a lack of action by government officials and the lack of enough activists to push them to address these health issues adequately. "There are some great activists working in AIDS and several leaders in Congress have done good things," said Reyes-Teran, "but it's all been a drop here and there." The Mexican government applied for Global Fund money, but its application was rejected. There is new funding through a program backed by the National Institutes of Health, and the Pan American Health Organization (PAHO) is active on the AIDS front.

Meanwhile, a lack of activism has contributed to the poor levels of treatment for rural residents. "This is the most difficult thing, to mobilize people to demand care," Belmares-Sarabia observed in Puerto Escondido. "I see the absence of treatment options as the biggest problem, because prevention itself is very limiting."

"Right now activism is stalled," complained Reyes-Teran, referring to the national movement. "I think it's been corrupted a lot too. The groups are not working well together now. They are fighting among themselves when they should be united in pushing the government for money to fight AIDS." Recently, for example, a schism within Frenpavih led to the creation of a second network called Vanpavih (Vanguard of People Living with HIV).

AIDS activists in Mexico have been small in number, but they have fought hard, despite limited resources. Today, aside from networks like La Red Mexicana in the capital, the divided twins Frenpavih and Vanpavih, and the national AIDS program, there are small local groups like those working on Oaxaca's coast. Although there are many sharp leaders in the AIDS arena, the fight "is all too fragmented," complained Reyes-Teran. "We need to unite." He gave high marks to Carmen Soler, a physician heading the AIDS program in the federal district who's been a strong advocate in pushing the Fox government and civil leaders to do more.

Tackling Stigma and Homophobia

It hasn't been easy to mobilize Mexican civil society to fight AIDS. The Catholic Church is a strong force in Mexico, and its opposition to homosexuality contributes to the closeted life of many gays and bisexuals. "It's true that many gays stay hidden, even here in the capital, where it's easier to live openly," said Luna in 2002. "Here you have to be careful because [HIV cases] in men who have sex with men are strongly linked with bisexuality," as are those in women affected by bisexual partners. "The identity of gays is different. In Mexico, the one who penetrates is not gay, the one who is penetrated is gay." That could help explain the apparent absence of

AIDS cases linked to gays in Oaxaca, he added. "In Oaxaca, there could very well be the perception that none are gay, but they are still sexually active."

"Here there is bisexuality and gay men who are married, and the other closeted gays who don't want to come out," agreed Reyes-Teran. "I don't know if it's machismo that's limiting this, or the relationship of individuals to the church." What he does know is that there are gay men with AIDS in states like Oaxaca. "There are a lot of very poor gays who don't have access to treatment, who don't want to know their status, who don't fight. They prefer to be unknown, hidden."

Reyes-Teran also feels that class divisions are somewhat to blame for a lack of activist attention to the needs of rural people with HIV and AIDS. Now that middle-class, HIV-positive gay men in the capital have access to treatment, he said, they've become complacent.

The ones who have treatment don't care about the fact that AIDS is affecting those poor people in Oaxaca. You are dealing with something you'll find in the Third World, which is the virus of a lack of conscience and the virus of ignorance. That makes it really hard to mobilize people. We have a lot of politics around AIDS, a lot of people and NGOs who are affected with those viruses.

"The people asking for treatment in Oaxaca can't have a more proactive attitude because they aren't educated," agreed Luna. "They have the mentality that doctors are supreme beings and they can't ask." Treatment education, funding, and support are critically needed to strengthen local HIV-positive and AIDS groups. That's what his organization spends its time doing now.

La Red Mexicana began in 1985, but continues to operate on a tiny budget, boosted with funds from foreign groups like the UK-based International AIDS Alliance, as well as from Canadian groups. The organization had a tiny staff of eight in 2002, including Luna and a web-master, and relies on volunteers – often friends of the duo. In 2002 there was no sign outside the apartment where La Red Mexicana is located, and none on the office door – a precaution against prejudice from neighbors, said one activist.

Over the years, the group has focused its activities on education and health promotion for people living with HIV and AIDS. "We are educators, we produce materials," explained Luna "One of our areas is treatment and managing disease – how HIV is transmitted and so on. But we also do workshops on sexuality, empowerment, issues of disclosure, nutrition – all the issues that affect people living with this disease."

The group also gathers and distributes recycled drugs for people who don't qualify for government programs or receive care through the social security system. "Although the government of the Federal District has a [HIV drug access] program, many people here are not with social security, so they have no alternatives but our program," Luna explained. About 70 percent of workshop clients access social security, but none of those using the drug bank. "It is the only medicine bank of its kind," he added proudly. "We just gather it and give it freely to others, without any exchange of money. So we participate in a minimal way in access to treatment, but it is nothing compared to the enormous need in Mexico." In June 2002, around 100 people were getting recycled drugs through the bank.

Aside from the bank, Luna said some individuals were accessing drugs through clinical trials sponsored by drug companies, but here there were problems. "The trials are done for limited periods, the people don't realize what they are about and that they are not ethical," he explained. "It's just drug companies using people." He cited examples of clients who had accessed drugs through a trial, but none after it was over. "The patients don't know the consequences of entering a trial; they just give their signature. At first, they like it because they get an exam and good monitoring and they are happy. But after, no . . ." Unfortunately, activists have been too few to effectively take on the drug companies. And physicians by and large were not advocating on behalf of patients to insist drugs be provided after the completion of trials.

"It reflects how activists lack information or arguments to establish a dialogue equal to that of the authorities," said Luna. "There are too few people in positions of leadership to really discuss policy regarding treatment and use of HIV drugs."

Model Clinics in Mexico City

Behind its well-guarded walls, the National Institute for Respiratory Infections in Mexico City is indeed a world apart. It is one of ten federal health institutes, on a par with the National Institutes of Health in the US. At IRIN, Reyes-Teran provides patients with state of the art HIV care and conducts HIV/AIDS clinical trials. The institute has the biggest HIV case-load of any public hospital, because PCP pneumonia is the top killer of Mexicans with AIDS. TB is also high on the list.

Nearby there is a cancer hospital where women with HIV are seen. Children are treated at the Pediatric and Infants Hospital. Others are seen in the myriad branches of the public and private health sectors. "We don't know how many people are getting treatment," said Reyes-Teran. "There are many organisms, and many people get treatment through NGOs." Nor do doctors meet formally to compare notes. "There hasn't been a way for all doctors working on AIDS to come together to assess the national situation, as of yet," he said. "That's a problem."

In the capital, "The majority of those who should get treatment are getting it," according to Reyes-Teran. There are now 2,500 patients coming to see him annually, and he has 300 patients on therapy, up from 150 a year ago. They are doing well.

"Things have been changing here," he said. "Not a patient in this institution was getting HIV drugs four years ago. Now all my patients get them. It doesn't cost them anything. As soon as we were able to offer treatment, as we've seen in other countries, OIs dropped, and survival increased significantly." To date, the main problems have been similar to those experienced by US patients: difficulties with adherence and drug side-effects. "We've had anemia and liver-associated problems with some drugs like indinavir, and hepatitis with protease drugs that has been fatal in rare cases in this institution," Reyes-Teran reported. Unlike other countries, he stressed, "The incidence of hepatitis B and C in our population is low."

Women: Lagging in Care

Down the street, Volkow-Fernandez has had similar success with HIV therapy in a growing cohort of HIV-positive women at her clinic within the cancer hospital. Many early female cases were the result of exposure through blood transfusions. Others were among paid donors who sold their blood to commercial blood products centers and, as happened notoriously in China, received HIV-contaminated pooled plasma in return. Most of these women have now died. New patients are exposed through heterosexual sex, mostly with their husbands.

HIV testing of pregnant women is not mandatory in Mexico, but routinely offered and accepted in bigger centers. So is prophylactic therapy to prevent mother-to-child transmission (MTCT). Having children remains a paramount concern for HIV-positive women, and a hot topic in support groups. Off the record, some activists in Mexico say that illegal abortions are still common among HIV-positive women unable to access drugs, though that is now changing. At Coesida in 2002, Velásquez-Rosas had not seen that problem in Oaxaca. Only twenty-two pregnant women had tested positive there by June 2002, and all of them had received MTCT prophylaxis. Most of the children were born HIV-negative, but Velásquez-Rosas warned that post-natal transmission of the virus through breastfeeding occurs.

In other health centers the problems are myriad. "The main problem, apart from absolute lack of access to drugs for many people, is the infrastructure for health-care which for follow-up care is really bad for many diseases," Reyes-Teran said. As in Oaxaca, the lack of HIV diagnostic tools limits proper monitoring. Coinfection with TB, including multidrug-resistant TB, also remains worrying in HIV patients. Between 5 percent and 8 percent of Reyes-Teran's coinfected patients have pretreatment resistance to two TB drugs, rifampin and isoniazid, the same level as his non-HIV TB patients. "Vigilance of the liver is very important," he stressed. "But there are few centers who do strict monitoring like we do."

Like Belmares-Sarabia, Reyes-Teran has noticed the rapid progress of HIV in many patients: "We believe the evolution of the virus is faster in Mexico than in other countries like the United States. In our [pretherapy] cohort, three-quarters of our patients evolved to have AIDS in less than five years." He is now doing research to find out if genetic factors could be involved. He is also studying nutrition and immune responses in patients on therapy.

Like Volkow-Fernandez, Reyes-Teran believes that political activism, both domestic and global, is the only way to improve the situation in Mexico rapidly. Infrastructure problems exist, but they can be addressed; the health system can be improved. But too little will come from the present administration if things continue as they are. "There needs to be a raising of the consciousness of public officials," he said. "We need a national strategy. The way things are going now with the health authorities, I don't think we can effectively confront and control the AIDS epidemic in Mexico. We are likely to have a greater problem [than in the US] with the improper use of medicines and the emergence of multiple-drug resistance." As in the US, Mexicans on antiretroviral treatment develop resistance to their medicines the longer they stay on therapy, prompting a need to switch to substitute drug regimens. Since drugs are in poor supply, patients get their hands on whatever drugs are available. The lack of treatment and erratic use of drugs may contribute to an increase in the rate of drug resistance nationally.

Reyes-Teran pointed out that little was known about the rate of spread of resistant viruses in Mexico. "There isn't a single study to determine primary or secondary resistance in Mexico." Because people are treated in the different institutions that make up the public health system, and by private doctors, with different protocols, he predicted that varying patterns of resistance will emerge in these treated populations: "I think resistance will increase. So I think it's critical to maintain control of the course of the epidemic and the development of secondary resistance."

Reaching Across Borders

One source of cash and other help could be Mexico's northern neighbor. "I think organizations in the US should help us because the problem of resistance is going to penetrate the US," predicted Reyes-Teran. "It's in our common interest." In the wake of 9/11 and falling tourism in Mexico, he added, "Immigration has increased as a result of poverty increasing, and they are going to export the virus, there can be no doubt."

Barring major change, he remained pessimistic about the current treatment situation for Mexico. Given the existing AIDS budget and limited new sources of funding for fiscal year 2003, access to antiretrovirals will increase modestly in 2004, he predicted, but not in time for those on waiting lists for the drugs. "I think there will be some improvements: clinically, in prevalence, in the quality of life with patients who can get the drugs who will feel better, etc. But we will give suboptimal care compared to what we should give. The situation is not improving enough," he said. "Our goal should be to improve as much as we can, and this is the gap right now. This is preventing me from being an optimist with regard to controlling the virus."

On August 5, 2003, President Fox announced that Mexico would now foot the bill for Mexicans with HIV who can't afford antiretroviral drugs by the close of the year. But Fox didn't indicate how many more patients would receive the drugs, nor where the money would come from. Activists remained concerned about how quickly these words would translate into funds for vulnerable communities like the indigenous women of Oaxaca.

"We just have to keep fighting," concluded Reyes-Teran, who was keeping up pressure on health officials to deliver on their promise. "So maybe you can write something to let people know. We desperately need things to change in Mexico and we need people to help us. The situation is very serious."

8

UGANDA:
SPARING THE NEXT GENERATION

The Great Lakes region of East Africa is a naturally rich, verdant zone that encompasses the Rift Valley, long viewed by archeologists as a geographical template of human evolution. Along the beds of Lake Victoria and Lake Tanganyika, archeologists continue to hunt for well-preserved fossils and specimens of pre-hominids.

Lake Victoria forms a triangular border that knits together Uganda, Kenya, and Tanzania. Next to Uganda is landlocked Rwanda, and below it Burundi, which shares the waters of Lake Tanganyika with its huge Western neighbor, Zaire, and with Tanzania to the south and east. To the north, Lake Albert sits between Uganda and the much larger Democratic Republic of the Congo. In the south, Lake Nyasa flows out of the tail of Tanzania into Malawi and Mozambique.

AIDS began very early here, and quickly transformed the capitals of several countries into mini-epicenters of a fast-moving virus: Kampala, Nairobi, Kigali, Dar es Salaam, Bujumbura, Kinshasa, Lilongwe.[1] Today, much of the global attention to AIDS in Africa has focused on the hardest-hit sub-Saharan countries. That has obscured the devastating impact AIDS has had on East Africa, where it affected not only vulnerable and socially marginal groups such as sex workers, but government officials, teachers and other members of Africa's educated, professional class. The region is now harboring what epidemiologists call a mature AIDS epidemic, one which is moving into its third decade and shows few signs of slowing down.

One exception is Uganda, which has gained worldwide acclaim for its success in slowing down HIV's spread due to a high level of engagement by civil society and the government's own prevention efforts. There, adult HIV seroprevalence rates have dropped from a peak of 18 percent in 1995 to around 5 percent at the end of 2001.[2] The Bush administration has touted the Uganda prevention model, one that stresses sexual abstinence and monogamy, as a model for the world.[3] Ironically, Uganda bears the sad distinction of having more AIDS orphans than any other country in Africa. In this country of 21 million, one in every ten people is a child orphaned by AIDS.[4] That's an important reason why Ugandan civil society responded so strongly to the threat of AIDS, and why public health officials there were quick to embrace a program to prevent mother-to-child transmission (MTCT) of HIV.

I traveled to Kampala, the capital of Uganda, in September 2001, shortly after my fact-finding trip to central Haiti. I'd been to the region twice before, to Kenya and Tanzania, traveling both times into the interior of the Great Lakes region. I was in Kampala, attending an AIDS conference on September 11, when the terror attacks took place in New York.

I had several questions in mind for Ugandan officials. I wanted to determine if, in fact, Uganda had really succeeded in curbing new infections and stabilizing HIV, as government statistics suggested,[5] or if instead their epidemiological picture somehow reflected the enormous cumulative death toll and a kind of saturation point for the spread of the virus.[6] So many Ugandans had died and were already exposed to HIV; perhaps the rate of new infections wasn't keeping pace with the initial exponential explosion of the virus?

I was hoping that Ugandan forecasters were right about their progress. If they were, I wanted to know more about how Ugandan communities had managed to counter the prevailing stigma that shrouded AIDS everywhere else I'd been on the continent, and about the prevention strategies they used to convince so many Ugandan youths to abstain from having sex before marriage.

I attended three overlapping regional conferences that allowed me to meet many of the leading doctors, organizers and government policy-makers working in AIDS, as well as community activists. The first brought together clinicians and researchers from the Great Lakes region, the other was an international conference on prevention of mother-to-child transmission (PMTCT) of HIV, attended by many other African scientists.[7] These meetings spotlighted recent *progress in AIDS prevention and treatment, and the obstacles facing government officials.*

I was particularly interested in looking closely at Uganda's nascent MTCT program, to see if it might continue to reproduce the success of the national prevention effort. I also wanted to know how well pilot MTCT programs could serve as a stepping-stone to adult treatment, a new concept called MTCT-Plus.[8] I wanted to hear what local HIV-positive women and their spouses and families felt about MTCT programs, which provided therapy to prevent infants from acquiring HIV but failed to provide drugs for ailing mothers – and fathers. I got a lot of information during a week-long satellite MTCT conference that brought together 100 Ugandan women from across the country, and a small number of men, to discuss how Ugandan groups needed to respond to the challenge of mobilizing local communities to take up MTCT and, they hoped, antiretroviral treatment.[9]

As I quickly learned, Ugandan women were furious and desperate about their lack of access to treatment – and determined to access it not just for themselves, but for their husbands, relatives and other members of their communities. They linked their own exposure to HIV to a lack of women's empowerment in Uganda. As new activists, they vowed to use the AIDS issue as a vehicle to push for better rights for themselves and their daughters. I realized that a positive offshoot of the AIDS crisis in Africa is the global attention it focuses on women's issues, which is helping African women to fight against long-standing legal, political, social and cultural inequities. As Uganda shows, AIDS is a female pandemic, and women are at the forefront of this battle.

Kampala

In much of the world, the stork is regarded as a symbol of fertility. Not so in the capital of Uganda, where the giant marabou stork with its huge black wings and pink gullet is viewed more as a Grim Reaper, a symbol of death and decay. These large creatures are all over the capital, perched ominously like vultures in the trees, atop giant construction cranes, on telephone wires. They even alight on cars parked at the side of the road, and fly so low that residents instinctively duck when one goes overhead.

A scavenger, the marabou arrived here in the mid 1980s to feast upon piles of refuse that built up during two decades of civil war, including the successive reigns of Milton Obote and his notorious protégé, dictator Idi Amin, who ruled from 1971 to 1986. Up to a million Ugandans were murdered during this terrible period, their bodies lining the grassland shores of Lake Victoria where the marabou like to nest. Many others lost their homes and livelihood, dying of hunger and disease. These included the first victims of AIDS, which was then called "slim disease" because of the rapid weight loss that it triggered.

In 1996, when current president Yoweri Museveni took power, Uganda was politically, economically and socially in tatters. It was also reeling from the fast-moving HIV epidemic. Like the marabou stork, HIV flourishes in such settings of poverty and civil instability.

Ask around Kampala: few families are untouched by HIV and AIDS. The situation is worst in the countryside, where entire villages have perished. The high death toll has affected not only the poor, but a wide swath of society, including professionals, soldiers and policemen.[10]

AIDS has disproportionately attacked women and their children. National infection rates among those in their early twenties are twice as high in women as in men. Girls aged fifteen to nineteen are deemed four to six times more likely to have HIV than boys – a trend reported in other parts of sub-Saharan Africa, and Uganda continues to have more AIDS orphans than any other country in the world. Many of them are HIV-positive children who have lacked access to education and other support. To their credit, many Ugandans have opened their doors to take in orphans, but the demand far exceeds the supply of parents and families to help these children. Many have died – a national tragedy that is still shrouded in silence.

Early Success in Prevention

Given this stark picture, it is rather surprising to find Uganda viewed today as a model of success in HIV prevention, as well as a litmus test of what more can be achieved by hard-hit African nations battling AIDS. In 1992, 16 percent of Ugandan adults were estimated to be HIV-positive; by 1996, that number had fallen by half. Other studies offer a more striking success story: according to a May 2003 WHO report on Uganda's progress, the country had a nearly 30 percent seroprevalence rate, which had fallen to

below 10 percent in two decades.[11] Newer statistics show an HIV prevalence rate of 6.1 percent for 2001. Credit must go to the government's
National AIDS Control Programme, set up by the Ministry of Health,
which has emphasized mass education about HIV and condom use, as well
as voluntary counseling and testing (VCT). Although AIDS remains highly
stigmatized and feared, polls suggest there is a broad awareness of the
disease and the ways it can be contracted, though such awareness remains
more common in Kampala than in the countryside.

The national picture remains very sobering. In a keynote address at the
September 2001 African Great Lakes Conference on Access to HIV AIDS
Care and Support, leading HIV researcher Peter Mugyenyi noted, "The
current HIV rate is unacceptably high and appalling and would constitute
a state of emergency in developed countries."[12] A million Ugandans were
already infected by HIV, and they had limited access to antiretroviral medicines, said Mugyenyi, predicting that "[n]ew infections will continue to
spread from the huge infection reservoir, most of whom do not know their
serostatus." That included a large number of women passing HIV on to
their offspring. The Ugandan government has found that the present rate
of mother-to-child HIV transmission is 28 percent. Out of a million live
births per year, 100,000 test HIV-positive, according to Dr. Laura Guay of
Johns Hopkins University and Makerere University in Kampala.

In 2000 the government announced a major national program for the
prevention of mother-to-child transmission (PMTCT using anti-HIV
drugs like AZT and nevirapine. By 2004, it hopes to offer all pregnant
women attending government clinics a comprehensive package of voluntary HIV counseling and testing, maternal care and STD prevention, and
for those who test HIV-positive, a PMTCT regimen. The services offered
will also include antimalarial and antiparasitic treatment.

The program will utilize two PMTCT regimens. The first is "short-
course" AZT. AZT will be administered to pregnant women from the thirty-
sixth week of pregnancy until a week after delivery, with a liquid dose of
AZT for the newborn. The alternative regimen is a single dose of nevirapine
to a mother going into labor, and a single liquid dose for her baby within
seventy-two hours after delivery. Both regimens are deemed safe for mothers
and infants. Combined with an effective counseling and testing program,
they have proved quite effective in reducing maternal transmission.[13] The
groundbreaking HIVNET 012 study carried out in 1997 at the antenatal

clinic in Kampala's Mulago Hospital, for example, showed that nevirapine can reduce maternal transmission of HIV by 50 percent.

The Ugandan PMTCT program is backed by a five-year donation of free nevirapine from the German manufacturer, Boehringer-Ingelheim. Additional financial support has come from the Gates Foundation and USAID, among others. The first reports show that implementation of the program is steady. But serious barriers have emerged that raise concerns about the PMTCT effort's ultimate ability to protect babies from HIV.

The government's strategy consists of integrating the PMTCT program into the admittedly weak national health infrastructure of government hospitals, and family planning and rural antenatal clinics, where voluntary counseling and testing services are already offered. In 2003, only a half-dozen government hospitals in Uganda offer VCT, so the new program provides an opportunity to build up the national health infrastructure. The PMTCT sites are initially limited to several in Kampala district, including Mulago Hospital – the largest medical center in the country – and hospitals in Galu and Arua districts. By early 2004, the government expects all districts to have sites up and running.

Since only 40 percent of Ugandan women are estimated to deliver their infants in hospitals – the remainder in private clinics or at home with midwives – the number of pregnant women seeking care from the public sector should increase. There is also talk of introducing PMTCT-Plus.

Early Results

At the Third International Conference on Global Strategies to Prevent Maternal to Child Transmission in Kampala in September 2003, Dr. Saul Onyango, the director of the PMTCT program, reported that 19,700 pregnant women had been counseled for HIV in the hospitals that now offer VCT; over 70 percent had accepted testing. Of that number, 2,026 were HIV-positive. "Our biggest encouragement is that after one year of implementation, almost 20,000 mothers know their serostatus," said Onyango. "That is a good starting point. We hope they can bring their friends and peers aboard, but also get into services."

Given Uganda's limited national health budget of $12 per person, the PMTCT program represents a major investment. In addition to counseling and testing, an antiretroviral regimen, and monitoring and treatment for STDs, pregnant women are given vitamin A, folic acid and iron supplements to maintain their health. "Mother and infant will also be followed during the first two years of the baby's life. All of this is costly," Onyango noted. "Coordination, training, sensitization, putting in supplies, monitoring, evaluating the whole program – all of these must be put in a system that is very weak. Community education, mobilization and sensitization is another challenge."

As he sees it, implementation will be relatively simple in urban areas where there is some infrastructure, but harder in remote areas where clinics lack even basic medicines, equipment and doctors. This is partly due to a government policy of decentralization of the health sector, which has resulted in "cost sharing" – or competition for scarce funds between urban and rural agencies and programs – and more layers of bureaucratic red tape.

New Data Send a Warning

A key component of the government program is a clear-cut recommendation that HIV-positive mothers either exclusively breast-feed or exclusively use replacement formula for the first six months, then immediately wean their infants to solid foods. That recommendation is controversial – culturally, economically and medically.

Breast-feeding is an intimate activity for mothers that is directly related to bonding with a newborn. Many studies have documented the beneficial effects of breastfeeding on the emotional development of infants, as well as the high nutritional content of breast milk. Although infant formula represents the safest option to avoid exposure to HIV, it is not always practical for mothers. Many are poor and cannot afford formula, which also requires preparation and clean water. In such cases it may be safer for the infant to be exclusively breast-fed. Breast milk is more sterile and provides more complete nutrition than its alternatives. Mixing formula with dirty water is dangerous to an infant, who may then be exposed to pathogens. Research suggests that mixed feeding leaves the infants more vulnerable to GI tract infections and to HIV, which takes advantage of inflammation in the lining of the digestive system.

Socially and culturally, there's also a controversy over the promotion of infant formula to women in developing countries by large corporations such as Nestlé and by international agencies. Supporters of breastfeeding have argued that infant formula represents a Western norm adopted by women in the United States and other industrialized countries, one that is at odds with cultural practices and social values held by Africans and others in more traditional societies. The concern fueled a global campaign to stop the promotion of infant formula by international aid groups in the 1970s and 1980s, and led to a reconsideration of the critical value of breastfeeding in the context of culture and tradition, as well as health and economics.

The government's new infant feeding guidelines for HIV-positive mothers are based on a review of recent trial data presented at the 2001 Global Strategies meeting by co-chair Dr. Francis Mmiro. He found that mixed feeding – occasionally replacing breast milk with formula, soft porridge or other foods – is linked in Uganda to a higher risk of HIV transmission through breast milk than either exclusive breast- or bottle-feeding. Mixed feeding also carries with it a higher rate of infant mortality.

There's plenty to worry about. Dr. Anna Coutsoudis of the University of Natal in Durban, South Africa, estimated that, based on studies to date, the overall risk of MTCT through breast-feeding is 15 percent if a baby is breast-fed for two years. The infection rate over the first six years is not known. Out of 700,000 children worldwide who contract HIV through MTCT, up to half acquire it through breast-feeding, Laura Guay estimated.

A Delayed Risk

Amsterdam researcher Joep Lange and colleagues, conducting the PETRA PMTCT trial in Uganda, South Africa and Tanzania, presented preliminary results at the Global Strategies meeting that were sobering. These clearly showed that the initial benefits of using anti-HIV drugs to prevent maternal HIV transmission are lost over time due to postpartum transmission through breast milk.[14]

The PETRA study compared three PMTCT regimens with placebo. Arm A consisted of short-course AZT-3TC from week thirty-six to labor, with postpartum AZT for mother and infant; Arm B tested AZT-3TC during labor and postpartum for infant and mother; and Arm C used AZT-

3TC only during delivery. (A placebo arm was stopped in September 1998 when it was clear that AZT worked well to reduce MTCT.) Arms A and B were both effective at first in reducing MTCT, whereas Arm C was not very effective. Lange remarked that "very little benefit remained after 18 months" with any of the regimens. In short, PMTCT was failing due to transmission through breastfeeding.

The Next Step: Postpartum Transmission

The exclusive breast-feeding recommendation is somewhat controversial in itself, but the real problem is that many mothers cannot adhere to it. The obstacles are varied, a major one being fear of revealing one's HIV status.

Dr. Michele Magoni is an Italian HIV doctor who oversees one of the Ugandan PMTCT facilities. "We opened a [PMTCT] site and there the test kits are available, but only 10 percent of the women are tested and go there for antenatal counseling, and so few receive the testing," he said. "At the end of the day, almost none have received the prophylactic treatments."[15]

The problem, his team realized, was its failure to address women's fears of disclosure and its consequences. Magoni remarked, "In the first year and a half of activity, we did not move enough on community mobilization because it was a pilot project. We have to deal with the stigma."

A pilot PMTCT program in Abidjan, Ivory Coast, revealed other barriers besides fear of disclosure, including difficulties with staff or clinic procedures, disbelief of HIV results, and doubts about AZT's efficacy.[16] In Uganda few people know much about anti-HIV drugs, including nevirapine. Limited educational material is available in local languages, and illiteracy is high in rural areas. Pregnant women worry about taking drugs that might cause problems for the fetus or unknown side-effects. When they do learn about nevirapine, they wonder about drug resistance and efficacy.

"Are women going to be able manage MTCT?" asked Milly Katana, an outspoken HIV-positive activist who helped organize the satellite PMTCT conference and works with the grassroots National Guidance and Empowerment Network, one of several networks for people living with

HIV. "Some will, but not all, and I fear it won't be easy. I think many of the women would choose formula if they could, because they don't want to risk passing on the virus," she said.

> But first of all, is formula going to be available for free for that whole time? Look at the problems we have just in getting other things. Also, it is difficult for women who have to go to work, or poor women who are in the bush, to use formula because it requires cooking equipment. They won't always be able to keep it up without a lot of support.

The issue is more than the costs of exclusive bottle or breast-feeding. "Already," Katana said, "the women are expressing fears of rejection should they openly declare their HIV status, and health workers say the women are afraid that the [PMTCT] treatment will stigmatize them." Such fears were openly discussed at the Focus on Women satellite meeting, where many HIV-positive women admitted they hid their status from their husbands and partners. To them, being forced to adopt an exclusive feeding choice means having to explain why. "Women come back from these antenatal clinics and are blamed for bringing HIV into the home," said Jane Nabalonzi, a member of the Society of Women and AIDS in Africa. "They are afraid their husbands will beat them, or kick them out of the house. So here we are asking them to do something to protect their baby that makes them vulnerable."

Another problem is that the recommendations are seen by many as foreign. "Culturally, we have the habit of mixed feedings in Uganda, and we supplement with porridge and other things. So this is something new that must be adopted," Katana explained.

Early results from the pilot PMTCT feasibility study at Nsambya hospital in Uganda do not ease her concerns. There, a short course of AZT and nevirapine was offered to women who tested positive late in their pregnancy. Out of 462 HIV-positive women, 240 accepted a PMTCT regimen and 198 had delivered their infants by the time of the Global Strategies conference. One hundred and sixty-two women received AZT and seventy-eight nevirapine. At the sixth week after delivery, 63 percent of the treated mother–infant pairs returned for follow-up care; at week fourteen, that number had fallen to 44 percent; and at month twenty-eight, it had dropped to 8 percent.[17] That makes it hard to know what the transmission rates are after birth.

Mobilizing the Community

One suggestion for avoiding the disclosure issue is to distribute PMTCT medications to all pregnant women, regardless of their HIV status. This is an idea pioneered in Tanzania by Axios International, a public health technical assistance organization. Despite covering all pregnant women, the universal approach saves money by sidestepping HIV counseling and testing. Activists and even Onyango point out that there are ethical problems inherent in indiscriminately distributing medication. This approach also ignores the critical role counseling and testing play in prevention and in helping women access care. It clearly leaves the baby vulnerable after birth.

HIV-positive women have a better idea: Why not treat them with anti-HIV drugs? "What's the point of saving the child if it's just going to become an orphan?" asked Cissy Ssuuna, an openly HIV-positive nurse and VCT counselor at Mulago Hospital. "Why don't they care about keeping us alive and healthy so we can give our children a future? It may be cheaper to use nevirapine, but not if the parents die."[18] As she noted, studies show that three-drug regimens given to pregnant women can lower viral load and effectively prevent any transmission to the fetus. They keep protecting the infant after birth and help the mother. Treatment also lowers the risk of sexual transmission.

Government officials don't disagree with the science, but they cite the prohibitive cost of anti-HIV combination therapy and Uganda's weak infrastructure as real obstacles to adult treatment. Still, the momentum is building for PMTCT-Plus, which will provide for long-term treatment of mothers. For now, though, the government is looking at medical means to protect newborns. Ugandan pediatric PMTCT clinical trials are under way that provide infants with nevirapine for up to twenty-four weeks after birth. Uganda is also proposing a neonatal HIV vaccine trial, the first such trial outside North America.

On a social level, the Ministry of Health is focusing on community mobilization to sensitize people about HIV. It hopes to involve HIV-positive advocates like Katana and Nabalonzi in peer education and the setting up of support groups to help women manage safer feeding options. Speaking at the Global Strategies women's satellite conference, Onyango urged participants to become key players, along with their spouses. He asked, "Can some of you people be lay counselors, so we can increase the number of people actively involved in the program? You are the ones who can reach these women and their partners."

As Onyango stressed, "Getting to the spouses is a real challenge." The PMTCT program will now actively target men by encouraging partners of HIV-positive women to come to the antenatal clinics, traditionally the province of only women and their infants. Pre- and post-test counseling will be offered to both partners, in order to help families confront issues around disclosure.

Acknowledging men and their role reveals a hard lesson the government has already learned.[19] Success in PMTCT is not going to be a simple matter of providing pills or counselors. It requires tackling deep-seated gender dynamics and empowering women to have more control over their lives.

The women's HIV networks have started moving quickly on that front. In October 2001 a new coalition was announced called the Women's Treatment Action Group (WTAG). Led by HIV-positive women, it plans to push not only for access to PMTCT and PMTCT-Plus, but, as Nabalonzi says, for more input into the national agenda: "As mothers and as women, we are going to have to fight, and fight hard, not just for our own survival, but for our families and our communities. We have no other choice."

"The husbands are a real problem," she confirmed. "Many husbands have two wives, and sometimes these wives do not even talk to each other about HIV, even if one of them is HIV-positive. They cannot afford to tell their husbands. That is the reality we are going to have to confront." Some conference participants knew men with HIV who had moved from other areas to "start fresh" after the illness or death of their first wives, and then remarried – never disclosing their past.

A number of HIV-positive, married women at the conference said they had always been sexually monogamous with their husbands, but that their husbands had obviously not been faithful.[20] "We have a double standard here in Uganda where it's accepted for an African man to have other women, but not for the woman. If she does it, they say she is a prostitute," said Nabalonzi.

Other women complained about the myth that HIV is primarily being spread by sex workers and prostitution – an incorrect assumption in their case. Of course, there's plenty of informal commercial sex and prostitution in Africa. With high unemployment and low education, sex work is a viable option for women who need to support families. It's also true that prostitutes have been hit very hard by HIV and AIDS in Uganda and elsewhere. But to conference participants, marriage – not sex work – is a major, and hidden, battlefield of AIDS.

Spotlight on Domestic Abuse

Two years later, much has changed in Uganda, but the role of men, the vulnerability of women, and the lack of gender equality remain critical obstacles impeding progress against AIDS. In Uganda, as in South Africa, Zambia and other countries, sexual violence remains a major cause of transmission of HIV, and little is being done to stop it, either by the government or civil society. The rape of children, and especially orphans who are street children, is a phenomenon that has recently emerged and been branded another hidden epidemic fueling HIV infection in African children.

In August 2003 Human Rights Watch issued a report documenting the widespread domestic abuse and rape of Ugandan women by their husbands.[21] Within marriage, the report noted, Uganda has no laws against domestic violence. A 2001 survey of fifty Ugandan married women showed that 41 percent had experienced domestic abuse, and thirty-five of the fifty had been physically forced to have sex with their husbands. The others were verbally threatened to do so. Many women are beaten for refusing sex with their husbands or partners. Some women cannot negotiate condom use; others are forced into sex as a marital obligation.

The issue of marital rape continues to be linked to the high rate of sexual violence directed at women across Africa. In South Africa, media attention has centered on the escalating cases of gang rape, along with marital rape, that have increased HIV's spread. The incidence of rape is also much higher in black women than white women there, and the rape of orphaned girls is also a critical issue cited by women's rights advocates. These issues are directly the result of a lack of women's empowerment, and of social and family laws that give men, and especially husbands, economic power over their wives, particularly in relation to property and inheritance. Women can't easily leave their abusive husbands without risking homelessness and other forms of disinheritance or social shunning.[22]

The Human Rights Watch report concluded that Uganda's AIDS

programs "incorrectly assume that women have equal decision-making power and status within the family." It referred to Uganda's much-heralded ABCs – abstinence, betrothal and condom use; an approach to HIV prevention that President Bush has touted as a good model for the world. In Uganda there is a connection between the rise of HIV cases linked to sexual violence and pregnancy, and the increased demand for MTCT prevention services. It's also linked to the growing number of orphans.

Behind all these statistics are young and older women – married, monogamous, faithful – who were socially pushed to marry young to have children, who saw no reason to use condoms with their husbands, and who were often exposed by their husbands – not as a result of having had multiple sexual partners or their failure to be sexually responsible, as has long been assumed, but because they adhered to the sexual "ABCs." What's needed now, say women's advocates, is an urgent focus on the deep-rooted familial problem of "D" – domestic inequality between spouses.[23]

"The Ugandan government's failure to address domestic violence is costing women their lives," said LaShawn Jefferson, director of the Women's Rights Division of HRW. "Any success Uganda has experienced in its fight against HIV/AIDS will be short-lived if the government does not address this urgent problem." It called on the government to pass laws prohibiting domestic violence and marital rape, and to change family law and other policies that now spell inequality for women, including married women.

It should be noted that polygamy is practiced in Uganda and in some other countries in Africa. At the satellite conference I attended, some women admitted they knew their HIV-positive husbands had not informed their other spouses about their serostatus. These women were afraid to confront their husbands or tell the other wives, fearing they would be blamed, beaten or kicked out of their homes.[24]

"These problems are not new – we are just paying attention to them because of HIV," said Florence N. (a pseudonym she requested, fearing public disclosure of her HIV status), a Ugandan woman attending the Focus on Women meeting.[25] "The problem is that it is accepted for men to beat their wives," she added. "Here it is seen as a wife's duty to have sex with her husband. She can't easily refuse him." Several women at the forum publicly disclosed that they had been exposed to HIV by their husbands – men who had known their HIV status and had hidden it.[26]

Some Ugandan authorities dispute the conclusions of the Human Rights Watch report. Dr. Elizabeth Madra, head of the Health Ministry's AIDS control program, said domestic violence was a factor in the spread of HIV, but not a major factor and not the cause. A parliament member, Kagole Kivumbi, said women were already protected under existing laws against violence in general. Uganda's Minister of Gender, Zoe Bokoko-Bakoru, said the legal reforms suggested in the report had already been approved by the Ugandan government and would be enacted by the end of 2003.

Laws are an important tool, but so is political leadership – and not only from the top, but across civil society. Revising inheritance and property laws to give married women greater equailty means challenging cultural practices and traditional beliefs that are patriarchal in nature. Such attitudes aren't likely to change easily. As a powerful leader in Uganda and across Africa, President Museveni could use his considerable voice to denounce sexual violence and marital rape; but will he?

Uganda's leaders – indeed, African and global leaders – need to make that connection for themselves, and begin seriously addressing the thorny issue of gender dynamics that underlie HIV's spread – male sexual violence, condoned by society. Health officials need to do more to reach men with educational messages about AIDS and to include them in the national AIDS and MTCT programs. Until men are on board, women's access to testing, care and treatment will remain limited.

War and Rape

The link between war, rape, displacement and the spread of HIV in women has been documented in the Great Lakes region, as well as in countries like Bosnia, Haiti, and Sierra Leone. The most egregious example is the mass rape of women that took place during Rwanda's 1994 civil war.[27] For 100 days in 1994, Hutu nationalists slaughtered and mutilated close to 1 million Tutsis, and some Hutus who opposed "ethnic cleansing." They also raped 250,000 mostly Tutsi women and girls.[28] Today, 70 percent of the rape survivors have HIV; many are shunned by family and friends. In 2002, half of these women were very ill and some had died due to lack of access to HIV treatment. The rapes produced 30,000 pregnancies, and many of these orphaned "children of shame" are also HIV-positive. The attackers included PWAs who were allegedly taken out of hospitals and formed into "battalions" of rapists.[29]

Tragically, this history may be repeating itself next door: in August 2003, human rights workers reported that thousands of Congolese women were arriving in health clinics having been raped by Rwandan soldiers and other warring groups. Considering the very high HIV rates among these soldiers, a new wave of HIV is expected in the Congo which also threatens Uganda and other neighboring countries.

Positive Steps

On a more positive note, there have been many advances in Uganda on the AIDS front as a whole. At the community level, WTAG members had completed trainings in twelve districts by early 2003. More importantly, key members who needed drugs have personally accessed treatment, reassuring their leadership. "That is a big victory because many of us were sick," said WTAG's Ssuuna.[30]

"What I know is that literacy has tremendously increased and we, as frontline workers, are receiving more and more inquiries for support to access treatment," said WTAG's Katana, who is also Uganda's community liaison to the Global Fund for AIDS, Tuberculosis and Malaria. In her opinion, VCT services had only slightly increased, though. "Places out of the city are integrating VCT services, similarly to PMTCT. But for both, we are nowhere near access to VCT within a radius of two kilometers [from Kampala] which is a reasonable walking distance [for those seeking testing]." She also found gender dynamics to be a thorny issue, proving hard to overcome. "There are major cultural and economic barriers to break," said Katana. "Men are at work. Getting them into clinics, especially when they are not sick, is difficult."

In 2001 the Mailman School of Public Health at Columbia University launched a pilot MTCT-Plus initiative aimed at offering treatment to 10,000 pregnant women. It is backed by considerable money from the Rockefeller Foundation and eight other private foundations.[31] It involves twelve sites in eight countries – all in sub-Saharan Africa except for Thailand. That includes two sites in Uganda that are enrolling patients: Mulago Hospital and St. Francis Hospital, both in Kampala. The basic tenets of the program are family-centered care, provision of HIV clinical care and treatment with antiretrovirals, psycho-social support and a strong evaluation component, according to Dr. Wafaa El-Sadr, who heads the program.

The MTCT-Plus initiative has taken some time to get off the ground. Initial efforts focused hard on the issues of community mobilization and treatment preparedness, for both new staff and target communities. By March 22, 2003, 220 women were enrolled. By May the number was up to 400. Now that the programs are up, El-Sadr expected the numbers to increase quickly.

Among the new approaches that have come from Uganda is group counseling. In the US, VCT sites have stressed individual counseling, but due to the demand in Uganda several programs have found that group counseling works in a pre-testing context. Being in a group helps many women speak openly about their experience and, according to counselors, allows them to draw support from other women. Any women who test positive are then given individual post-test counseling.

Uganda has also made significant strides on the PMTCT front. The US Centers for Disease Control (CDC), through their new Global AIDS Program fund the MTCT program in Mulago.[32] Nationally, the government is continuing to extend PMTCT and MTCT services to smaller cities and rural areas. In 1998 UNAIDS backed five pilot treatment programs that are now being expanded.

Expanding Services

Years ago, UNAIDS, along with the CDC, USAID and other agencies, also helped develop comprehensive HIV services in ten districts, which have provided a framework for the current national scale-up effort. Now that the Global Fund for AIDS Treatment and Malaria is in place, Uganda has succeeded in getting a grant for a major expansion of treatment. For now, though, the government does not provide the drugs free, and provides no subsidy to patients using them. Most patients cannot afford the medicines. In 1997 an estimated 900 people were on therapy; by 2000 this had doubled. As drug prices fell, 3,000 people were estimated to be on treatment at the end of 2001, a number that had jumped to 10,000 by the end of 2002.

That number should be compared with the number of new cases since the Global Strategies meeting, an increase from 1 million to 1.2 million as of November 2002. Cumulatively, 947,552 had died by then, according to government statistics. The economic cost of AIDS remains very high: AIDS cost over $702 million a year in lost wealth in 2002, while malaria cost $348 million. "Comparing it with how much we earn from coffee, this loss is several times bigger," President Museveni told other African leaders at a meeting of the Commonwealth Regional Health Community for East, Central and Southern Africa, which gathers every three years.[33]

The government has steadily built up its treatment effort and is now field-testing new treatment guidelines built along WHO guidelines for resource-limited settings. In a first phase in 2000, it increased the number of treatment centers from five – all in Kampala – by adding three others outside the capital. By May 2003, twenty-five sites had been accredited to provide antiretroviral treatment in Uganda, and twenty-three were offering the drugs. In regional hospitals, six were providing antiretroviral drugs, including Aura, Mbarara, Kavale, Lira, Masaka and Gulu. The government hopes to provide antiretroviral treatment in eleven regional hospitals by the end of 2003, and in twenty health center IVs[34] (clinics run by medical officers) by the end of 2005.[35] By the end of 2006, all health center IVs are scheduled to provide antiretroviral treatment.[36]

That spells a significant expansion of testing and counseling services, since VCT sites are an entry point for treatment. The government is now setting up HIV testing sites at all health centers. It has also moved to develop its diagnostic and laboratory services. In government health units, HIV testing is free; in private laboratories, it cost between $3 and $5 as of May, 2003. There were some twenty public testing sites run by the Ministry of Health in Uganda. CD4 T-cell tests are available in eleven regional hospitals, at a price of $30 to $50 (as of mid 2003). Viral load tests cost $100, but this was also expected soon to change. For now, viral load tests are not considered routine, and are only performed when necessary – usually when patients are failing therapy.

A key ally in the national plan is TASO, the leading AIDS organization, which is doing intensive community mobilization to educate and prepare communities, as are smaller networks like NACWOLA – the National Community of Women Living with AIDS in Uganda. Both have chapters in rural areas. A number of HIV-positive women belong to both groups, and to WTAG, which has expanded its MTCT education to reach midwives in rural villages, where public health services are limited.

Using Generics

Uganda has also made good use of generic AIDS drugs. In May 2003 it licensed three Indian suppliers – Cipla, Hetero and Ranbaxy – to market their drugs in Uganda. Five other generic companies are being evaluated. In all, eighteen brand-name and eight generic drugs were available in Uganda.[37] The drugs are supplied by two main non-profit organizations, the Joint Clinical Research Center (JCRC) and Medical Access Uganda, Ltd., and procured by a non-profit outfit, Medical Access Uganda Ltd. Non-antiretrovirals are procured by two non-profit organizations, the Joint Medical Stores and the government-owned National Medical Stores, in addition to private distributors. This has allowed Uganda to purchase low-cost medicines and establish a distribution system to get the medicines to district and local health centers, avoiding any shortages.

Compared with many other African countries, Uganda's government has proved it will take the lead on the AIDS front, and will push hard to access available money and programs from sources abroad. President Museveni's status as a Friend-of-George-W.-Bush, and Uganda's growing reputation as a prevention model, will also help public health officials there push forward their national plan. The Bush money will be used to further beef up prevention and the MTCT efforts.

Not all is well, though. A proposed domestic patent law could prevent Uganda from importing generics from the Indian companies – something activists are actively fighting. Meanwhile, there is a gap between the government's plans on paper and the reality of access to drugs on the ground.

"A few more people are getting the drugs, and that is a positive step," concluded WTAG's Cissy Ssuuna, as she looked back at what had changed in recent months.[38] She is one of the lucky recipients. In 2001, during the Focus on Women conference, she was ill and cobbling together treatment courtesy of recycled drugs donated by friends and activists abroad. Her daughters worried that she would die. Today she is getting drugs and care from a local program, and has regained her health. She's also received scholarships to attend major AIDS conferences and is sharing her newfound information with other women in the community. Several orphaned children she has helped to keep alive are now being treated at Mulago hospital, and are flourishing.

But every day she sees all the others who aren't so lucky, as part of her job as a hospital nurse who cares for HIV patients, mostly women. In rural areas the number of pregnant women lacking access to nevirapine is high. "There are so many people who are dying, and are just going to die while we wait for the medicines to be delivered," commented Ssuuna. "It continues to be a tragedy when we see the drugs are cheaper now and we still can't get them to these people. We just have to keep pushing and pushing. But I'm afraid it won't be fast enough."

9

MOROCCO'S BOLD EXPERIMENT

Is Islam an obstacle or a tool in the fight against AIDS? This question has been at the heart of debates over the AIDS epidemic in North Africa, the Middle East and other regions where Islam is a dominant religion. In 2003, the incidence of AIDS appears far lower in North African countries. Some analysts feel religious taboos on sexual topics block prevention efforts, while religious laws and practices stigmatize HIV-positive individuals.[1] Others claim that Islam, with its traditional segregation of men and women and its ban on homosexuality and extramarital sex, has helped to counter the spread of HIV in the Arab world.

The impact of religion on HIV control is an issue relevant for all countries. But the debate over Islam, and especially Islamic fundamentalism, has taken on greater importance of late. This is partly due to political events in general, including the US-led War on Terror, which is focused on hard-line Islamic groups. Such groups recently gained power in Morocco, both at the local level and in parliament. As in other countries, they seek to impose strict Sharia – orthodox religious law – on citizens, a move that would roll back rights for women. This could seriously affect how Morocco responds to the threat of AIDS.

Like many Arab countries, Morocco has a low level of HIV infection, but the real scope of the epidemic isn't known. Given North Africa's strategic location, sandwiched between Western Europe and hard-hit sub-Saharan Africa, there is fresh concern that the HIV epidemic could take off here and quickly spread. Some experts worry that this is happening now, and is being ignored by political leaders. Their concern is based on past and current reports that suggest AIDS is proliferating in the Eastern Mediterranean, defined as the Middle East and West Asia.[2]

There, HIV/AIDS cases more than tripled in the three years leading up to 2003, jumping from 220,000 cases in 1999 to 700,000 by February 2003. Here, too a fast-growing percentage are women: in 2000 alone, female HIV rates jumped from 17 percent to 32 percent of the national total. These are the officially reported figures. But regionally, HIV testing is very limited, while stigma and ignorance of HIV and AIDS are high. So the real number of those affected is certain to be much higher. At a recent Cairo conference focusing on the regional epidemic, delegates reported that AIDS patients preferred to die without treatment than reveal their AIDS status.

For these reasons, treatment stands a chance of having a big impact on the region, since the first step in accessing care is testing. That may increase the demand for HIV services, only to reveal the extent of the epidemic. Regionally, the number of AIDS deaths has already started to fall, as some governments begin accessing treatment. But the high cost of drugs is still an impediment. In 2003, the average cost of the cheapest three-drug cocktails on the market in North African countries was around $1,200 a year, a huge decrease from $12,000 in 1996. But even at $100 a month, treatment is out of the question given how many people are living below the poverty line in this region. Experts say Morocco, Lebanon and Iran have the best health infrastructures to combat AIDS, followed by Tunisia.

That's one reason I wanted to go to Morocco. Another was because it is a country that has shown leadership around the epidemic. I met several Moroccan physicians at the Fourteenth International AIDS Conference in Barcelona, and saw their reports documenting Morocco's early efforts to turn back its small but growing epidemic.[3] They told me Morocco was contemplating the use of generic drugs in defiance of big pharma companies. They had secured seed funding from the Global Fund to embark on an ambitious national AIDS plan, and Morocco's political leaders were beginning to jump on-board. If their plans come to fruition, Morocco could provide a model for the region that will help policy-makers around the world measure the impact of treatment on HIV prevention and control in countries with a low incidence.[4] Could early treatment help Morocco shut out HIV? Will countries where AIDS has turned up go on to become the greatest beneficiaries of the global AIDS effort?

Like its neighbors, Morocco suffers from widespread poverty. Despite pockets of thriving urban industry, unemployment hovers at 25 percent and illiteracy is high – around 40 percent for men and 70 percent for women. Child labor is endemic, as is homelessness among uneducated, rural youths who migrate to urban areas looking for work and take up prostitution or drug trafficking to survive. Women also have a subordinated status compared with men. In Morocco and Algeria, Berber tribes of the Atlas region represent its oldest inhabitants, and are a poor, nomadic population. They are also a group that has pushed for greater civil rights and equality.

The Royal Kingdom of Morocco is led by 39-year-old King Mohammed VI, a youthful, moderate leader who has carefully balanced secular policies and Islamic law, and maintained an open attitude toward the West. To most outsiders, Morocco has long enjoyed a reputation as one of the more stable and democratic Arab states. But in truth, Morocco has remained a traditional monarchy, with political power tightly held by the King and his advisors.

For many years, the King has kept political opposition groups at bay, including a growing sector of orthodox Islamic groups, by integrating them into his government, and so diluting their power. As political tensions increase in Morocco, what will become of the nascent AIDS effort?

The Middle Atlas region of central Morocco is a beautiful, mountainous area pockmarked by dark volcanic lakes and forests of giant cedar, oak and cork. It has long been home to the Berbers, Morocco's oldest inhabitants, a majority group in the Islamic Royal Kingdom. For centuries, desert caravans stopped here, heading west across the Sahara toward the great oasis of Tafilalt in the south. Today, the Berbers' black-brown tents still dot the foothills here, testimony to their enduring, nomadic way of life.

Other Berbers have settled down on the outskirts of small villages and cities. Unable to afford modern housing, some live in primitive but large cave dwellings hand-carved from the rock. During the day the caves provide cool respite from a broiling sun; at night, the chilly mountain air still seeps in. These cave homes lack running water or toilets, yet sometimes include other modern amenities – electricity, portable cooking stoves, television sets. The walls are typically covered with thick, decorative hand-woven rugs that make them oddly cozy, and help ward off the dampness and cold of the mountain air, as well as rodents. Throughout this region, it's common to see men and women using hand-held wooden spools to spin wool into thread.

In the past two decades, a growing number of Berber have migrated to nearby Sefrou, a small walled hamlet. Today, many tourists visit the old city of Fez, which is just an hour away, but the modern world passes Sefrou by. Like Fez, it's a picture-postcard setting, with a minaret-laden mosque and a maze of narrow streets and small shops that lead to a central *medina*, or square, where the *muezzins* call the Muslem faithful to prayer.

Like many remote villages across Morocco, Sefrou also represents a kind of ground-zero in the global AIDS war. Here, Moroccan health officials hope one day to measure the success of a bold new experiment, one designed to prove the theory that AIDS treatment can not only bridge HIV prevention efforts, but actually serve as a prevention tool. Advocates believe the coupling of treatment with expanded HIV testing and counseling services to cities and rural areas like the Middle Atlas will spur those who are now afraid to get tested. It will help reach the most vulnerable groups and those with the fewest services, including Berber communities, and help physicians identify patients at earlier stages of infection. Health officials will then be able to target prevention efforts to stem any outbreaks that emerge. By offering prophylactic treatment to newly or acutely infected individuals, they may also help counter the spread of the epidemic.[5]

The Embryonic Epidemic

By initiating a national treatment plan now, Morocco is in the enviable position of contemplating whether it can stop AIDS in its tracks. The country appears to have a tiny epidemic – the Ministry of Health estimated only 1,152 AIDS cases at the end of March 2003, and 15,000 to 20,000 HIV cases. But since few people are now tested for HIV itself, no one really knows how big the epidemic is. One harbinger of an expanding AIDS epidemic is the dramatic rise in other sexually transmitted diseases. Up to 600,000 cases are recorded in Morocco annually. That would suggest HIV cases could in fact be much higher here than is realized.[6]

The first AIDS cases in Morocco occurred in the mid 1990s among gay and bisexual married men, and also a small number of intravenous drug users who had spent time living in European countries. Heterosexual transmission is becoming increasingly common, putting women and girls, who are socially disempowered, at greater risk. A key reason for this is the stigma surrounding AIDS, which is linked to the taboo subjects of homosexuality, bisexuality and promiscuity. Male homosexuality is outlawed in many Arab countries, but it remains common in Arab societies where men and women are socially segregated. Typically, bisexual and gay men live closeted double lives, and bend to family and community pressures to marry and have children. Once they are exposed to HIV, they may pass the virus on to their unsuspecting spouse – or spouses, since under Islam, Arab men may have several wives. This pattern is being reported in Morocco and other North African countries, which makes it harder to grasp the scope of the regional epidemic.

"If this situation appears less dramatic than in other regions of the world, it is still very worrisome," said Professor Hakima Himmich in Casablanca. Himmich is the dynamic head of the Association de Lutte Contre le SIDA (ALCS – the Association to Fight AIDS). She is also a key figure in the national treatment effort.[7] "There is mostly silence about AIDS, and a lot of discrimination, so you understand why people hide it." The introduction of HIV testing services and targeted education will help, but for now deeply rooted social and religious attitudes are the big stumbling block.

AIDS prevention programs have proliferated in Morocco, albeit mostly in larger cities. But Himmich criticized the absence of national and mass-media educational campaigns about AIDS on the radio and television, which could help counter ignorance and stigma. Given the high rate of illiteracy in rural areas like Sefrou, the media could play an important role. But that would require more openness about sexuality. Although Morocco has an independent press, and internet use is steadily increasing, the media is subject to censorship by state and religious authorities, and references to sexuality are routinely monitored. In Fez, for example, black markers or paint are used to cover up images of scantily clad women on Western movie posters.

"The obstacles are not at the level of the Ministry of Health," Himmich stressed. "Up to today, there has never been a national prevention campaign. There is no political engagement because the epidemic has just started," she explained, warning that "if we don't push them, we'll have what was seen in other countries – 10 percent of the population infected before they wake up. We want to try to avoid that."

Treatment is a way to keep the epidemic down, Himmich believes. "I think stigma can change with access. The minute a mortal disease becomes a chronic one that you can treat, this is where you will see the change happen. It's clear that you can't have an effective prevention strategy without access to care for affected people." But there is a paradox: although she is convinced Morocco can help to confirm the theory that treatment access strengthens prevention efforts, she's not sure how to offer concrete proof of success if HIV remains rare. "I don't know how to show it works so that it can serve as a model, because people could say, 'Well, you didn't have many cases because the epidemic started late, and you are a Muslim country.' How do you measure something that doesn't take place? . . . How can you validate such a model? It won't be easy."

Integrating Islam

Until recently, Morocco's religious leaders either stayed silent on the subject of AIDS or denounced prevention efforts, arguing, for example, that condoms promote infidelity. One well-known leader publicly declared that belief in Islam was enough to protect the faithful from AIDS.[8] As far-right groups gain influence, so do their messages.

"Sometimes we fall upon someone who is open, but most of the time they just say the response should be abstinence," said Himmich, who deemed this message "totally counterproductive." But she was the first to agree that, in the future, prevention messages can succeed only if they are integrated into Moroccan culture. "We won't have the same prevention discourse here as in France or Sweden – that's clear. We're going to keep our society in mind, which is Muslim and North African and has its characteristics that we must respect, in order not to shock the public." But she admitted that this is easier said than done.[9]

HIV education and prevention programs are currently focused on groups at high risk, including sex workers, men who have sex with men, drug users, and youths – the latter including street children, who often come from rural areas and turn to prostitution or drug trafficking to survive when they arrive in cities. But Himmich and other health experts are particularly worried about women and girls, knowing they are highly vulnerable to sexual exposure to HIV. Under Islam, women are relegated to second-class status as citizens, and men are given decision-making power in many arenas. The result is that women in Morocco lag behind men in accessing education and services, including health-care. That includes Berber women, who are often very poor.

Sex Workers and Their Husbands

Although Berber tribes of the Middle Atlas make up a majority of Moroccan society, their customs, language and nomadic movements have historically kept them on the economic and social margins. In Sefrou, Berber women spend their days sitting outside the former shops of Jewish merchants who fled to Israel when Morocco became independent in 1956. Until recently, they survived by working as prostitutes, turning the old Jewish shops into mini-brothels. Among the Berbers, sex work is not highly stigmatized, but is viewed as something of a family trade passed along from mother to daughter. Regardless of Islam's bans, these women rarely lacked for clients.

All that changed in the spring of 2002, when radical Islamists vying for political power in the Royal Kingdom succeeded in outlawing prostitution in Sefrou. Almost overnight, the Berber women lost their source of income and became destitute. "These women have no future," declared a young Muslim resident, who served as my unofficial chaperone during an afternoon's visit to Sefrou. "We reject them because they are not pure and no one will marry them. And if they can't make money for their families, they are of no use to anyone."

The question remains: How many Berber sex workers have HIV? What about their husbands and male clients? Without widespread testing, no one knows for sure. A study by the Ibn Roch Infectious Disease Hospital in Casablanca, one of two specialist centers treating AIDS patients, found that 65 percent of married women with HIV surveyed were exposed by their often older husbands. Many of the husbands had ultimately fallen sick and died of AIDS.

"I hate to say it, but the biggest single risk for Moroccan women with HIV has been their husbands," stated Himmich. "That fact makes it even harder for us to confront the problem, because the husbands are in denial and they blame their wives. So you see, it's really a social problem that affects the whole family and community." Doctors at Ibn Roch hospital confirmed that women lag behind in getting tested and accessing care.

"We've had a problem with certain patients about telling their wives," said Adnani Kadmiri Said, head of the ALCS's treatment education program. "Sometimes they bring the wife, but what can we do? We can't force them to bring the wife, not easily." Ignorance of AIDS remains a big obstacle for men and women. For example, one HIV-positive man admitted to ALCS counselors that he had deliberately sought out young virgins for sex and marriage in order to cure himself of AIDS – illustrating a myth prevalent elsewhere in Africa.

A growing number of divorced women turn to sex work after being abandoned by their husbands and families, said Himmich. Under Moroccan law, which reflects Islamic Sharia religious law, a man can divorce a woman simply by publicly declaring "I divorce thee" three times. Women do not have this legal right, despite efforts by Moroccan feminists and other progressives to reform marriage and family law. Meanwhile, studies by Himmich's group indicate that female sex workers are exposed by their clients – not the other way around. To date, her studies show that almost half of HIV-positive prostitutes in the country are divorced or widowed, and are struggling to raise their children alone. They rarely use condoms with clients, who generally refuse to do so.

The plight of sex workers may be contributing to another problem. Random testing in an orphanage in the south in 2002 had turned up a surprising number of HIV-positive infants, said Himmich. "That means that there are sex workers who are positive and give birth and abandon their infants," she grimly concluded. Since HIV testing is not routinely offered to pregnant women in public hospitals or private institutions, there is no way of knowing how many other children may be exposed.

All of this impacts on the kind of care that individuals may be getting in health centers far from the capital or bigger cities. Right now, patients arrive in hospitals with symptoms of HIV illness, meaning they've been harboring HIV for some time. By the time they see doctors, their health is precarious. Without drugs to treat either HIV or opportunistic infections, doctors have had a hard time keeping these patients alive.

First Steps

To its credit, Morocco has moved quickly to put its treatment plan into practice. Luckily, it holds several aces in its hand, a major one being money. In 2002, Morocco won a $ 9.24 million grant from the new Global Fund to fight AIDS, Tuberculosis and Malaria.[10] That pays for a national plan that will extend existing HIV testing and prevention from the big cities out to rural areas, and target the most vulnerable groups. It also pays for free antiretroviral drugs and HIV care for patients who need them. The plan is being carried out under the direction of the Ministry of Health, with key NGO allies like the ALCS, the Pan-African AIDS Organization (OPALS), AMSED and the Moroccan League Against MST. It builds on an infrastructure created by these groups over the past decade.

The main leadership has come from pioneering physicians like Himmich, who is viewed as a force of nature by her admiring colleagues. "She's ten of us in a single woman's body," joked Dr. Mustapha Sodqi, an affable physician and ALCS member. "Without her, I don't know where we'd be with the AIDS situation."

The ALCS was set up in 1998 as a voluntary agency that provides prevention and other services in eleven cities, with its national headquarters in Casablanca. It cites a list of early victories, some shared with the other NGOs and the Health Ministry: early educational and prevention campaigns in Casablanca, Agadir, Marrakech and Fez; forums in schools, prisons, the army and police; launch of an AIDS hotline; support groups and legal assistance to people with AIDS; and the establishment of eight anonymous, voluntary HIV testing centers.[11]

The Access Battle

Before 1999, Dr. Sodqi explained, the ALCS provided 80 percent of the medicine for opportunistic infections used to treat patients at Ibn Roch hospital and a hospital in Rabat. For years Ibn Roch relied on donated drugs to make up for chronic shortages. In 1999 the Health Ministry contributed money for two AIDS drugs – AZT and 3TC. Patients paid for the third drug themselves, until a grant from the French Therapeutic Solidarity Fund (FSTI) provided

2.7 million dirhams (approximately US$260,000) for this. The ALCS also managed to convince insurers to cover the cost of HIV care for workers.

In 2000, GlaxoSmithKline provided a two-year grant for patient treatment education; a French foundation is now picking up the tab. Other French NGOs such as AIDES provided donations of medicine and supplies to the ALCS during the initial lean years, and have promised further support. ACT UP–Paris activists have also worked closely with the ALCS and Himmich to advocate access to treatment for Moroccans with HIV/AIDS. But the cost of medicine remained too high for poor patients, including such OI therapies as ganciclovir for cytomegalovirus, fluconazole for fungal infections, and interferon for hepatitis. Most tests were free for HIV patients at Ibn Roch, but not all. Elsewhere, hepatitis B and C testing was not available in public hospitals.

As the global battle for treatment access heated up in 2001, the ALCS joined with Médecins sans Frontières (MSF) to explore the availability of generic HIV drugs. Instead Moroccan officials secured a deal for sharply discounted brand-name drugs through a UNAIDS-backed Accelerated Access Initiative designed originally for sub-Saharan Africa.[12] But even at $200 a month, discounted three-drug regimens cost more than the average $150 monthly salary of the ALCS clients who are employed – and most are not. As Himmich discovered, the discount deal was in any case less than it seemed. GlaxoSmithKline, Boehringer Ingelheim, Merck Sharp and Dome, and Bristol-Myers Squibb – all dropped their prices, but Roche refused to meet with the ALCS, she recalled.

In July 2002, days after the Fourteenth International AIDS Conference in Barcelona, the ALCS and MSF co-hosted a forum in Casablanca to determine whether Morocco was ready to pursue generic HIV production. The answer was a qualified yes, from key figures like the Health Minister and local generic drug manufacturers like Gallenica. Major international players were at the conference too, including representatives for Indian, Thai and Brazilian generic companies, the WHO, and activists from ACT UP and Health GAP.[13]

How quickly the government moves depends on many factors. Morocco recently requested a technology transfer and help from the Brazilian government, which pioneered state production of generic antiretrovirals. The main obstacle, say Health GAP activists, is the attitude of the US government, heavily influenced by multinational drug companies who oppose the use of generics. Here, the HIV issue may run into problems with Morocco's bilateral trade relations with the US, and other patent issues overseen by the World Trade Organization.

By late July 2002, 130 people were receiving antiretrovirals, and 182 were on a waiting list. By May 2003, that number had more than doubled to 354, with 186 soon to receive drugs. With the much-needed influx of Global Fund money, the Health Ministry promised to provide free anti-retroviral drugs to all patients through 2003. It will also beef up the HIV diagnostic capacity of provincial hospitals. The ALCS is using some of the money to study the sex work problem in seven big cities, to fund prevention programs aimed at men who have sex with men, and male prostitutes, and prevention efforts targeting workers in the textile and agricultural sectors. The government has also increased its national budget for HIV prevention and treatment. European donors and other agencies promise to throw additional money into the pot. These funds will help provide treatment education and training to both health professionals and patients, and to build up the overall public health system. At the same time, medical groups like MSF are continuing programs that provide STD screening and care to sex workers.

So far, so good. But with expanded HIV testing, Morocco can also expect its patient population to expand. The end result could be future drug shortages if funding isn't sustained.

The Face of AIDS

Nothing underscores the plight of people with AIDS like impending blindness, progressive madness and death. On the same July weekend that health officials were debating generics, three people died of AIDS at the Ibn Roch hospital across town, including a pregnant woman.[14] Although doctors are more adept at treating HIV patients there, many patients are still referred late. "We offer them antiretrovirals, but to be honest, triple therapy hasn't done much for these severely advanced cases when they arrive with [cerebral] toxoplasmosis, etc." said Dr. Rajaa Bensghir, chief of Ibn Roch's infectious disease day-clinic. Physicians often fail to diagnose early cases, in part because tuberculosis, malaria and parasitic illnesses produce common symptoms such as fever, diarrhea or weight loss. Hepatitis B and C are also common. That very weekend, Dr. Bensghir noted, two other patients were going blind from CMV, and she had no ganciclovir to give them. "It's heartbreaking," she admitted.

By comparison, those who are diagnosed early enough and treated as necessary are doing well. At the Barcelona conference, several reports showed that prompt treatment benefited Moroccan HIV patients. In one three-year study evaluated by UNAIDS, anti-HIV therapy quickly lowered viral loads in 219 symptomatic patients, a trend that held for 120 weeks. CD4 cell counts increased on average from 150 to 350 cells/mm^3. Hospitalizations dropped by 84 percent, along with opportunistic infections. But not all people benefited: twenty-six died, three abandoned therapy, seven had treatment interruptions, and a few failed their regimens. Drug side-effects were common, though mostly minor. They included gastrointestinal problems, elevated lipid levels – including a few cases of lipodystrophy – and liver toxicity. Adherence was also very high.

"Access to [HIV drugs] in a country with limited resources is possible provided that it is innovative and truly actively committed," concluded the study authors. These results suggest that Morocco's treatment effort will quickly benefit the remainder of those now waiting for therapy. And as the general public learns about this success, it can help dimish fears of testing. Both of these are goals that Himmich's team plan to move towards.

Daily Problems

Today, most HIV patients at Ibn Roch hospital are either from the Casablanca–Rabat region or the southern cities of Marrakech and Agadir. Those living in the north go to the infectious disease hospital in Rabat, though many end up at Ibn Roch anyway. Children are usually referred to a pediatric hospital in Casablanca. In contrast to two years ago, patients on therapy are now monitored at Ibn Roch's outpatient day-clinic, freeing up hospital beds. There, Bensghir heads a small team of doctors and nurses, with outside specialists on call. Lab work is performed at the clinic, including CD4 and viral load tests. Patients return monthly for check-ups. If they live far away, they are sent back to their referring physicians for follow-up. This is not ideal, admits Bensghir, since local doctors aren't trained to monitor patients on HIV therapy.

A lingering problem, aside from side-effects, has been a big pill burden for patients, because certain doses of drugs are lacking. "With Retrovir [AZT], which comes in 500mg and 600mg forms, we have just the 100mg tablet, so we give them five pills a day," Bensghir explained. "That's just one of the three drugs." That will now change as new regimens arrive. As she points out, the access gap has a direct effect on the daily quality of life for patients on therapy, and it effects adherence. Getting access to new fixed-dose generic combinations will certainly improve that situation.

A lack of pediatric drugs, including liquid AZT, has long been another problem. Fortunately, there have been few maternal HIV cases at the center so far. Over the years, the ALCS provided HIV transmission prophylaxis, initially AZT plus 3TC, to pregnant women who tested positive. In 2002 only AZT was available. For some time, pregnant women with symptomatic HIV who required combination therapy have received it. After delivering, mothers receive free infant formula to avoid transmission through breast-feeding. To help these women avoid disclosure of their HIV status to family or the community, ALCS counselors tend to suggest a white lie. "They simply say, 'We don't make enough breast milk,' and this explains why they can't breast-feed," said Dr. Bensghir, grinning. "That is a common problem for women. But it works."

Elsewhere, stigma and discrimination continue to face those trying to access care. The ALCS has confronted dentists and surgeons who won't treat HIV-positive patients or refuse to do C-sections on pregnant women. Until recently, the agency was forced to provide extra sheets, gowns, gloves and other materials to gynecologists in other hospitals. "We've had some training in regional hospitals, but it's not enough," said ALCS educator Said in 2002. "There's a lot of stigma, even among doctors. Education and training of health professionals is a real priority."

Now that the big money is flowing in, life is more hopeful for those requiring treatment. "In the beginning we had to choose which patients to start on therapy. We were confronted by families: why this patient, why not this one?" said Bensghir. "That was an enormous problem. We'd really like to have treatment for all of them. It's hard to have an illness and be isolated. Some of my patients have been on treatment for three years. But the minute we begin talking they are in tears, even if they are in good health. They are really suffering. We have to manage to help them."

Shifting Political Winds

Where does this leave the destitute Berber women of Middle Atlas? As the national effort grows, HIV and STD testing should begin to reach these vulnerable communities, and with it access to care. But in Sefrou, as in the rest of Morocco, the political climate is also changing. Some of this is connected to the recent rise of Islamic fundamentalism in Morocco, and to outside events like the 9/11 terrorist attacks in the US. As the political climate changes in Morocco, so might the political muscle of the mullahs, and the political will of the monarchy.

In September 2002, Morocco's Party of Justice and Development, an Islamic far-right coalition, scored an historic breakthrough in legislative elections, gaining forty-two of the 325 seats in the parliament's lower house. The victory was especially impressive because the PJD only ran candidates in half the country's districts, and it has changed the political character of parliament. It was also rightly seen as a blow to the King's power. The PJD is now the third-largest political party in Morocco, and as an official party it recognizes the monarchy.

At the same time, other reforms moved forward. In that same September election, women gained thirty-five of the seats in the lower house, due to a new quota system requiring that 10 percent of new deputy seats go to women. But with the rising power of the far-right mullahs, AIDS activists worry that a religious backlash could hamper the nascent national AIDS effort and reverse gains in women's status.

Based on the events that followed, they have reason to worry. On May 11, 2003, Moroccan suicide bombers attacked five targets in Casablanca, killing forty-three people and injuring eight foreigners – a shocking event that Moroccans view as a national wake-up call.[15]

Days after the sucide attacks, the *New York Times* reported that Morocco's King had openly allied himself with Bush and the US War on Terror, and had helped the Central Intelligence Agency to pursue "terror suspects."[16]

The economic situation in Morocco has also worsened following the 9/11 attacks in the US. As in America, Europe's borders have been more tightly sealed to prevent illegal entry – an ostensible anti-terrorist move that has made travel to Europe harder, especially for seasonal migrant workers in Morocco. Drug trafficking and use are also fueling the spread of

HIV, nationally and regionally. Morocco remains a trans-shipment point for opium and heroin destined for Europe. Where drugs thrive, so do crime and prostitution, and HIV also finds its niche. Coastal cities like Tangiers have long been havens for drug trafficking, attracting immigrants seeking entry to Europe via Spain, just across the narrow Straits of Gibraltar.

Uncharted Waters

With the monarchy under attack for its pro-Western reforms and its cozy relations with Bush and the CIA, relations with the US remain very touchy. Will the King seek more protection from the West, or more independence? In the months ahead, the Royal Kingdom and its embattled monarch face important political and economic decisions that will provide clues about Morocco's course.

In the arena of the War on Terror, the US needs all the progressive Arab allies it can get, so Morocco has political capital. Will that translate into bold positions in the arena of its bilateral trade with the US? In this area, Morocco is far the weaker partner. With tourism down, Morocco needs access to US and European foreign investment and export markets, as these affect its ability to confront the Bush administration or big pharma companies in the arena of trade and generic drugs.

For now, Morocco's long-term reliance on outside funders to pay for treatment is a problem that needs resolution. Given its industrial capacity, Morocco is well poised to manufacture its own generic drugs, or to support private companies like Gallenica. It could quickly gain capacity at least to repackage drugs, and, with a little technical help, to make finished pills and even export them to neighboring countries. That's why Morocco has been talking to the pioneers of state generic production – Brazil and Thailand – and why Himmich is pushing health officials to support this move.

But others in Morocco are eyeing the larger economic picture. In November 2003, Moroccan and US trade negotiators announced a bilateral free trade deal between the two countries that was commended by the Bush administration. AIDS activists quickly denounced the impending deal, charging that it would prevent Morocco from accessing or producing generic AIDS drugs.

The economic picture is also tied to current political tensions in Morocco.

Although it's difficult to gauge how the current religious–political battle will affect national prevention efforts, here are some easy predictions. At the local level, in places like Sefrou, the mullahs are already putting arch-conservative policies in place. If hard-line Islamist groups gain more power to shape national policies, the AIDS prevention battle will become difficult. If orthodox Sharia laws are implemented, women and girls will suffer, and their access to care and education will decrease; it won't be as much of a priority to reach out to prostitutes. Instead, these groups may find reasons to avoid seeking services from public programs. The situation could become dangerous for gay and bisexual men, given the harsh penalties religious conservatives reserve for homosexuals. Those now being encouraged to come forward for testing will have reasons to hide. It won't be easy to talk about condoms or safe sex on national television or in public education campaigns. Progressive Moroccans may find fewer powerful allies within government for their innovative programs targeting sex workers, men who have sex with men, and drug users. The new women deputies in parliament may have less power.

That's the grim view. Countering it is Himmich's optimism and the talent she and colleagues have successfully shown in battling AIDS so far. As the War on Terror changes our world, so does the global war on AIDS. Morocco is getting outside support and attention for its pioneering efforts to stop AIDS. A nascent grassroots movement is beginning, and it is linked to a regional movement of a new generation of people with HIV, who are ready to defend their right to survive and thrive. Steadily, they will help to counter the reigning stigma and silence. Amid the prevailing political crisis, then, the wider Arab world is waking to the problem of AIDS, and Morocco is at the forefront of that awakening.

Will Morocco's grand plan – treatment as a bridge to prevention – succeed in limiting the spread of AIDS? With outside money coming in; with leaders like Himmich advising the Global Fund; with high-level government cooperation; with NGOs willing to mobilize communities, Morocco is well positioned to have an impact on the spread of AIDS. In the short term, the picture may appear to be getting worse, as more people are tested and the true face of the epidemic emerges. But if the AIDS effort works, they're likely to gain access to treatment and supportive services – as long as Sharia law doesn't disrupt the plan. At the tip of North Africa, Morocco remains a bright spot of hope on the planet, and a model for the Arab world.

10

AIDS, APARTHEID AND SOUTH AFRICA: THE CHALLENGES OF SURVIVAL

In July 2000, the world's attention became riveted by the horrifying magnitude of AIDS in southern Africa when thousands of South Africans led the largest ever AIDS protest march on African soil, through the streets of Durban, site of the watershed Fourteenth International AIDS Conference. The march was dubbed the most important since the famous anti-apartheid protests here. Many familiar faces from that earlier movement joined AIDS activists from the Treatment Action Campaign and its now-famous leader, Zackie Achmat, a Cape Malay, former prostitute and gay activist who is openly HIV-positive. They included Nelson Mandela of the African National Congress and his second wife, Graca Machel, herself a well-known politician; his ex-wife, Winnie Mandela; union leaders of COSATU, and Anglican Bishop Desmond Tutu. They also included many politicians, a broad stripe of the country's civil society, and long blocks of citizens wearing white T-shirts that boldly proclaimed in purple block letters: "HIV-positive."

As many in the world now know, South Africa's AIDS epidemic is the biggest in the world, though countries like Botswana have a higher percentage of their population that is infected. An estimated 5 million South Africans have HIV, and over 1,000 people a day are becoming exposed.[1] In 1999, over 40,000 babies were born with the virus, due to lack of access to AZT to prevent maternal transmission; GlaxoSmithKline was offering the drug at US$50 a year per person at that time – out of reach for most citizens.[2]

In the absence of medicine to treat people or to prevent maternal transmission of HIV, the epidemic has surged to the point where forecasters predict a half-million AIDS-related deaths in South Africa alone by 2010, and the World Bank recently predicted the country's complete collapse within two decades unless emergency measures were taken. Today, new cases are increasingly among females and young people: in hard-hit areas like the mining center of Carletonville which suffered the highest rates of HIV in the country in 2000, up to 30 percent of miners were HIV-positive, while 70 percent of young girls aged fifteen to twenty were exposed. Most young women contract HIV through unprotected sex, including a high degree of forced sex and marital rape with husbands and partners, but gang rape and prostitution are also factors. HIV is high among commercial sex workers, and due to poverty, women also engage in informal transactional sex for money.

Other hard-hit sectors include agricultural workers and soldiers; a recent estimate said a quarter of South Africa's military has HIV. The migration of people seeking work, the long absence of miners and soldiers from their families, and the movement of troops all contribute to the spread of the epidemic.

What all this means is that in the decade since Mandela took office in 1994, later handing the reins to Mbeki to continue the job of rebuilding a democratic South Africa, AIDS has come along to destroy the country's dreams.

This particular history is not, however, accidental. Instead, there is a direct link between spiraling AIDS and four decades of apartheid – a racial system of structural violence aimed at keeping the white minority, and particularly Afrikaners, in power. A key reason why so many black South Africans have died and are facing death from AIDS and other diseases of poverty like TB now is because they were deliberately denied the fundamentals – basic education, healthcare, housing, jobs and services of every kind – for so long.

In 2000, when I visited the sprawling shantytowns of Soweto outside Johannesburg, tens of thousands of residents still lived in packed city blocks of small cardboard and tin shacks separated by muddy walkways. They lacked potable water, plumbing or regular electricity. Instead, they contended with rats and hunger and joblessness, struggling to raise children in neighborhoods where street violence had become endemic. Alongside HIV, rates of other STDs, TB, and malaria were and remain sky-high.

These are all legacies of apartheid. They are the reasons why AIDS has affected blacks far more than whites; why sexual violence plays such a big role in spreading HIV to women; why a generation of youths have become AIDS orphans. Apartheid is the reason why few doctors or clinics or drugs exist for black residents, whether in suburban Soweto or in rural areas, including the remote, formerly segregated "homelands." Instead, many still rely on traditional healers. There are over 300,000 'inyangas' and 'sangomas' in the country, and they use herbs and traditional potions to treat diseases, including AIDS.

It's important to use the lens of apartheid to understand why Mbeki and his closest aides adopted a policy of denial of HIV, and refused for so long to provide drugs for citizens, even when these were offered for free. These anti-apartheid activists were shaped by years of exile and resistance to white rule. They had good reason to be suspicious of the belated concern of governments and leaders who, not long ago, supported the white racists in South Africa and cared little for the fate of its black majority. The catastrophic failure of Mbeki's administration to respond to the threat of AIDS is thus an aftershock of apartheid. It doesn't excuse Mbeki's actions or his administration's failure to protect millions from illness and death; they will likely forever be judged for what TAC deemed their "culpable homicide." But the frame of apartheid does reveal how profoundly this recent history shapes the future in South Africa.

I've introduced the issue of apartheid to provide a social and economic context for judging the country's response to AIDS. That includes not only access to treatment, but also its effort to develop and test a vaccine or microbicide to protect the uninfected. Thanks to its relative wealth, South Africa has the scientific infrastructure to carry out such high-tech clinical studies, but its success will hinge on the involvement of affected communities. Here, Mbeki is hardly alone in being suspicious of the agendas of Western drug companies and scientific researchers.

Unfortunately, thousands of South Africans participated in earlier clinical HIV drug trials, but were denied treatment once the studies were complete. White doctors who oversaw the trials were handsomely rewarded by drug company sponsors.[3] It's thus no wonder residents will need to be convinced of the potential benefit of participating in any further clinical research.

There is also an egregious aspect of South Africa's apartheid history to blame. It concerns a South African Defence Program of Chemical and Biological Warfare (CBW) known as Project Coast, which was carried out in the 1980s and early 1990s by the apartheid-era government. The program was led by a former special forces army brigadier named Wouter Basson — nicknamed "Dr.

Death." He happened to be a top cardiologist who served as a personal heart assistant to then-Prime Minister P.W. Botha and to this day continues to practice medicine – much to the outrage of others who have demanded he be barred. Beginning in 1997, and as late as 2001, South Africans were treated to regular front-page headlines that detailed Dr. Death's horrible Mengele-like experiments. He and colleagues stood accused of mass murder against hundreds of anti-apartheid activists by the use of an array of lethal pathogens including plague, cholera and anthrax – and HIV. Evidence in the case against Basson was provided by a few living survivors to the Truth and Reconciliation Commission (TRC). Basson's activities drew international coverage through a CBS Frontline documentary in 1998 and a later New Yorker piece in early 2001.[4]

The allegations included that the program developed a sterility vaccine to use on black South Africans, used toxins and poisons for political assassination, released cholera strains into the water sources of certain South African villages, and provided cholera and anthrax to Rhodesian (now Zimbabwean) troops for use against anti-apartheid guerilla rebels exiled there. In 1979, the world's largest anthrax outbreak took place in Rhodesia, killing eighty-two people and making thousands ill. By contrast, HIV was reportedly deemed a poor candidate for a weapon since it took years to cause illness and death, according to court documents and witness testimonies. This cloak-and-dagger story read like a seriously evil version of a James Bond-meets-Dr. Strangelove movie, revealing the perverted lengths to which the apartheid regime went to exterminate black opponents.

When I was in South Africa for the Durban AIDS conference in 2000, there were fresh details emerging from the TRC about Basson's activities. Prosecutors had implicated high government officials, including Botha, and there were allegations that the CIA and several other international intelligence services had links to South Africa's CBW program. A number of South African AIDS activists mentioned the case to me, wondering what Americans thought of the news. Did I believe that the CIA had helped create AIDS? They were deeply worried that Basson would escape punishment because he seemed to have dirt on many people still in the government. When he later got off scot-free, their cynicism deepened. It only got worse when he was taken back into government service by Mandela's administration – a move designed to keep Basson under close watch, said insiders.

Why bring this up? There are serious crimes and serious damage that have been done to South Africans around HIV and AIDS, some in the name of science. Such crimes have given real ammunition to those who see government conspiracies in the global AIDS pandemic, and these individuals are not restricted to South Africa. In the US, and particularly among African-American communities, there is a deep mistrust of the government and its agendas around medical research linked to the infamous Tuskegee syphilis trials. In relation to vaccines and microbicides, the scientific battle is really step two. Step one involves addressing the legitimate concerns and needs of a populace deeply scarred by apartheid and enduring racism, by unethical white researchers and drug company representatives, by the campaign of misinformation about HIV and AIDS waged by Mbeki and the dissident crowd, and by their own fears and lack of information about a raging epidemic. For that reason, the central challenge remains that of community mobilization, and the ethical burden of proof lies with those who want to conduct such studies, given this recent history.

The Perinatal HIV Unit (PHRU) of the University of Witwatersrand is housed inside the Chris Hani Baragwanath hospital in Soweto, and is considered a premier site for community-based HIV programs combined with clinical research. The hospital treats a huge HIV-positive population. The unit is also led by two physicians who were anti-apartheid activists and who pushed colleagues to undertake clinical studies that would provide stepping-stones for local community access to HIV MTCT and adult treatment programs. They also clashed with Mbeki and government officials who opposed access to treatment for South Africans. "We were able to do what we have because the community is totally behind us – we are part of the community and we listen to what they want," remarked Glenda Gray, a pediatrician at Chris Hani. "It hasn't been easy, but it's not hard because we have had that unity."[5]

Now that the government has backed universal treatment, the landscape will be dramatically altered. But a look at the evolving situation in Soweto offers a glimpse of the task at hand as new vaccine, microbicide and clinical drug trials are being launched. What's changed in the wake of Mbeki's change of mind are the doomsday forecasts, replaced by a cautious hope that South Africa can now do what it did with apartheid: against all odds, overturn a destructive force and declare a new day.

Soweto's Vaccine Dreams

At a short drive from the modern metropolis of Johannesburg, the bustling, impoverished township of Soweto was the site of fervent anti-apartheid activism in the 1970s. Today Soweto is the largest residential area in South Africa, a place where the smoke from cooking-fires at dusk leaves a haze over the new housing projects that stand beside the tin and cardboard shanties of squatter settlements. Less well known to outsiders is that Soweto is also home to the PHRU housed at a well-established HIV research and clinical trial facility. Chris Hani Baragwanath is said to be the largest hospital in the world. It is a recent entrant into the HIV vaccine and microbicide arena.

The PHRU began with the efforts of its two directors, obstetrician James McIntyre and his colleague Glenda Gray. The two have been working in the AIDS care field for over a dozen years, and stood strongly beside Zackie Achmat these last years in championing access to treatment and taking on the Mbeki camp. Alongside their clinical and research work, the duo helped draft South Africa's early National AIDS Plan – in particular the chapter on perinatal HIV. Before their scientific careers began, they were political activists involved in desegregation of the health sector and in helping the ANC formulate health policy. "We've always been part of the AIDS community," said McIntyre when we first spoke in 2000 about the PHRU's work. He was also co-chair of the national AIDS consortium for many years. Added Gray: "People trust us. You have to earn that trust."

They started by setting up a perinatal HIV clinic in 1991, "as a response to bad treatment," explained Gray, who added that HIV testing of mothers in their hospital actually dates back to 1987. It was one of the first facilities in South Africa set to offer HIV testing and counseling in a maternity setting. It was also among the first to emphasize STD management and to train midwives and counselors in outreach to the surrounding community – activities which grew out of early links with local NGOs.

In 1996, the clinic expanded to become a research unit of the University of Witwatersrand, and produced a steady stream of scientific and policy work around HIV and reproductive health. Besides its hospital setting, which provides clinical services for many thousands of HIV-positive women and their babies, the Unit and its close collaborator at the Chris Hani, the Reproductive Health Research Unit (RHRU), have carried out a variety of phase I, II and III trials of agents to treat and prevent AIDS. Through these other joint studies, the PHRU has worked with a wide range of multilateral and national agencies, major pharmaceutical companies and scientists around the world.[6]

By 2000, it already had a research staff of nearly 100 people conducting large, scientifically rigorous trials. Most importantly, it had built up community involvement, support and outreach programs, and become a passionate advocate on behalf of the community it served. Much of the needed infrastructure for vaccine trials was thus already in place.

The PHRU's international reputation was launched through early clinical trials of treatments to prevent mother-to-child transmission of HIV. It was one of five clinical trial sites for an African study called PETRA that compared the success of different AZT regimens in lowering maternal HIV transmission. The PHRU also participated in the South African Intrapartum Nevirapine Trial (SAINT), which proved that nevirapine offers a cheaper, more effective alternative to AZT.

In both cases, the community played an important role in shaping the trials. "We've never had a top-down approach that a lot of researchers have," said Gray. She cited placebo trials as a case in point. In September 1997, the *New England Journal of Medicine* published an editorial that strongly criticized the PETRA study for including a placebo arm, since a fourteen-week course of AZT given to HIV-positive pregnant women was already known to reduce MTCT – although the duration and price of this treatment put it out of reach for the developing world, including South Africa. "The moment there was a furor about it we called the community, the NGOs, the people in the trials and we discussed it," Gray said. "We allowed them to decide." The consensus: go ahead. And the results: unambiguous validation of the shorter, cheaper regimen – and a community's empowerment.

Given Mbeki's later opposition to AZT and nevirapine for use in MTCT programs, these trials are all the more important, since they were conducted by and with South African civil society. There could be no charge that outsiders were imposing foreign study results.

To Gray, these trials also reaffirmed the crucial importance of serving the community throughout the research process. "Our mother-to-infant trials were a success because we run good support groups," she said.

Aside from quality medical care, the PHRU has long offered mental health services, counseling for men by male counselors, and milk at half the retail price, to name a few perks that come with participation in research studies. In 2000 the unit embarked on another nevirapine trial, backed by a R4.5 million (US$690,000) grant from Bristol-Myers Squibb's "Secure the Future" project. At the time, a South African government report found that MTCT treatment would save up to 50,000 lives a year, and save the country R270 million ($45 million), but Mbeki was blocking MTCT. The Soweto group forged ahead after securing endorsements "at every single level within the health service nationally," said McIntyre.

Again, the community provided them with a moral compass. "Now that we have gone to the communities," Gray told me in 2000, "their response is, 'What took you so long?'"

Still, these trials did nothing to endear McIntyre and Gray and their colleagues to administration officials. Instead, they were viewed as enemies by the Mbeki crowd, who began courting the AIDS dissident community. What's interesting is that, prior to this time, Mbeki and his then-Minister of Health, Nkosazana Zuma, had championed a domestically made drug called Virodene, claiming South Africa had found a local weapon against HIV and AIDS. When the regulatory Medicines Control Council tested the drug and branded it useless, Mbeki and Zuma tried to abolish the agency.

As they did with AZT, this camp has attacked the use of nevirapine, which was registered for use there in 1999 and for which there is considerable evidence of safety and efficacy from international clinical trials. In August 2003, the dissidents succeeded in pressuring the MCC – its equivalent to the FDA – to demand that Boehringer Ingleheim, makers of nevirapine, submit new efficacy data within ninety days or face withdrawal of the drug there. The move sparked a fresh furor over the government's opposition to MTCT programs.

In response, McIntyre presented data at the South African AIDS Conference in August 2003 showing that 100,000 South African women had received nevirapine in the past two years, and that "no serious safety issues had been found."[7] Because the use of the drug was not in controlled research settings, it wasn't possible to measure efficacy in this group accurately. In 2002 alone, 14,000 mothers in KwaZulu Natal, 8,000 at his hospital in Soweto, 8,000 in western Gauteng, and 8,000 in Western Cape were given nevirapine. The latest results from an ongoing study of 600 pregnant women showed that a single dose of the drug protected 89 percent of infants from getting HIV.

Vaccine Plans

The escalating incidence of new HIV cases in Gauteng province, especially among women, spurred the duo to begin HIV vaccine work. Together with two other groups, they mapped a proposed consortium that could test HIV vaccines, and looked for ways to make it happen.

In 2000 they joined colleagues to launch the South African AIDS Vaccine Initiative, or SAAVI. Its initial goal was to develop an affordable, effective, preventive vaccine by 2005 that would work against HIV subtype C viruses prevalent there. Under the direction of Dr. Salim Abdool Karim, an esteemed South African scientist, preparatory work began in the rural community of Hlabisa, 300 kilometers north of Durban, the first site chosen for a potential phase III vaccine trial.

Since then, a number of groups including the Soweto team have worked on vaccine preparedness, an umbrella term that covers such things as establishing facilities for HIV testing and elaborate T-cell work, training personnel, setting up an ethics review board and clear procedures for approval of clinical trials, and community involvement in the process.[8]

Building on this effort, the South African Microbicide Research Initiative (SAMRI) was launched in spring 2003. It aims to test safe, effective microbicides that can prevent sexual transmission of HIV. Given the high rate of new infection in girls and women there, this effort is particularly critical.

Outreach to Communities

To get started, the Soweto group obtained a small grant from the International AIDS Vaccine Initiative to flesh out the vaccine trial preparedness plans. That included more detailed planning for cohorts, or study populations, a small expansion of their on-site laboratory, additional training of counselors and nurses, and more community outreach and mobilization.

The group has already done preliminary work to probe community attitudes about HIV, relying on Florence Ngobeni, the unit's seasoned community coordinator, to lead the effort in 2000. A poised, outspoken, HIV-positive woman, Ngobeni provided a role model, sounding board and advocate for many women who were afraid to reveal their HIV status. Incorporating vaccines into their community work has meant tackling a new set of issues, from educating people on HIV vaccines and probing the informed consent issues they raise, to making decisions on treatment and care in the context of vaccine trials. And if there's one thing Ngobeni said she'd learned as an outreach worker, it was never to assume she knew what communities would say or feel when it came to HIV.

In June 2003, the MCC approved the Soweto group's participation in the country's first vaccine trial (HVTN 040), after it was approved by the US Food and Drug Administration. The Chris Hani Baragwanath hospital is a member of the HIV Vaccine Trials Network, or HVTN, a global clinical trials network established by the US National Institutes of Allergy and Infectious Diseases (NIAID) to study potential candidate vaccines. Four South African groups collaborated in preparing for the HVTN 040 trial: the University of Cape Town, the National Institutes of Communicable Diseases, the Medical Research Council in Durban, and SAAVI. It will also be tested at the MRC and four US sites. The vaccine will be given to forty-eight HIV-negative participants at each site.

The trial will evaluate a candidate vaccine called AlphaVax 101, made from a weakened strain of Venezuelan equine encephalitis and derived from the subtype C HIV viral strains common to Southern Africa. The vaccine has generated considerable interest among vaccine researchers because it targets both arms of the immune system – cell mediated immunity and antibodies – and appears to elicit broad-based immune defenses to HIV. In August, the MCC approved a second trial of a vaccine called HIVA.MVA, which uses a modified version of the vaccinia Ankara, the basis of the small-pox vaccine, and derived from subtype A HIV strains found in East Africa. This vaccine is also being studied in Uganda, Kenya and England. The trial is sponsored by IAVI and will enroll 111 volunteers in South Africa and Europe. Another vaccine is also preparing for clinical trials in South Africa, pending regulatory approval.

In 2003, the European Union launched a new program to foster partnerships among groups preparing large-scale clinical trials that could also boost the capacity of African sites to conduct vaccine studies.

Women and Vaccines

Among the many questions that vaccine researchers hope to answer in the future is how well they can protect women compared with men. In the US there is a growing body of evidence that shows HIV affects women and men differently. For example, women initially have HIV viral load levels up to 50 percent lower than men, though both progress to AIDS at the same rate. The question is important for vaccine developers, since viral load levels are a crucial measuring stick used to evaluate the efficacy of candidate vaccines that don't block infection, but block progression of HIV disease.

On the immunology front, there are observed, but poorly understood, gender differences that could also influence responses to HIV and to vaccines. Recent studies done with a herpes vaccine (HSV-2), for example, showed signs of efficacy in women, but not at all in men. These issues may be particularly important to South Africa, since studies from Carletonville and elsewhere that show genital herpes is a major co-factor in HIV infection among miners and sex workers. Researchers are also interested in understanding why some women with undetectable viral load levels transmit HIV to their partners, while others don't. Similar observations have been made in men. They point to our need to understand factors that affect not just immune control of HIV, but what constitutes *infectivity* – how infectious a person may be – and sexual vulnerability to HIV – why and when some people acquire HIV. All of this information could help us understand how a vaccine that lowers viral load could also affect transmission.

The New Frontier: Microbicides

Compared with research into vaccines, clinical research into microbicides – gels, creams and other barriers to sexual transmission of HIV – is in its infancy, but a number of promising products are being tested in phase I, II and now III trials. Early studies conducted by the RHRU unit, among others, helped prove that nonoxynol-9 does not fully protect against HIV transmission – an important finding.

Interestingly, the South African government has fully supported microbicide research – so far. The government's Health Minister, Manto

Tshabalala-Msimang, pilloried by TAC for her open opposition to HIV treatment and AZT for MTCT, was on hand for the launch of the new national effort to prevent sexual transmission of HIV. "The development and marketing of an effective microbicide could have a greater impact on the well-being of our country's women, and consequently on the children they bear," she said in a press statement.[9]

Under SAMRI's umbrella, South Africans are investigating the efficacy of microbicides with condoms, and with devices like diaphragms used to prevent pregnancy. Carraguard is a seaweed derivative that appears to block HIV, according to a study sponsored by the Population Council; it is also being tested in a phase III trial in several South African sites that will involve up to 6,000 HIV-negative, non-pregnant women; it is being studied in Thailand as well. The Soweto unit is testing a product called ACIDFORM when used with a diaphragm, and comparing its effectiveness with the anti-spermicidal lubricant KY Jelly when used with a diaphragm. In Durban and Hlabisa, groups are testing BufferGel and PRO 2000/5, other leading microbicide candidates.[10] In these sites, vaccine and microbicide trials are taking place simultaneously.

Back in Soweto, the community is pushing ahead on all fronts. "We've come a long way in terms of what is good science and what is good ethics," said Gray in 2003.[11] "Our patients are sophisticated enough to understand the research process, and our researchers are good enough to conduct good science."

11

CARLETONVILLE:
RESEARCH IN THE EYE OF THE STORM

In the mining community of Carletonville, an hour from Johannesburg, HIV rates were the highest in the country in 2000. Small-scale education and prevention programs there, aimed at miners and sex workers, have revealed the challenges and possibilities of reaching and caring for these highly affected, transient groups. The mining industry is leading the global private-sector response to AIDS by initiating HIV workplace treatment and prevention programs. Due to the devastating impact of AIDS on this sector, treatment has become a matter of necessity to prevent the realization of a recent forecast of death for the mining industry in southern Africa if AIDS is not stopped. These companies have an important role to play in helping governments respond to the threat. But the take-up of nascent corporate treatment programs has been slow, due to stigma and workers' fears of being fired.

Carletonville is among the first sites for AngloGold's new treatment program. Every day, some 70,000 migrant miners work grueling shifts in the largest gold-mining complex in the world. Many emerge after sunrise from the bowels of the mineshaft and spill into the cramped quarters of ten single-sex male hostels nearby, where up to fifteen miners share a room. Before sleep, they often wander over to makeshift foodstalls or to the shebeens *— informal shacks where home-brewed beer is sold along with sex by commercial prostitutes. It is in these "hot-spots," as they are known, that the HIV epidemic took off in the early 1990s, fueled by the intertwined factors of poverty, alcohol, violence, and the miners' fatalistic attitude about their own survival.*

"The miners say, quite correctly, that in 10 years the rocks or dust will kill us, so why should we worry about HIV?" explained Brian Williams, a South African epidemiologist working in Carletonville in 2000. "Their attitude is, in the meantime we might as well have a good time." That was before treatment became available. Now the race is on to see how successfully highly affected commmunties can take on the challenge of surviving AIDS.

The Economic Picture

South Africa's gold mining operations have long been the engine of South Africa's economy. The country is the largest producer of gold in the world. Johannesburg, for example, was built up from diggers' camps that sprung up in the region after gold was first discovered in 1886. The industry has long relied on contract labor to fill its workforce, and a key feature of this work is the transient and migratory nature of miners' lives.

In Carletonville and Soweto, the industry built rows of barracks of single-sex hostels for miners who lived in harsh, crowded conditions far from home. In the 1980s and 1990s, there were political protests to demand better housing and conditions for miners. Not suprisingly, sex workers tend to gravitate to the mines and their concentrated populations of single men. There are twelve mines in the Carletonville district, a 25-kilometer-square area that includes the historically white town of Carletonville (population 20,000), the largely black township of Khutsong (population 150,000) and smaller residential areas where migrant squatter settlements have also emerged as HIV trouble-spots.

Williams began working there in the mid 1990s, when he was hired to study overall health conditions among miners. What he found was a sky-rocketing HIV epidemic that flourished in a setting of poverty, danger and sex, along with rampant, untreated STDs. HIV prevalence was at 4 to 5 percent then. By 1998, 22 percent of the mineworkers he sampled had HIV, while an astonishing 50 percent of the 24-year-old local women tested positive. For local males, the peak came later, but the outcome was similar: 8 percent were positive by age twenty, and by age thirty-two that figure had climbed to 45 percent.[1]

Among Carletonville's commercial sex workers, some 70 percent were infected in 2000 and that number has climbed. Combine this with the fact that 90 percent of the miners are migrants – some from the neighboring countries of Lesotho, Mozambique and Botswana – and it becomes clear why and how HIV spreads so fast from such mining towns.

The Cost of Neglect

South Africa's mines are considered among the most dangerous in the world in terms of job safety. For many of the estimated 500,000 miners who are black, and who were long denied jobs in other sectors under apartheid, digging for gold and other metals offers a means of economic survival, but at a high cost in terms of health and quality of life. Many suffer from tuberculosis and other pulmonary diseases related to occupational exposure to gold dust and other irritants. AIDS makes these illnesses worse. In April, Anglo estimated that 80 percent of its employees with TB were HIV-positive.[2] Deaths in this group have tripled in the last four years. Recent reports show that AIDS-related deaths were also double those of work-related injuries.

A South African agency estimated in 1997 the average annual AIDS-related cost per patient to be R45,000 ($6,429), but that shot up to R70,000 ($10,000) in unmanaged patients. These costs take many forms, including employee absenteeism, sick days, hospital costs, days lost attending funerals of loved ones or caring for a relative – all of which results in lower productivity and, the bottom line for all businesses, diminished profits. A recent study commissioned by the South African subsidiary of British Petroleum, for example, found that workers with AIDS had taken on average 27.5 more sick days than other workers. Each death from AIDS equaled four days of a managers' time, and resulted in twenty employees losing five days of productive time. For each worker that died, the cost of recruiting a new worker was 15 percent of an annual salary. Many of the dead are managers. In Zambia, for instance, over two-thirds of deaths among managers are due to AIDS. That has made it harder for companies to replace their ailing workforce.

In 2000, the Debswana Diamond Company tallied the cost of AIDS care to be 10.7 percent of its payroll. By the early 1990s, life insurance payouts had increased sevenfold in Zimbabwe, where 60 percent of death claims from employees were from AIDS. There, 1 million people died of AIDS between 1984 and 1990. Such figures do not factor in the impact of sickness or death on the workers' families and dependents, since many workers are the primary breadwinners for extended families. Nor do they reflect the negative impact of AIDS on local buying power or the consumer market for company products.

Cost-Effective Treatment

As one of South Africa's biggest companies, AngloGold employs 44,000 people there, including contractors and their employees.[3] Over a quarter are estimated to be HIV-positive. Until recently, the company offered employees a comprehensive range of education prevention and care services for HIV, but shied away from paying for antiretroviral drugs, despite mounting pressure by unions and workers.

As the rate of workers' funerals mounted, the company undertook a feasibility study of the impact of HIV on its operations, and considered how to introduce a treatment program. It found that providing HIV drugs to its workers with AIDS would add $4 to $6 to the cost of producing an ounce of gold. But if no action was taken, the cost could rise to $9 per ounce. AIDS treatment was a critical business matter: the workforce is sick or dying, and workers cannot be trained fast enough to replace them. The cost of doing nothing had become too high.

On April 8, 2002, AngloGold offered antiretroviral therapy to 200 Carletonville miners at a company cost of $1,500 per employee per year. Three thousand workers needed treatment immediately, based on their health status. In July, it took the next step, signing a comprehensive agreement to provide HIV care for workers with five unions at a special ceremony at the company's West Wits operations near Carletonville.[4] Based on models from two actuarial companies, the HIV/AIDS program budget may be 8 percent to 17 percent of the company's payroll. Broken down and spread across all employees, the HIV program cost $17 per employee in 2002, for a total of $743,000. When community programs were added, that figure jumped to $971,000. Such figures pale next to the projected death of the South Africa's mining industry if AIDS continues unchecked.

"We believe, given the stage of the epidemic in this country, which is at a very advanced stage, treatment is the only short-term intervention," said Dr. Brian Brink, Anglo's chief medical officer at Anglo American LLC, its parent company, which has 124,000 employees.[5] "From AngloGold's perspective, HIV/AIDS is something that has to be managed – and it can be managed," the company's public affairs manager, Alan Fine, told reporters.

AngloGold has set clear, measurable goals for its HIV program. It hopes to have 820 workers on treatment by the end of 2003, train enough peer educators to achieve a 1:100 ratio of educators to workers, distribute two condoms per worker a month at each site, and offer voluntary counseling and testing to 4,000 workers – about 9 percent of its workforce.[6]

Most recently, GlaxoSmithKline was providing discounted drugs for the program at two-thirds the market price – $104 (R840) per person per month for a three-drug regimen. As locally produced generics arrive on the scene, the cost of treatment could fall even further, making treatment even more cost-effective. But there will also be a growing demand for voluntary counseling and testing services, based on figures showing a surge in testing when the company began its pilot treatment program.

A Focus on STDs

AngloGold clinics also offer treatment for sexually transmitted diseases, and these serve as entry points for the HIV program. In early 2003, over 2,000 employees and their partners were referred and treated at the clinics. Working with local NGOs in private–public partnership, they also provide home-based care for workers who retire due to illness, and supportive services for miners returning home.

Again, services vary, and stigma remains a serious barrier. It's one thing for a company to offer services, another for workers to access them. Several years ago, South Africa initiated a campaign called "Love Life," aimed at encouraging HIV-positive individuals to come out and provide role models for others. A woman named Gugu Dlamini was stoned to death by members of her community after declaring her status on public television on World AIDS Day.[7] That killing symbolized the fear and violence that have long surrounded HIV and AIDS, and made it difficult for people to come forward for testing and services.

"I have been humbled by the degree to which people are afraid to reveal themselves even to people who love them," said Eric Goosby, MD, executive director of the Pangaea Global AIDS Foundation of San Francisco, who worked with the Clinton Foundation's team to help South African health officials draft the new national treatment plan.

> You have a situation where people are getting physically attacked and beaten by people they have known their whole lives. It's a level of disincentive to revealing your status that is much higher than in other places. I honestly believe the stigma will only be addressed after a critical percentage of people known to the community are demonstrating the benefits of antiretroviral care – that's when it will diminish.[8]

A critical challenge now facing AngloGold is how to work closely with local communities to help counter the stigma and fear of discrimination that face workers with AIDS and their families, both on the job and at home. That's harder to do when you won't invest money to pay for treatment of families, too. At this writing, AngloGold's HIV program does not cover spouses or staff who retire. That has been protested against by workers, who contend that the company has a responsibility to their families. Letting husbands live and wives and children die is bad policy, they charge. It's an evolving dialogue, since family members will now be covered by the government's free national plan. Of course, it may take years for the government's plan to reach all communities.

The company does back the community-based Mothusimpilo HIV/AIDS Outreach Project ("Working Together for Health" in Zulu) HIV/AIDS program in Carletonville.[9] In 2002, the project provided peer education, condoms and treatment to 4,000 commercial prostitutes in Carletonville. Their program also strongly emphasizes screening and control of STDs.

Training Peer Educators

The Carletonville AIDS program was started in 1997, after local AIDS activists began pushing for a local response to the crisis. In a 1995 meeting, Williams met with mining and union officials, miners, community leaders, and professional colleagues, such as Catherine Campbell of the London School of Economics and Liz Floyd, director of the AIDS program in the greater province of Gauteng. The Mothusimpilo project was launched in August 1997 to develop a sustainable, community-based intervention to evaluate the impact of STDs and HIV in Carletonville.

With US$1 million in grant money from USAID and the British Department for International Development (DFID), they reached out to others with a stake in the local community, such as national and provincial health departments, mine management, research organizations and local NGOs, a strategy meant to ensure community "ownership" of the project. Their immediate goal was to provide syndromic management of STDs while working closely with traditional healers. They also wanted to recruit miners and "hot-spot" sex workers into a sustainable HIV peer education and condom distribution project.

The first phase of their work involved assessing community needs and identifying potential outreach workers. Next came the epidemiological surveys of HIV and STD rates. Once a year, they did anonymous cross-sectional surveys of 1,500 people aged fifteen to thirty, including 1,000 miners and 100 sex workers from the hot-spots. The surveys included screening for HIV and STDs (carried out at the South African Institute for Medical Research in Johannesburg) and administering an extensive questionnaire adapted from one used by UNAIDS for its multicenter studies elsewhere in Africa.

When they began there was little AIDS awareness in the Carletonville community; in its place was fear, stigmatization and denial. "No one was interested in HIV," Williams said bluntly. Nor did anyone know much about community attitudes and behavior around HIV. "So we spent the first two years talking to sex workers, and learning a lot," he explained. What was urgently needed, they found, was HIV support groups, counseling for rape, alcoholism and pregnancy, and job training and housing assistance – areas where local NGOs had a role to play.

With four major ethnic groups in Carletonville, the team also learned how to tailor educational messages in culturally sensitive ways, and to scrutinize how those messages are received. By recruiting and training miners and sex workers, they have developed a committed team of outreach workers. "It's very basic stuff," Williams says of the peer training program. "You give them a two-week course on STDs and physiology, and at that level it's working."

The key to success is their focus on peer-to-peer outreach. The engagement of the community in potential studies also allows them to take charge of the scientific agenda. "The challenge is how do you make science really work in the Third World," said Brian Williams. "The point is to work very closely with the local community and look at good science in the context of real people's lives. Any projects that aren't rooted in an established community or give lip service to community involvement are simply asking for trouble," he added.

Their biggest success has come from the intense focus on STDs. "We've had a fairly dramatic effect because the women realized early on that they were no longer getting STDs," he says – a major incentive for community involvement in the project. Tens of thousands of condoms later, the safe-sex message is spreading and is being carried into high schools by youth peer educators.

Yet success had not been uniform in 2000: while the highest-risk women had developed a very active program of peer education, reported Williams, "peer education among mine workers has been less successful, mainly because the industry is unwilling to allow men time off work to be trained." He was more hopeful about school-based interventions – the project's new frontier, born out of the early, unexpected findings that adolescents, primarily females, have such high rates of infection.

New Prevention Strategies

The clear link between treatable STDs and HIV has also been incorporated into their strategy. In 2000, with the backing of USAID and the Population Council's Horizons Project, the Carletonville team initiated Presumptive Periodic Treatment (PPT) of STDs, using a mobile health unit to treat those at high risk for STD re-infection before they become symptomatic. A similar program at the gold fields of the Free State province showed that PPT of sex workers had led to a substantial decline in STDs among mineworkers.

The PPT program's initial results were already encouraging in 2000. "STD rates are going down dramatically in sex workers," reported Johannes van Dam, deputy director of the Horizons Project, which funds the PPT program.[10] To him, the program's other achievements are the "enormous increase in condom distribution" and the greatly increased awareness of HIV/AIDS in the community at large.

Perhaps the biggest measure of success was the local community's desire to manage the Carletonville project. "It has always been our expectation that the intervention site be taken up by local groups," said van Dam. "That shows they have become self-sufficient." While it took some time for the various players to sort themselves out, they did secure support from local mining companies to fund continuing activities, and local municipal authorities have signed on. Among their 2000 plans were studies to examine the effect of male circumcision on HIV transmission and studies of who young girls are having sex with, and why – an attempt to find out "where the chain of infection is vulnerable to intervention," said van Dam.

The Bigger Picture

The battle taking place in Carletonville is an intensified microcosm of what is beginning to be seen elsewhere – in parts of rural China, Russia, Nigeria; each with mini-epidemics that affect local and national economies. Like Africa, Asia and Eastern Europe also face catastrophic forecasts about their human and economic future due to out-of-control AIDS.

In sub-Saharan Africa, where 30 percent of adults have HIV, per capita growth in the region has dropped by 1.2 percent annually. It's estimated that five countries – Botswana, Mozambique, Namibia, South Africa and Zimbabwe – will lose up to a third of their workforce by 2020. By then, according to the International Labour Organization, the population of the twenty-nine hardest-hit nations in Africa will be 9 percent smaller due to AIDS, and their workforces will be 12 percent smaller. If HIV treatment can be quickly delivered, these numbers will radically change. But maybe not right away, since more people will be expected to access testing as these services are expanded.

AIDS is now the paramount threat to every economic sector in Africa, disproportionately affecting skilled workers in blue- and white-collar jobs, including miners, teachers, farmers and health and security workers. The most affected industries are mining and extraction, followed by agriculture, construction, tourism, transport and security. (In the public sector, HIV rates in the military and police are also very high.)

Take the case of Botswana, where nearly 40 percent of adults are HIV-positive. Life expectancy there has dropped to thirty-seven years. A 2001 survey by the Debswana Diamond Company in Botswana found that 60 percent of employee deaths were due to AIDS, and the majority of workers were thirty to thirty-four years old.[11] Almost 30 percent of workers who agreed to testing were HIV-positive. Rural residents who do agricultural work are also affected. Around the world, 7 million farm workers have died of AIDS since 1985, and another 16 million will die unless they access treatment.[12]

Mobilizing Business

Of course, no one knows the real scope of AIDS in most poor countries, since HIV testing is limited in many countries and, given the prevailing stigma of AIDS, many workers avoid getting tested. Only 1 percent of South African firms had assessed the impact of AIDS on their companies in 2002, according to Andrew Sykes, chief executive of consulting firm NMG-Levy. In Nigeria, a recent survey from the Joint United Nations Programme on HIV/AIDS (UNAIDS) showed similar foot-dragging: AIDS was not cited as a management concern in 230 Nigerian manufacturing firms, although the epidemic is raging there.

"The truth is that businesses have not done 10 percent of what they could be doing," said Richard Holbrooke, ex-ambassador to the United Nations. Holbrooke heads the Global Business Coalition, a non-profit group that is pushing companies to confront the epidemic and backs private–public HIV initiatives.

> Frankly, most of them have had their heads in the sand. Now we see that it's starting to change because it's been proven to be more cost-effective to put good AIDS programs in place. The message is beginning to get through. It's not just treatment; it's a comprehensive package that includes prevention and education. You end up doing the right thing morally because you take care of your workers and you also save your company money. There is that initial investment that can be costly, but in the end, it pays off.

AngloGold's move is part of the growing response of large corporations to AIDS. It also represents the hope that many governments have about the potential contribution of the private sector and businesses to the fight. The automotive giant DaimlerChrysler estimated that averting one new HIV infection among its employees saves the equivalent of three to four annual salaries. "It's hard to put a dollar amount on it, and it depends what element of the [AIDS workplace] program you're dealing with," said GBC staff member and South African physician Neeraj Mistry. "Companies have expressed it as a dollar amount per employee per year for all HIV-related activities. But they've also looked at the cost of not doing anything. A lot of models have shown a distinct benefit to actually providing care."

The GBC Role

The entry of corporations into the global AIDS arena has been slow, but is beginning to pick up momentum. Back in 1997, Holbrooke was tapped by his friend Kofi Annan, the UN Secretary-General, to help mobilize the private sector's response to AIDS in Africa. Annan steered him to the nascent GBC, whose initial members were drug companies like Merck, GlaxoSmithKline and Pfizer, and several corporations active in AIDS such as Levi Strauss, MTV, Viacom, MAC Cosmetics and The Body Shop. The latter pioneered corporate AIDS awareness campaigns and programs in their workplaces and via mass-media campaigns aimed at the general public.

Today, the GBC has expanded to become an alliance of 130 international businesses, with over 4 million combined employees in 178 countries. The coalition's central goal remains simple yet ambitious: to act as an umbrella advocacy group, catalyst and hub for businesses worldwide, helping them to develop humane workplace policies and an overall plan of action around AIDS. That includes identifying local resources and potential allies. Many of Africa's biggest employers are GBC members.[13] "Our strategy was first to look at the really big employers: mining, oil, extraction industries," explained Ben Plumley, who was executive director at GBC, on loan from UNAIDS. "Our second priority has been textile industries with large numbers of workers. Essentially you have champions of industry in every sector and you work with them – it's peer-to-peer advocacy." Looking ahead, he added, "I think the oil industry is now poised for a significant response. There is direct leadership by BP. They are addressing it head on, with prevention, testing and treatment, but also by looking at trucker routes and informal settlements and trying to learn some of the lessons of the mining industry."

A Historic Challenge

Given the magnitude of the epidemic, there is no historical precedent for what's being asked of businesses in confronting AIDS. In many ways, the challenges to the private sector are similar to those for the public sector: African countries are hobbled by weak economies and health infrastructures, low literacy rates (especially in rural areas), a lack of AIDS education, and a high death toll among professionals. These all impact on companies doing business in these countries.

Many companies have limited experience in directly providing medical services for their employees. Those with their own medical programs still need to establish or upgrade drug procurement and monitoring systems, as well as train doctors, nurses and technicians in HIV care and diagnosis. Most companies have forged new private–public partnerships with community-based and government agencies to help them. But in high-impact areas, such organizations need help to develop the technical and human capacity to deliver HIV services, including testing, counseling, nutritional and home-care programs.

On the plus side, businesses have unique resources to offer the public sector and affected communities. Large beverage companies like Coca-Cola and Heineken have transport and communications systems, trucks and drivers, warehouses and even clinics. Their trucks can serve as mobile billboards for HIV education, their supply systems and warehouses can procure, store and deliver medicines to area health centers, and their bottlers can provide clean water to communities.

Private–Public Partnerships

With many programs just commencing, no one knows the total number of workers receiving HIV treatment in Africa or Asia. Several companies have garnered praise for pilot treatment programs that rely on the new private–public multisector partnership model. In 2001, DaimlerChrysler paired up with the German Technical Cooperation Agency (GTZ) to offer comprehensive HIV care to some 23,000 workers and their families at three sites in South Africa. GTZ provides the technical program expertise, while

Medscheme, a South African insurer, provides medical services through its "AID for AIDS" (AFA) program.[14]

Heineken has adopted another model, creating its own local infrastructure for treatment with help from outside experts. It teamed up with the Dutch non-profit group PharmAccess, led by AIDS expert Joep Lange, MD, head of the International AIDS Society, in order to set up a drug procurement, delivery and monitoring system for medical treatment. The company flew doctors and nurses from its clinics in Africa and Asia to the Netherlands for HIV training. HIV patients are now treated on-site, and the firm has implemented Directly Observed Therapy, or DOT, to bolster adherence to treatment.

Heineken is the largest employer in Rwanda, where, it has partnered with the Pangaea and Clinton Foundations to help the government there roll out a national AIDS plan.[15]

Other sectors are starting to follow the lead of the mining companies in South Africa. In August 2003, trucking industry leaders announced a plan to work with government officials in order to set up seven clinics and training centers along national routes used by long-distance truckers, another hard-hit population.[16] These centers would provide AIDS education, testing and counseling to truckers. A 2001 study found that 56 percent of long-distance truckers in KwaZulu Natal Midlands were HIV-positive; in one stop in Newcastle, 95 percent of truckers coming in for testing were HIV-positive. The trucking industry's goal is to reduce HIV rates by 20 percent among long-distance truckers by 2004. Here, too, prostitutes who also work along the trucking routes need to be targeted, and would benefit from this type of initiative.

Slow on the Uptake

Not all has been smooth on the road to workplace treatment. Behind the scenes, the cost–benefit debates have often been fractious, and the low ground has been taken in moral debates. Plumley admitted that some workplace prevention plans he's seen are distinctly inadequate.

Coca-Cola, for example, drew the ire of activists around the world for a phased treatment plan that initially offered HIV drugs to 1,600 corporate employees in Africa, but not to 58,000 workers at forty independent Coca-

Cola bottling plants across Africa. The US-based activist group Health GAP launched a media campaign to protest the policy and staged a colorful protest at the International AIDS Conference in Barcelona in July 2002.

In September 2002, Coca-Cola announced a cost-sharing scheme with bottlers to subsidize 90 percent of treatment costs for the bottling plant employees and their families.[17] But months later, Health GAP spokesperson Sharonann Lynch complained that Coca-Cola was moving too slowly. "Nothing's really happened since the announcement," she charged. "No workers have gotten treatment." On March 31, Coca-Cola released a statement saying that its HIV treatment program had enrolled all forty bottlers. But the company did not provide any hard figures on workers who had actually started therapy.[18]

A different problem surfaced for the South African mining companies: government opposition by the Mbeki administration. Under pressure, DeBeers initially put its HIV treatment feasibility project on hold, angering workers, unions and activists. In fall 2002, it finally rolled out an AIDS care plan that provides 90 percent coverage of HIV drugs for its 90,000 workers.

Slow Roll-Outs

With so many players, funds and programs materializing, how many workers have accessed treatment? Not many so far. It's proved difficult to change human behavior overnight.

Botswana provides a good example. An estimated 38 percent of the 1.7 million adults there are HIV positive, and the army has been heavily affected as well. Less than 5 percent of the Botswanans had been tested as of 2002. A year earlier, a national treatment program called Masa, or "Dawn," began with $50 million each from the Bill and Melinda Gates Foundation and Merck & Co. It involves the mining company Debswana, among others. But few workers were taking advantage of the program.

"We assumed once we started giving out the drugs, people would flock to get tests," said Benedict Moyo, one of Masa's program managers, in late 2002. "No way. Everyone still thinks: 'AIDS isn't me. It's the other guy.'"[19]

Again, the problem is stigma, said Ernest Darkoh, MD, a physician who manages the Botswana program and is a former management consultant for

McKinsey & Co. "We're making astounding progress, and it's astoundingly inadequate," he added. "We've got all the guns blazing, machine guns, shotguns. But we're overwhelmed. The reality is just staggering." He conceded that people are waiting until they are very sick to get treatment, if they come forward at all. "Donors may help deliver drugs and resources to Botswana, but fears and beliefs about AIDS will take longer to change," he said.

In December 2002 the virus was spreading at a rate of five new infections per hour, with 75 deaths a day. In June 2003, Botswana's government released figures showing that only 9,000 people had been tested at six health clinics, where the government plans to provide free treatment to 110,000 people. The program will be rolled out to seven sites by the end of the year. While this represents one of the most rapid roll-outs in a developing country, it can't keep pace with the runaway epidemic.

"Finance is but one of a series of bottlenecks that developing countries will face when it comes to implementing effective national health programs, be they HIV/AIDS related or not," stated Darkoh in a mid-2003 update. "Capacity is largely the sum of past commitments and no amount of money can instantly rectify a heritage of underdevelopment. The reality is that HIV/AIDS simply exacerbates the pre-existing structural and systematic deficits, while creating new ones as incidence continues to increase."

"The concern at the moment is that employees are not taking advantage of the services," agreed Plumley, who had visited Botswana and seen the problems up close. "Take-up of these services is very, very slow. Time and again, it's, 'If I come forward, I'll be sacked.'" Stigma is also the reason why many employees said they would prefer to see their own physicians and be referred to off-site clinics.

"The most important thing is for companies to make it absolutely clear that people who come forward for testing and accessing services for HIV aren't going to be discriminated against," added Plumley.

New "Co-investments"

In May 2003, as the WHO was revising its 3×5 global treatment plan, the GBC and its partners in the International AIDS Treatment Coaliton organized a meeting of technical experts and policy makers to identify practical mechanisms to help scale up both workplace and national treatment programs. Ten "first-wave" countries were identified as sites for immediate action.[20] In December, the GBC announced a new "co-investment" initiative, involving nine major companies who will help expand pilot HIV/AIDS programs in several countries.[21] It aims to reduce the public costs of initiating national treatment programs and provide management capacity and business training to public agencies and to NGOs doing HIV outreach to affected communities. In South Africa, Anglo American and Eskom will pool their resources over areas where both companies have mines and power plants.

The Mothusimpilo prevention project offers an example of what can happen when there is commitment and financial investment in grassroots programs that train HIV-positive individuals to lead the local effort. In it, peer-based outreach and support groups are helping to break down stigma. The Carletonville experience shows that the ideas and strategies for stopping AIDS can and must come from within local communities if they are to succeed and become self-sustaining projects. Corporate co-investment or private–public partnerships may offer new avenues for money and resources for the public sector, but these resources need to be directed at HIV-positive groups at the grassroots level. It's the old political saying: think globally, act locally. It's time for that lesson to trickle up to the global level.

With much of the infrastructure in place in Carletonville, the mines also represent a possible site for future vaccine studies. With teenage girls at such extreme risk, "they are one of the groups you want to test a vaccine on," said van Dam in 2000. "By the time they are adults, it will be too late," Williams agreed, suggesting that vaccine advocates begin tackling the thorny ethical issues of testing HIV vaccines in adolescents. That calls for building upon groundwork laid by the Mothusimpilo project to assess community attitudes towards vaccines and clinical research trials.

Promising First Steps

In December 2003, Anglo's Brian Brink provided an update on the company's treatment program. Only 10 percent of workers out of the company's total estimate of 30,000 HIV-positive employees had enrolled in its HIV "wellness" program – still a slow roll-out. A thousand were getting antiretroviral therapy, an encouraging result, Brink stated.[22] "The best indicator of this is that 94 percent of them are at work, and by and large in the mining industry, that is tough (physical) work." About 8 percent who clinically qualified for treatment declined it – some because they worried about side-effects, others because they worried the treatment would not work. So far, treatment adherence rates were very high – 90 percent – while less than 2 percent of patients had serious side-effects. "My overwhelming impression is that this treatment really works," said Brink. "One can only speculate how many would be dead without [it], but my own feeling is about 30 percent."

Back in Carletonville in 2000, every day without progress towards a vaccine seemed like another step towards the dark scenario projected on Williams' computer, in terms of both the current number and the exponential rate of increase in infections. "You're sitting in Carletonville where nearly 70 percent of all 25-year-old girls are HIV-positive and they are going to die in the next five to ten years," Williams said then. "We need something unbelievably drastic if we're going to save even half of them. If you cannot protect them, then everything is lost. It's an almost unimaginable situation."

Today, there's a ray of hope in Carletonville and the rest of South Africa. It lies in low-cost treatment and access to care, but also in HIV prevention, in clinical research, and – most importantly – in the mobilization, training, and peer-based education of miners, long-distance truckers, sex workers at the *shebeens*, and teenagers in school – a grassroots army at the front-line, ready to take up the challenge of survival.

12

RUSSIA'S POST-PERESTROIKA PANDEMIC

Since 1991, when Communism fell in Russia and elsewhere in the eastern bloc, AIDS has become an out-of-control epidemic in many states of the former USSR, alongside other diseases like tuberculosis. HIV has increased at a faster rate there than any other region in the world, and there are fears it will spread to Central and Western Europe.

I visited Russia in the spring of 2003, accompanied by a colleague who reports on HIV vaccines. We were quickly initiated into the nuances and peculiarities of Russian officialdom by several Russian friends who are journalists, and by local AIDS activists. Although the Soviet state is officially dead, the average citizen still encounters Byzantine layers of bureaucracy when it comes to day-to-day life. I quickly came to appreciate what individuals go through to navigate the complex, badly fractured public health system in order to access HIV services. It's not easy for doctors or researchers or program managers either: the government is broke, wages are very low, and there is little support for those hoping to initiate innovative programs.

At the time of my visit Western newspapers were reporting that the epidemic in Russia had exploded, but it remained a hidden, stigmatized disease.[1] I knew AIDS activists and outside health experts were actively pushing the Vladimir Putin government to provide leadership and funds to pay for treatment to those with AIDS, with limited success. Russia's huge size and population make the challenge of delivering AIDS therapy quite daunting. The majority of affected individuals are heroin users, many in prison, where TB is also a huge problem. Sex-trafficking is another link to the epidemic among women in Russia.

I was interested in how frontline doctors were grappling with the task of treating and caring for active drug users with multiple co-infections, who survive on the streets when they aren't in prison. How well were health professionals themselves coping? What tools were available to them? Did hospitals have basic drugs and equipment? How were doctors trying to integrate HIV and TB treatment into harm-reduction and drug-addiction programs? What successful models or strategies were emerging, if any? How difficult is it to treat and monitor such patients? And what about access on a national level? Outside cities, were people with HIV accessing care in the snow-swept villages of Siberia? Was testing even available there?

What I found was a country and government preparing to grandly celebrate the 300th anniversary of the imperial city of St. Petersburg, formerly Leningrad, one of the most beautiful cities in the world. Friends who are AIDS activists were openly critical of the millions being spent by Putin, a native son of St. Petersburg, to spruce it up and sweep out the homeless and addicts in order to welcome important foreign visitors to the party – money that is desperately needed to treat those dying of AIDS in hospitals and on the streets.[2] I saw a country and society still steeped in Soviet culture and attitudes, one where many people are struggling to find work and make ends meet. Russians, I found, are just beginning to open their eyes to the massive, still-hidden AIDS problem; one that many link to exposure to the West and to Russia's recent war in Afghanistan, which opened fresh avenues for the heroin and flesh trades.

I met talented doctors, scientists, public officials and activists with HIV who have succeeded in persuading other world leaders of the severity of Russia's problem, but not yet their own. What I didn't anticipate was the scale and severe impact of alcoholism and drug use on the health of ordinary Russians, and the extent of unemployment and homelessness in young people. I was disturbed to see how many children have been abandoned by their alcoholic and drug-using parents, how young they are when they enter the drug cycle and begin sniffing glue, and, in a short time, have contracted HIV through survival sex. I was surprised at the level of isolation of people with HIV, given Russia's proximity to Western Europe, where AIDS activism is so strong. I also didn't expect to see so clearly the links that exist between Russia's recent political history, its economic policies, and the continuing spread of its brush-fire epidemic.

On a windy afternoon in early May, the neighborhood of Krasnoselski in St. Petersburg looks a bit gloomy and desolate – a portrait in gray. Although it's a relatively warm day by Russian standards, the damp air coming off the nearby Baltic Sea is chilly enough to cut through layers of clothing, preventing city residents from lingering out of doors for long. Just off a highway leading out of the city stand several massive, unadorned low-income residential apartment complexes, towering like sentinels above barren plots of land dotted with garbage – a scene from an urban wasteland. There are few residents to be seen, no children playing outside; just a RV trailer parked along a side road near the apartment complex, with several people huddling outside it, smoking and chatting, before stepping back inside.

The trailer is a mobile clinic that belongs to Humanitarian Action, a new non-profit organization affiliated with the French humanitarian agency, Médecins du Monde (Doctors of the World), an offshoot of the better-known Médecins Sans Frontières. The trailer parks here every afternoon, at one of two mobile needle exchange sites that are viewed as the frontlines in Russia's battle against AIDS. A short time after its arrival, people quietly begin slipping out of the surrounding apartment buildings to make their way over. Inside, space is so cramped that counselors and nurses must move their legs to let clients enter. Most stop at a small window where, after giving only their first names, they hand over used syringes in exchange for fresh ones. Over 230,000 syringes are given out a year by the program, and 98 percent are traded for used ones.

The program is one of forty-three harm reductions programs in the twelve-member Commonwealth of Independent States (CIS) region, backed mostly by money from the US-based Open Society Institute and its Soros Foundation.[3] The AIDS Foundation East-West (AFEW), an international humanitarian organization that grew out of MSF-Holland's projects in the CIS region, sponsors their work.[4] It was established in December 2001, and has initiated a wide range of prevention activities in Russia, Ukraine and Mongolia, and is the lead NGO working on HIV in prisons.[5] Other groups like the Canadian Russia Project and the WHO are active in Russia.

Inside the trailer, new clients step further back for an intake check-up by a nurse or doctor, and for pre- or post-test HIV counseling and blood tests for HIV, tuberculosis and hepatitis. Many clients have all three. They leave with referrals for follow-up tests and care at the city's AIDS program or the specialist AIDS ward at Botkin hospital. Some are referred to TB hospitals for X-rays and treatment, or to STD services at the VD clinics, or, for women, for gynecological and obstetrical care. More and younger clients are getting pregnant, and few have access to prenatal care. While not a full-service medical provider, the program provides a necessary bridge between groups at high risk of contracting HIV and Russia's sprawling public health system.

"We are a syringe exchange point, but we noticed the need for care and treatment is very great in this population," explained Alexander Tsekhanovitch, who heads the mobile program.

> We feel that our program is not a polyclinic or an ambulance-on-wheels; it is a step between real life, or the street, and the health services of the city. We try to organize a way, a route, and we try to connect them with real people. We bring them in touch – patients and doctors. Before we started here, there was no [single] connection between official services and these vulnerable groups.

At the same time, he conceded, "what we are doing is very limited.[6]

Many of the clients live on the street and have an array of needs: food, jobs, housing. At the top of the list is treatment for drug addiction, which many ask about, but which is seriously lacking in Russia. Methadone use is outlawed and there are few rehabilitation programs. Most clients shoot heroin; many are hardcore addicts. Like sex workers, they tend to avoid anything official, including city health-care services, fearing arrest or discrimination – for good reason, noted Tsekhanovitch. "The general attitude toward drug users is very negative. The basic policy has been to lock them up. It is the same with prostitutes. Now you are adding HIV into the mix. I hate to say this, but many people would be just as happy to see them all die."

No Safety in Numbers

Harm reduction projects were just getting off the ground in 1999, a turning point in the epidemic, say health officials. Since that year, their statistics show, it has exploded at a rate they call an E-curve, with annual new infections more than doubling the entire caseload of the previous period. Up to now, the bulk of those affected have been drug users and sex workers, who typically turn to prostitution to support a drug habit. In this huge country of 143 million people, an estimated 2 to 4 million Russians use drugs; in some regions, 60 percent are already HIV positive. The drug problem has increased crime, and many have landed in prison, where HIV testing is mandatory.

Today, 37,000 out of nearly 900,000 prisoners are HIV positive. Many are released with new infections of drug resistant tuberculosis and hepatitis – shadow crises of the AIDS problem.[7] Meanwhile, HIV rates are high in the army.

Over the past year, Russian government warnings have started to match doomsday forecasts by frontline AIDS groups that describe the epidemic in catastrophic terms – a giant waking bear no one can fully grasp, never mind contain. Russia officially claims 230,000 HIV cases and 800 AIDS cases, including 191 children. Six hundred people have died over the years. This spring, Vadim Pokrovsky, MD, the country's top AIDS scientist and head of the federal Center for AIDS Prevention and Treatment in Moscow, put Russia's HIV caseload at 1.5 million, with four to eight hidden cases for every documented one.[8] These numbers are based on some 2 million mandatory HIV tests carried out in the general population annually for a decade. But critics say the official numbers are flawed. Before 1996, only 600 cases were detected.[9]

HIV statistics vary wildly because no one knows how big the most affected group – intravenous drug users – really is. What's most clear is the exponential spread of HIV in this group. According to one 1999 survey, once HIV prevalence reaches 10 percent in networks of Eastern European drug users, it can rise to 40 percent and 50 percent in a few years. Factor in a difference of 1 or 2 million drug users and you understand why the numbers game matters so much.[10]

Compared with elsewhere, the epidemic in the former Soviet bloc has a very young face, reflecting its youthful population. Nationally, 80 percent of Russian HIV cases are in people under thirty, and 20 percent are teenagers. In the Central Asian Republics, half of all cases are in people under twenty. It is also increasingly rural. The epidemic was first concentrated in Moscow and St. Petersburg, but has spread to poorer, remote regions, including vast Siberia. In Orel Oblast, a largely agricultural province in central Russia, there was a forty-fold increase in HIV between 1998 and 2001, the overwhelming majority in young male intravenous drug users. There, local authorities put a fairly effective surveillance system in place, but elsewhere there's less information about how fast HIV has moved. According to Open Society reports, HIV has grown faster in Eastern Europe than anywhere else in the world for the past three years.[11] That's fast enough to have prompted a US political analyst to predict recently that the epidemic in Eurasia, if unchecked, could one day surpass that of sub-Saharan Africa.[12]

An immediate concern is also HIV's spread from regional hotspots like Russia and Ukraine, to Central Europe in one direction and to China in the other. In Ukraine, where the epidemic began with an outbreak in 1995 (as it did in Belarus), 1 percent of the population is already infected. Here, too, drug use is the primary route of transmission. As of mid 2003, intravenous drug users in the European newly independent states of Russia, Moldova, Belarus and Ukraine accounted for 88 percent of HIV cases, and 80.1 percent of cases in the Baltic States (Estonia, Latvia, Lithuania).[13] That's more than nearby Poland, for example, where just over 60 percent of cases are among intravenous drug users. And it contrasts sharply with the picture in Hungary, the Czech Republic and Slovakia, where fewer drug users have HIV, though there are many drug injectors there too. Romania has a serious epidemic that affects children, including many orphans who were infected in the late 1980s and early 1990s through tainted blood.

The countries and regions less touched by HIV are the European states of Bosnia, Herzegovina, Bulgaria and Croatia; and in the CIS region, the Caucasus (Armenia, Azerbaijan, Georgia); and the Central Asian states (Kazakhstan, Kyrgyzstan, Tajikistan, Turkmenistan, Uzbekistan), where less than 0.1 percent of the population is affected in most countries (the rate is 0.2 percent in Armenia). Since HIV testing is limited in these regions, however, it's impossible to say, of course, how accurate these statistics are.

The Impact of "Shock Therapy"

Russians brand AIDS a disease of *perestroika* – rebuilding – the word that came to symbolize not only its embrace of capitalism, but what some wryly call the freedom and sins of the West. The fall of Communism in 1991 opened the door to free-market and radical "shock-therapy" financial reforms that produced profound economic, social and political upheaval in a region with entrenched poverty. In Russia, the privatization of national industries led to the collapse of the already bloated, corrupt public sector, including the health system. There was a massive flight of capital – $130 billion dollars a year since 1993 – much of it into Swiss bank accounts.[14] Unemployment spiraled along with a 2,500 percent inflation rate, alcoholism, mental problems, suicide, homicide and crime in general. An underground economy sprang up, including the multibillion-dollar drug and commercial sex industries.

The impact of this on health-care in Russia was and remains devastating. Under Communism, the USSR had a centralized production and distribution system for medicine. In its place was left a badly fractured public health system where huge hospitals fell into disrepair and medical staff toiled without pay. Before 1991, the Soviet Union's Sanitation and Epidemiology services (SanEp) monitored deviant behavior and favored quarantine and mandatory treatment to control TB and other contagious diseases. It was repressive, but like many punitive health measures, cruelly effective – it kept these infectious illnesses in check.

In her 2000 book, *Betrayal of Trust*, a damning catalog of the recent collapse of the global public health system, *Newsday* journalist Laurie Garrett reports that a number of illnesses became endemic in Russia after *glasnost* and *perestroika*, including TB, syphilis, gonorrhea, hepatitis B and C. Resistance to antibiotics and first-line TB drugs was rampant. In 1996, the number of *narkomans*, or addicts, jumped a hundredfold while prisons became breeding grounds for MDR-TB. From that year on, one in five TB cases was resistant to treatment, according to Paul Farmer, who began working in Russian TB prison colonies then, as well as in Haiti and Peru.[15] By then, Russia was in heavy debt to the World Bank and International Money Fund, and a third of its workforce was jobless. Though Russian experts maintain that the fall of 1999 was HIV's turning point, it's likely the epidemic was surging along, undetected, in high-risk groups, riding on the coat-tails of MDR-TB and hepatitis.

Not everyone went broke either. Some people got very rich, including the feared Russian mafia. A cabal of political officials and private individuals became overnight tycoons in the financial free-for-all that marked the wholesale revamping of Russia's economic and political landscape. They included Anatoly Chubais, a smooth-talking Young Turk who, at forty-two, was First Deputy Prime Minister in 1992, earning the dubious distinction of being the chief architect of Russia's privatization. In 1998, as Russia's economy slid further into chaos, a *New York Times* article said Chubais "may be the most despised man in Russia." But Chubais had plenty of help. He was politically supported by Boris Yeltsin, the ailing, cigar-smoking, pro-Western leader. They were in turn embraced by the Clinton Administration and other supporters of free-market economics.

The activities of Chubais and his fellow "Klondike capitalists" are outlined in a skewering 1998 *Nation* article by Janine R. Wedel, an anthropologist who described how Chubais and cronies formed a close alliance with some of the best and the brightest Western economists at Harvard.[16] The latter included economist Jeffrey Sachs.[17] The Harvard Institute for International Development (HIID) quickly "acquired virtual carte blanche over the US economic aid program in Russia, with minimal oversight by the government agencies involved," wrote Wedel. Chubais' clan also lured other big money into the fold, including billionaire speculator George Soros, who bought a big stake in Russia's second-largest steel mill, and Sidanko Oil, whose reserves exceed those of Mobil Oil. "During the five years that the Chubais clique presided over Western economic aid and policy in Russia, they did enormous harm," concluded Wedel.

Those who champion free-market economics tend to view the shape-shifting events in Russia differently and place a lot of blame on Soviet leaders for failing to adapt to the challenges of modernization and Westernization. Yet few can argue with the present weakened state of Russia's economy and public institutions. Or its exploding AIDS crisis.

It's important to see the links that exist between economic policies, disease and weakened public health systems, as Farmer and Garrett so eloquently illustrate in their books. In Russia's case, radical privatization helped set the stage for AIDS, TB and other epidemics, including drug addiction. Such policies fostered poverty, which led to disease and increased Russia's dependence on foreign aid, thus its foreign debt. Focusing on these links provides insight into how these problems can also be solved.

It's equally important to note the ironies in the Russian story, which are multiple. For example, Harvard's golden boy Jeffery Sachs, accused by Wedel of wrecking Russia's economy, is now the darling of global AIDS activists and their allies in the anti-globalization camp. Speaking at the podium of the World AIDS Conference in Durban in 2000, Sachs delivered an impassioned plea to help Africa, urging world leaders and donors to create a "war chest" to pay for AIDS treatment for the developing world – a speech that earned him a sustained standing ovation. Sachs has also allied himself with fellow Harvard pioneers like Paul Farmer – an unrepentant, vocal critic of privatization and structural reform. The duo helped draft a collective Harvard "White Paper" of sorts that backed AIDS treatment and helped convince skeptical global policy makers and donors to untie the AIDS purse strings.[18]

It's yet another irony that ex-president Clinton, through the William Jefferson Clinton Foundation, has recast himself as an AIDS diplomat-at-large, and is playing a big role in helping to scale up and finance AIDS treatment programs in developing countries.[19] Turning back to Russia, it's ironic that George Soros has almost single-handedly funded the fight against AIDS there and pushed through radical programs like needle exchange. (For his part, Soros continues to champion free-market solutions for economically crippled nations, but has joined the anti-globalization debate. He doesn't want to dismantle the World Bank or IMF or World Trade Organization, however, but strengthen them, along with global health bodies like the WHO.)[20]

In Moscow, as elsewhere, money reigns supreme. In 1991 Soros and Sachs and their money bought radical privatization for Russia. A decade later, they're using their talents and contacts to address the economic and social problems linked to their earlier deeds.

An Unchecked Epidemic

In early 2003 the thing everyone most feared in Russia began to happen: the epidemic went mainstream. There were 500 to 800 new cases registered a week, and a growing percentage were linked to heterosexual transmission, not drug use or homosexual contact. Federal statistics capture the trend: in 2001, the ratio of male to female cases was 10:1; by May, it was officially 4:1. But at the mobile trailer site, the ratio is now 1:1, among new cases. The average age of girls exposed to HIV has also dropped over the past two years, being 2.5 years younger than boys. "This is a very dramatic situation because after that, the females are involved in sex work for drugs," said Dr. Vladimir Musatov, a clinical coordinator for the project, in May 2002.[21] He also heads the infectious disease ward at Botkin Hospital, the city's main AIDS hospital.

What this means is that a generation of teenage girls in Russia is getting hooked on smack early, then getting into sex work, contracting HIV and hepatitis, and having children, with ever-greater frequency. Throughout the region, a growing number of infants born to HIV-positive women who are active drug users have been abandoned, creating a crisis in relation to HIV-positive orphans. For now, these orphans live in hospitals, because no orphanages in Russia will accept them.

The Plight of Orphans

In St. Petersburg, HIV-positive infants who are orphaned are housed in two wards of Children's Hospital No. 3, a large, dilapidated institution that was being remodeled when I visited.[22] There are two adjoining pediatric wards for the infants, all under age two. Two nurses and a doctor were assigned to care for over two-dozen infants in each ward. The doctor earned $100 a month; the nurses complained that they hadn't been paid their paltry wages in weeks. There was no money to hire enough staff to simply hold the infants, which was the greatest staff need. The hospital relied on two volunteers from the community who came regularly. The ward had shortages of all kinds; before I left, the doctor handed me a list that included items like disposable Pampers. Just having those would free up the nurses to care for the infants, rather than washing soiled cotton diapers. In one ward, a veteran nurse in her seventies was mopping the floor of the ward, as there were no janitors on duty. She had worked at the hospital for 40 years.

The nurses on duty testified that women who abandoned their children after giving birth were usually active drug users; they rarely returned to inquire about the fate of the children. A number of children I saw suffered from fetal alcohol syndrome, or withdrawal from heroin or cocaine. They were lying in small iron cots, three, six or nine in a room, the cots crammed together, with little to distract them. There were few toys and few visitors aside from hospital staff. The ward nurses were skilled, compassionate, and devoted, but they could not cope with the needs of so many small infants. Some nurses had adopted babies from the ward after they turned out to be

HIV-negative. While HIV-positive infants remain in the hospital ward, those who eventually prove HIV-negative are placed in orphanages.

According to Galina Tyuleneva, the head of Children's Hospital No. 3, there is no money for PCR viral load tests that would indicate whether a newborn who tested HIV-positive at birth was actually exposed to the virus, or was merely carrying passive maternal antibodies that would be shed within 18 months. The only available tests were HIV antibody tests. The state's policy was to keep infants in the hospital ward until they tested negative; many did so after eight months to a year, and were then transferred to orphanages. A nurse on duty stated that the majority of the children turned out to be HIV-negative, but after months in the ward they suffered from a lack of physical and emotional stimulation, from spending hours lying in bed, from the absence of physical touching and being held. Many showed signs of delayed development common in infants raised in institutions.

Why is Russia keeping these infants in hospitals for months on end? Why not at least house them in a dedicated orphanage with access to medical services as necessary? I asked several health officials this question during my time in Russia. Considering many of these children weren't even HIV-positive, the policy is scientifically misguided. Tyuleneva informed me that the city and state budgets lack money to place the children elsewhere. In the past, some infants were sent to an orphanage for HIV-positive children at the federal Republican Hospital for Infectious Diseases, but they were full. There were no agencies taking such infants. Ordinary Russians were afraid or unwilling to adopt them. Globally, the immigration ban affecting HIV-positive individuals means the babies can't be adopted by potential families outside Russia either. Health officials there are aware of the crisis and hope to provide better care and services in the future for this small but growing population, but all concede the situation is terrible. A British charity, the Princess of Wales Foundation, has helped finance the remodeling of the ward and other improvements.

HIV is also on the increase among street children. At age nine or ten, they start sniffing glue, join gangs, and become exposed to HIV through transactional sex and rape by older children. By fourteen they're shooting drugs and passing on the virus. Outreach workers from Humanitarian Action are beginning to document these patterns of HIV exposure and transmission in this transient population.[23] They paint a scary picture of this still hidden mini-epidemic, where girls, particularly, are being infected at younger and younger ages. "We are talking about a situation that is unimaginable, even to us," admits Tsekhanovitch. "Up to now we have been a little afraid to evaluate the status of things."

A Dearth of Dollars and Rubles

How are Russia's leaders now responding to the crisis? Outside the Health Ministry, critics say AIDS is still not a priority for many political leaders. To date, President Vladimir Putin has yet to make a public speech about the threat, a step some feel would send a powerful wake-up message. Instead, AIDS activists contend that the government prefers counting bodies to curing them. As of summer 2003, Russia had no national AIDS treatment or prevention program. Instead, regional NGOs have led the charge.

According to frontline groups, the outlawing of methadone and drug maintenance programs remains a serious obstacle to HIV control efforts.[24] They add that the federal government has failed to invest a ruble in harm reduction programs, which are mostly foreign-supported. They contrast that to the billions the government has spent maintaining its army and fighting wars in Afghanistan, and now breakaway Chechnya. Moscow has money to treat AIDS, argue activists. But it chooses not to.

Right now, the federal AIDS budget is a paltry $3.7 million dollars. The average antiretroviral cocktail costs $7,000 a year. "If you have 230,000 people, you see that raises a big problem," said Dr. Pokrovsky, who has become outspoken on the need to increase the federal budget.[25] "About $2 million is directed to treatment out of this, and this will be enough only for several hundred. In a year, I expect, there will be many more patients and not a lot more money." He says $65 million is needed on education and prevention alone to confront the epidemic.

Antiretroviral treatment is free in Russia to those who qualify, but is strictly controlled, and provided only through municipal or federal AIDS centers. NGOs are generally allowed to do prevention work. In Moscow and St. Petersburg, a proof of city residency is required to obtain antiretrovirals; without this, one has to pay for treatment. By Dr. Pokrovsky's count in June, around 1,000 were getting a three-drug antiretroviral cocktail from the Moscow AIDS center, out of 20,000 HIV-positive people in Moscow. About fifty were on a waiting list for antiretrovirals. In the CIS states,

10,000 people were on treatment last year, out of 80,000 HIV-ill individuals who needed the drugs.

"In Moscow, it isn't such a problem to get the drugs," said Roman Dudnik of AFEW, "but it is a problem in other places. In the cities where the oil industry is richer and money is available, the AIDS centers are better set up and more treatment and testing is available. But in many regions, you can't do a CD4 or viral load test, so it's hard to know how many really need treatment."[26]

"With respect to antiretrovirals, it's a tragedy and an outrage," said Masha Gessen, an investigative journalist who covers Russian national politics.[27] "It's provided only to a few people and specifically to people who are registered to live in those cities and are not drug users. So that rules out 90 percent of the people who may potentially benefit." She has a friend from another region who recently sought antiretroviral drugs from the Moscow city AIDS clinic but, lacking residency papers, was threatened with deportation instead. Her views are shared by Gennady Roshupkin, probably Russia's best-known HIV-positive activist. "I am afraid that thousands of youth who [got] HIV infection in the last 3 to 5 years will die very soon, in the next years," stated Gennady, "because, for a lot of them, HIV specialists can't do anything."[28]

Since early 2003, the situation has started to improve, due to activist and NGO pressure and behind-the-scenes brokering by AFEW, the Open Society, UNAIDS and the WHO. With their help, Russian health officials began drafting a national plan and a grant proposal to the Global Fund for AIDS, Malaria and TB.[29] There were in fact two plans being submitted at that time – reflecting competing proposals by public health officials, on one hand, and, on the other an elite academic group led by Dr. Pokrovsky's father, who heads the country's medical academy. Russia also recently accepted a $50 million World Bank loan to fight HIV/AIDS, and a $100 million loan to fight TB. It will help, but comes at the cost to taxpayers of further foreign debt. The money will go to mass-media HIV campaigns, among other priorities. A national AIDS advisory council is also being formed that will include HIV-positive groups. In April, a first regional meeting of CIS AIDS activists was held in Minsk, with help from US activists from Gay Men's Health Crisis and other organizations. The subject: access to antiretroviral drugs, treatment preparedness and treatment literacy. All are positive signs of a growing grassroots response.

Unlocking the Doors to Treatment

The cost of drugs remains a huge problem. Though cheaper than in the West, antiretrovirals are far out of reach for most Russians. The state produces two drugs, AZT and a homegrown AZT derivative. As of spring 2003, it had registered twelve brand-name drugs; Trizivir was scheduled to be added to the list. With the pending Global Fund money, Russia could opt for cheaper generics, but activists worry they won't because, said Gessen, "Russia is hoping to become a member of the World Trade Organization, and doesn't want to be seen as taking a position against patents." Off the record, one top health official said that Russia would prefer to negotiate a steep discount on patented drugs from companies with whom they have established relationships.[30] "This is a political question," he admitted. At UNAIDS, Pedro Chequer is pushing Russia to revive its moribund pharmaceutical industry, and, like Brazil, manufacture its own generics.

There are other problems. The current public health system retains vestiges of its heavy-handed pre-*perestroika* bureaucracy. HIV testing is mandatory for prisoners, pregnant women, blood donors, soldiers and those needing surgery, but in practice it is routinely carried out on those seeking care from health clinics, often without their knowledge or consent. On paper, government AIDS programs include voluntary counseling and testing services but, said Gessen, "There is really no such thing as consent, regardless of what the government may say. There is no protection of the rights of people with HIV, who, for the most part, happen to be drug addicts and prostitutes – forget it."

Many citizens have obligatory medical insurance and, in theory, are freely treated at public hospitals and polyclinics that house a variety of specialists under one roof. Infectious diseases like TB are treated in separate clinics, as are STDs. Since HIV-positive drug users may be multiply co-infected with STDs, TB and hepatitis, that spells a lot of red tape to access care. Those released from prison or rehabilitation programs are often lost to follow-up due to an absence of adequate discharge planning programs.

Compared with city hospitals, which are rated as mediocre to terrible by Russians, the AIDS clinic at Botkin hospital in St. Petersburg receives good marks. It is a huge state facility with 1,200 beds which treats 38,000 in-patients a year, and 70,000 on an outpatient basis. Non-residents also receive care from an AIDS program at the federal Republican hospital on the outskirts of town, which specializes in treatment for HIV-positive children.

The AIDS unit at Botkin offers VCT services, clinical care, surgical services, HIV prophylaxis and antiretrovirals to qualifying patients. A special obstetrical unit exists for pregnant women, and AZT and rapid testing are offered to prevent maternal HIV transmission. So are abortion, and prenatal and postnatal care. Under treatment guidelines drafted by Dr. Pokrovsky, antiretroviral treatment is available to anyone with under 300 CD4 cells or a viral load above 60,000, and to those with HIV symptoms. AZT, 3TC and Crixivan comprise the standard first-line therapy.

Around 120 people began three-drug antiretroviral treatment at Botkin in 1999, and so far the results have been very positive. Fifty other people are on their waiting list. Those on treatment include former, but not active, drug users. There have been no deaths in the group, and people with serious AIDS cases have generally recovered. "Our experience is quite positive," said Dr. Musatov. But medicine, tests and materials are limited at the hospital, and patients sometimes pay for services. Although viral load tests are available, there is an emphasis on clinical monitoring and reliance on less costly T-cell tests. Across Russia, only a few AIDS centers offer viral load tests.

That's the positive news. Dr. Musatov acknowledged that, even with drugs, management of co-infected TB/HIV patients is an enormous challenge, and almost impossible in active drug users. Outside Botkin, things are worse. "The conditions in the polyclinic are really of quite a low level of training, equipment – especially laboratory equipment," Dr. Musatov confirmed, especially outside cities. "The really successful treatment of patients, to my mind, is in specialized hospitals."[31]

At the nearby Republican Hospital of Infectious Diseases, which houses the Pediatric HIV/AIDS Clinical Center of Russia, three departments care for children with HIV. Some belong to an initial group of 270 infants who contracted HIV in pediatric hospitals in 1989 through contaminated blood and equipment, an official scandal branded the Elista incident. Half the children are now dead; the other half began getting AZT in 1991, then dual and now triple therapy. Of the 130 survivors, 100 receive treatment. As a group, they constitute Russia's long-term survivors. Some spent much of their lives growing up in hospitals. A number were referred to the center from the pediatric ward of Children's Hospital No. 3, but now there is no more room for new children at the Republican Hospital.

"When we start to treat our children, they are very small, but they grow very quickly," said Yvgeny Voronin, MD, who heads the pediatric unit at Republican hospital. He's regarded as a strong advocate for HIV-positive children. But adherence is a major problem for children and their caregivers, he says. The drugs aren't working as well in some long-term survivors who've had HIV for thirteen years and received mono and dual therapy; some are resistant to most therapies. They have also developed side-effects such as metabolic problems and lipodystrophy.

In 1997, many AIDS centers began providing short-course AZT to pregnant mothers to prevent mother-to-child transmission (MTCT), and rapid testing to mothers during delivery who failed to get prenatal care. But only a few sites have rapid tests, and drugs are missing in many hospitals. In a controversial move, Dr. Pokrovsky says the government now plans to provide universal MTCT drugs to all pregnant intravenous drug users, dispensing with the need for consent or testing.

There are other policies that activists have denounced. In 2003 Russia's Prime Minister, Mikhail Kasyanov, signed an order identifying HIV and TB among diseases considered a national threat, which could be grounds for revoking work and residency permits for foreigners. Health Ministry officials have been grappling with how best to enforce the rules, though they have acknowledged that foreigners are not the major source of HIV's spread in Russia.

Love is the Drug

What does all this activity mean for those with HIV? To AIDS groups, widespread ignorance and stigma surrounding the disease are still paramount obstacles that cause discrimination and isolation of people with HIV. The vulnerability and instability of drug users, sex workers and street children makes these groups especially hard to mobilize. Although groups like MSF in 2001, and now AFEW, have backed mass-media campaigns to fight stigma and discrimination, many people here remain uninformed about HIV. A rash of news stories has helped to educate the public about the impact of the epidemic on Russia and the region, but activists say the disease is still very hidden.

Sergei, twenty-five, is a volunteer coordinator of a mixed support group that meets at Botkin hospital and is open to HIV-positive and negative people.[32] It is one of around ten support groups in the entire country. Sergei was serving his military duty in the north when he tested positive for HIV during routine screening for new recruits. When a doctor asked him if he had ever used drugs, he openly admitted it. He was immediately isolated in a diagnostic ward for twenty-five days, along with five other soldiers. "If you have this diagnosis, people are afraid of you as if you had the plague, or are a leper," he said. His group was fed separately, and only briefly allowed outside the isolation ward to smoke and talk to people. "People would pass by and peep into this window like we were animals in the zoo," he recalled bitterly. At 5 a.m. one day he was awakened, taken to the train station, and sent packing without food or money.

"Like everyone, I was afraid and I was totally isolated," said Sergei. "People are just told they are going to die and there is so much misinformation. For me, being with those other guys who had HIV helped. We supported each other. That's why I believe we have such an important role to play now." He said a close friend who was recently diagnosed with HIV just committed suicide. Another friend was on the verge of killing himself when Sergei met him. "These people feel desperate, like they are the only ones, . . . Nobody is helping them."

In September, the government issued new statistics showing that the military service had been unable to draft 5,000 potential recruits because they had tested HIV-positive.[33] By then, HIV cases linked to sexual transmission had gone from 6 percent to 12 percent, but most HIV cases were still linked to injection drug use. The official tally was 250,000 registered HIV-positive individuals, and a national estimate of 1.5 million probable cases.

"The first wish of every person is to get a magic pill," said Gennady Roshupkin:

> But from my point of view, in Russia now, we have more need for psychological support, for jobs, for AIDS prevention – even before treatment. The doctors and medical professionals concentrate on access to pills. But they have no skills or knowledge about how to work with a person who has to take a pill every day. Support is more important. It can't be forgotten. That's why support groups are so important. All of this is just beginning in Russia. It is the beginning of a movement, but we have so much work to do. As activists, we need to show all these young people how to live and stay healthy; not just survive, but how to carry on with their lives.

PART III

Rethinking Treatment

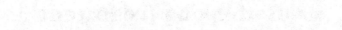

13

AIDS: A NEW MODEL FOR GLOBAL PUBLIC HEALTH

From Port-au-Prince to Fez, from Moscow to Oaxaca, the AIDS picture on the ground is shifting, very quickly in some places, but glacially slowly in others, as I illustrated in my field reports. The early success stories from Brazil and Haiti show that treatment advocates are right: it's possible to manage HIV and concurrent disease in the poorest settings, in spite of limited infrastructure, and these efforts are intrinsically linked to prevention. From a global public health perspective, treating AIDS offers an unprecedented opportunity to build up infrastructure and implement new models of care that will impact on the other global killers in developing countries: TB, malaria, dengue and other tropical diseases. And the lessons learned from fighting these diseases can also be applied to HIV and AIDS. By treating global AIDS, we will bring multiple resources to address poverty and other social and economic conditions that allow HIV to flourish.

As doctors in the field stress, disease and poverty work hand in hand, and we need to address non-medical issues related to poverty and social development if we expect the AIDS battle to succeed. Treatment programs may need to consider whether an affected community has access to a well for potable water, or a generator to keep the refrigerator running to store drugs or vaccines, or a road for a jeep that carries a mobile testing unit and a visiting doctor. In many ways, the task at hand represents battlefield medicine, requiring health workers and communities to do their best with limited or crude tools.

Those in the trenches have another plea: they want help to alleviate the suffering of those who are dying of AIDS without access to palliative care and pain medicines. With 6,000 people a day dying of AIDS in Africa, there is an immediate need to provide hospices and home care workers with pain medicines, which are sorely lacking.

In the pages that follow, I look at a variety of issues related to the medical and scientific challenges of managing HIV in settings of poverty or limited health infrastructure. Even if cost and access were not factors, the task of controlling HIV using the existing arsenal of antiretroviral drugs is very difficult, and raises many issues. For a non-HIV expert, these discussions may involve medical and scientific terms and concepts that are unfamiliar. I've tried to simplify the technical jargon for lay readers and have provided a glossary of commonly used terms at the end of this book. I've also attached several appendices of more technical material and in-depth discussions of treatment-related issues for medical and scientific experts and others interested in the nuances of managing HIV in the field.

Ultimately, these medical and scientific challenges represent the nitty-gritty details of a global endeavor that eludes us: developing a cure for AIDS. I decided to include this more technical chapter on treatment issues because I believe all of us need to be educated about this complex disease, not just the health experts. As global citizens, we are also responsible for providing solutions to this epidemic. To do so requires being able to participate in the global dialogue about treatment and science, as well as the politics and economics of AIDS. This philosophy has long been espoused by people with HIV who have had to learn to become experts in their own disease in order to survive.

2002–03: New Successes

At the 2002 global AIDS conference in Barcelona, early results were presented from a number of pilot treatment projects, including the Partners in Health effort in Cange, the PHRUs work in Soweto, the Cuban government program, MSF programs in Africa and Asia, and the ALCS effort in Morocco. They provided the concrete proof that AIDS patients in poor settings quickly benefit from simplified antiretroviral regimens and doctors who are trained in clinical management of HIV diseases. I've provided detailed updates on the Haiti experience. Its success is growing: patients are adhering very well, the roll-out is increasing. Tuberculosis, including drug-resistant tuberculosis, remains the daily challenge for doctors and patients, particular in those arriving with advanced HIV disease.

In Dakar, the government-funded Senegalese Initiative on Access to Antiretrovirals that began in 1998 also offered quick results. A three-drug regimen given to 470 treatment-naive patients with symptomatic HIV reduced viral load levels to below 200 copies after one month in 85 percent of individuals. Their CD4 T-cell levels climbed to 280 after the three-year cut-off of the study. The most common side-effects were anemia and poly-neuritis. After 39 months of follow-up, 86 percent of patients had taken at least 80 percent of their drugs, and only five had stopped treatment. There were twenty deaths during the follow-up period. This program relied on Dynabeads, the alternative method for measuring T-cells that a number of countries have adopted recently. Other countries reported similar progress in their pilot roll-outs, with few problems.[1]

A year later, the trend is still positive, though problems are cropping up in some programs. As an organization, MSF has garnered the most experience to date through ten pilot treatment projects that are being scaled up; some use WHO-approved generics or those imported from Brazil.[2] At the MSF clinic in Khayelitsha, a poor township in Cape Town, South Africa, the team led by Eric Goemare, MD, reports steady progress. In mid 2002, they had 360 patients on antiretrovirals and a 90 percent rate of adherence. Within six months, the average weight gain of patients was 8.8 kilograms, with undetectable viral load levels. Both adults and children are doing well in their program. MSF actions and success were critical in pushing South Africa's government to back treatment, despite opposition by Thabo Mbeki.

At the same time, the MSF project reported that 45 percent of women reported some side-effects, such as rashes, nausea, and headaches, laboratory abnormalities and elevated liver enzymes in the blood. These fairly minor adverse effects were judged "similar to those seen in other groups and should not be a justification to withhold HAART," concluded MSF.[3]

As of March 2003, MSF had 660 patients on therapy in South Africa, 607 in Malawi, 85 in Mozambique, 540 in South Africa, 615 in Thailand, 18 children in Ukraine (from 617 mother–child pairs), 270 in Kenya, 65 in Honduras, 436 in Guatemala, 260 in Cameroon, and 660 in Cambodia. They plan another nineteen treatment programs around the world. Their experience is a microcosm of what's been seen in myriad pilot projects, not just those I report on in this book, but in larger programs in Ivory Coast, Burundi and Benin, among others.

New Treatment Paradigms

Once money is in place, how well can treatment be implemented? As the chapters on Brazil, Haiti, Morocco and Mexico illustrate, treatment programs can quickly be implemented if communities are consulted and mobilized in advance to help deliver these new programs or services. If they aren't, the benefits may be limited. Bringing communties on-board after the fact is always harder. Doing it beforehand helps identify the barriers and social attitudes of communities that will lead to the success or failure of given approaches. Given the rapid roll-out, there may not be time or resources for advanced training, but the community dialogue can certainly begin, and there are plenty of actors and entry points for this to happen. It's a matter of prioritizing community education and ownership as the key ingredients in helping to counter stigma – the biggest barrier to access.

Unfortunately, there are limits to success when the national model is a centralized, top-down system, one that requires people to be residents or employed to access public health services, as is the case in Mexico and Russia and many other countries. That may rule out drug users or sex workers, or others such as seasonal agricultural workers who fall outside the system, yet represent the majority in need of HIV services. An alternative is the decentralized community model. Cuba's family-based system of care, which integrates HIV into primary care, is useful, even for countries with different political systems. It uses small teams – a doctor, a nurse, a social worker – assigned to care for a fixed number of people in a target community, but is applying a basic lesson: to locate and offer resources within communities, not far away from them.

That's a lesson the Gheskio group in Haiti is applying. By setting up health clinics that concentrate a wide range of services – primary adult and pediatric care, family planning and prenatal care, STD, TB, malaria, HIV testing and care – they make it easier for patients. PIH's *accompagnateurs* model also demonstrates the benefits of delivering home-based follow-up care to adherence. Some centers and programs don't label themselves as

HIV centers, to avoid the stigma of AIDS. All of these are examples of community-based care.

The lesson applies to prevention programs, too: Uganda's women coming in for prenatal or gynecological care get screened for HIV and TB and referred to MTCT programs. By adopting family-focused care, and doing outreach in workplaces to reach men and get them into prenatal clinics, Uganda is addressing the issue of men's decision-making power over the health of women in Ugandan society. This shift toward a family model also provides a way to engage both partners. At the same time, some programs have found that separate support groups for men and women are needed. Both sexes admit they cannot talk freely about sexual matters or their own sexual behavior in mixed groups. At the same time, Uganda's MTCT programs have seen how pre-test group counseling can help counter stigmatization of individuals.

The experience of Botswana is worth highlighting because it is further ahead in its treatment roll-out than many other African countries, but has hit early problems. Despite the massive infusion of outside donor money and strong support from the government, take-up is slow due to stigma. The lesson? More effort was and is needed to prepare workers for the arrival of treatment, to identify community partners, to engage and educate the families of employees. AIDS does not occur in a vacuum, nor does testing or treatment. Bringing in these services requires confronting stigma, not creating new problems for those who need help. Asking individuals what they need to manage HIV sounds like a basic first step, but it's one many programs still neglect to consider in their rush to act.

The Soweto and Carletonville programs show how community mobilization can help identify and address problems before or as they develop. As money reaches countries, there's still an assumption that money and drugs will spell immediate access or allow NGOs and small groups to begin rolling out treatment immediately. That's simply not true in many cases. They need support and financial resources to begin the more critical work of generating a community dialogue and forming partnerships before or as the programs begin.

Given that treatment will be limited and many people will be left out, who's going to decide who gets access? These are life-and-death matters. The answer to this critical ethical problem needs to come from affected communities and individuals with HIV, since they will bear the consequences of these decisions. By investing in communities and giving them resources to take up this challenge, those active in programs can ensure that solutions will come.

What's been missing in the global scale-up effort – what continues to be lacking – is a concrete focus on the steps that need to be taken to help groups at the grassroots level implement treatment, or link with incoming government programs. In the past few months, I reviewed a number of on-paper national scale-up programs. They tend to be strong in the arena of building up public health systems and the logistics of testing, but weak in the area of community mobilization. They refer to the critical role that must be played by local actors in communities, but provide few concrete examples, models or suggestions with the kind of detail they give to, say, a pooled drug-procurement model. And they often fail to consider the other programs that are needed to overcome barriers to access, such as roads to get to a clinic, or support groups for people being tested, or safe housing for women who suffer domestic abuse or have been raped and are now HIV-positive. HIV care and treatment are fundamentally tied to the social and economic conditions of people's lives. Governments and programs need to consider these issues as they relate to accessing HIV care.

The follow-up picture is also unclear. Many programs have already learned that once people get better on treatment, they need jobs, in order to eat and stay healthy. But being HIV-positive means they now face a degree of discrimination. Jobs, food, housing – these are also critical to long-term adherence and good health.

Many NGOs that were focused on HIV prevention are now turning to treatment, and are hoping to access money and drugs from governments or outside donors to set up these programs. But they haven't concretely focused on the logistics of setting up a treatment program beyond getting the drugs. They need to hear about how other groups are doing this, which ideas have worked, and why. They need to hear from activists around the world who can share their experiences about how to get people with HIV onto the planning committees and ethical review boards of new government, NGO and drug company programs and clinical studies. That's where governments and the WHO and large agencies can also be useful, in imparting this information to frontline communities, not just health officials or doctors or large technical agencies.

The Model: Trickle-Up, Not -Down

Botswanan officials have learned another important lesson, one that challenges the current approach to AIDS control favored by most countries. Since so few doctors and health workers exist in Botswana, particularly in rural areas, AIDS experts there have found that they lack enough people to deliver HIV treatment to communities. As a result, Dr. Ernest Darkoh, the Botswanan physician leading his country's treatment program, favors training non-professionals to deliver the drugs. "The magnitude of the problem in the developing world is such that, to the largest extent possible, people must treat themselves," said Darkoh to a global audience at the July 2003 International AIDS Society Conference in Paris. "We need to critically reassess our bricks-and-mortar approach. Antiretrovirals involve a patient taking pills constantly – are buildings really necessary? Don't community and individual-based models make more sense?"

At the Paris meeting, WHO officials suggested that they had learned this lesson. "The time has come for us as experts to stop talking about how complicated HIV treatment is," said Joep Lange, MD, IAS's president. "It doesn't have to be that complicated. And it's become a lot easier with simple regimens like a pill a day. We need to start getting that message out to people."

That kind of approach runs counter to Western experts' approach to HIV disease management, with its reliance on specialists to manage what is viewed as a complex disease. But as Botswana's Darkoh noted, many patients on HIV therapy in the US only visit their physicians every few months, after they've completed the initial period of counseling and testing for HIV and started therapy. As my country reports from Haiti and Brazil show, poor patients there adhere to regimens better than those in developed countries. The ultra-decentralized model also frees up the few doctors and nurses that are available in countries, so they can focus on the patients who most need their services.

Among the pioneers, MSF is proposing a more simplified treatment model that reflects a tiered level of care, starting with community health centers staffed by nurses and lay community workers, where HIV testing and treatment could be initiated using fixed-dose pills [4] These centers could provide basic care, treatment to prevent OIs, management of simple side-effects and adherence support. More difficult cases would be referred to district hospitals, where doctors could handle severe side-effects and OIs such as TB and crytococcal meningitis, and care for pregnant women. There, second-line substitute regimens could be offered, with laboratory tests including liver enzyme and CD4 tests. Even more difficult cases would be seen at referral centers in the capital or provincial facilities, where full hospital services and viral load tests would be offered, along with community resistance monitoring.

Instead of devoting the bulk of new funds to training doctors and nurses in city or district hospitals, or rebuilding hospitals and then expecting a trickle-down of services and care to rural clinics, governments should consider such alternative grassroots models. By immediately shifting needed resources, drugs and supplies to AIDS hospices and home-care providers, for example, governments could reach many critically ill patients who may never get to the district centers. A larger portion of incoming resources and money should be devoted to training hospice workers, and to helping people with AIDS and HIV become experts in their own care, along with family members and patients. These individuals are the human infrastructure needed to extend HIV services to their own communities, as peers – the Carletonville model. Once they begin to recover, they provide visibility to counter stigma and proof that treatment can work, as the Cange experience has shown. It's a trickle-up, not trickle-down model.

Shifting resources means shifting power and shifting our notions of who we regard as the experts. The question is, will governments, donors and Western scientists support that? How willing are health officials and doctors to empower HIV patients and hand over drugs to community lay workers? In India, doctors are treated as gods. The Western concept of patient empowerment and advocacy is not something doctors are that eager to embrace, according to those I interviewed in Mumbai.

"You will find great resistance to the idea of doctors becoming less important," said Dr. Ishwar Gilada, an enterprising physician who has provided AIDS leadership there. "They like to keep the information to themselves, and that is the truth about most of my colleagues." After all, he noted, having the knowledge means having a service to sell; it's about money, too. If patients don't need doctors as much, they won't have to pay for medical services. "I think that would threaten a lot of doctors I know," admitted Gilada. "Honestly, you'll find serious opposition." Empowering patients means regarding them as being capable of taking charge of their own health, or accompanying them – the PIH equity approach.

The point is that different settings call for different models, or could make use of different models. It really means being willing to reconsider what's needed when we think of material and human infrastructure to deliver HIV services and care at the grassroots level. Although there may be limited physical infrastructure for health-care, there may be multiple points of entry to deliver HIV services: churches, mobile child vaccination programs, markets, truck stations, beauty salons – anywhere people and communities regularly congregate. Given the stigma of HIV, they don't have to be billed as HIV services, but they do need to be integrated into people's lives.

As long as there are people, there are community resources. If you ask Darkoh, the real hurdle is often in our minds and fixed attitudes. If decentralized individual, family and NGO-based models were developed, then the army of a few becomes an army of many more. The various projects I profile in this book make that point over and over again.

The WHO's Low-Tech Treatment Guidelines

In 2002 the WHO, after extensive consultation, put forward a public health model for treating AIDS that greatly simplifies existing treatment guidelines and monitoring strategies.[5] Their minimalist model reflects a radical, pragmatic, and economical approach to the task at hand, one in which a near-complete lack of resources is a given for most of Africa – and the bottom line for starting treatment. This low-tech approach offers countries with a limited infrastructure of drugs, doctors, hospitals and laboratories a roadmap for introducing antiretroviral therapy, and lays out steps to build up their capacity as they go forward. In short, it's a stepladder. At the top of the ladder are the kinds of treatment options available in the best centers of Europe and the US. They're out of reach for much of Africa today, but are being put within sight in the future.

The low-tech model advocates simpler, non-protease regimens and syndromic, or symptom-based, clinical management of HIV. It dispenses with the more sophisticated tools like viral load tests, and even T-cell tests, required for starting therapy in the US. The WHO guidelines only require an HIV antibody test to confirm that people have been exposed to the virus.[6]

The alternative guidelines rely on basic blood tests, available in community clinics and in many district hospitals in the poorest countries, to monitor those starting antiretroviral treatment. Experts caution that the new guidelines are meant only as a rough guide to treatment. It will be up to doctors and nurses – and patients on therapy – to put them into practice and see how well they work. There is considerable debate among the experts over many topics in the evolving field of AIDS. One of the strengths of the WHO guidelines is that they point out the potential minefields facing clinicians and patients. They also draw attention to steps that could be taken to fill in gaps in our knowledge of how to treat AIDS in more complex settings.

The guidelines are designed primarily for senior policymakers and treatment advisory boards who are establishing national AIDS treatment programs in developing countries. But they will directly benefit clinicians and other health professionals who now lack training and experience in managing AIDS patients on therapy, as well as affected communities who have a frontline role to play in mobilizing individuals to take up testing and treatment. The main topics covered by the guidelines concern the initiation of antiretroviral therapy: when to start, what drugs to use, when to switch, how to monitor treatment, problems of toxicity and resistance, and specific treatment issues concerning women (including pregnant women), children, drug users and other special groups. These also cover potency, dosing, drug interactions, managing HIV–TB co-infections, and the difficulties of distinguishing symptoms of HIV drug failure from other conditions. (For a fuller discussion of the guidelines and other issues, see Appendix A.)

According to experts, there are several characteristics of an ideal HIV drug regimen that will be used in treatment-naive populations in developing countries, and in individuals with advanced illness.[7] The most important is that it is affordable. Without cheaper drugs, few will access them. They must be effective against HIV and easy to take, causing minimal side-effects. Since many individuals needing treatment now have AIDS, the regimens must be potent in patients with advanced disease, and should work in those with co-infections of tuberculosis, hepatitis, or malaria, and in women who may be pregnant or nursing. They should not interact with other drugs or complementary therapies used to boost the immune system. They should not cause long-term damage to health. They should be stable in tropical conditions or in freezing climates. And treatment should be available even when other resources, such as laboratory tests or diagnostic equipment, are not. Obviously, no HIV drugs fit the bill.

Instead, there are several new 3-in-1 "fixed-dose" pills made by brand-name and generic manufacturers, including Triomune and Trizivir. The two most popular are non-protease regimens that have proved to work well in treatment-naive individuals who are relatively healthy, but not always as well in those with AIDS. For the most severely ill, protease inhibitors provide extra potency, though they are also harder to take, and more expensive – thus out of reach for many. What's needed are more choices of fixed-dose combination (FDC) pills that combine different drugs and easy-to-use tests and equipment, which can monitor several diseases at once and be used by patients themselves, since doctors and technicians are scarce. All of that for pennies, not dollars, and certainly not hundreds of dollars. It may take years, but that is the wave of the future. The WHO is advocating the development of new FDC pills, but it's a political battle. Making such pills requires competing brand-name drug manufacturers to package their drugs together, sharing sales with their rivals. They would rather that consumers continued to use single drugs where they retain control of the profits.

Treatment Literacy

The low-tech guidelines assume that patients, families, and communities will play a critical role in treatment education and emotional support, to help individuals adhere to a taxing lifetime regimen. They reflect an awareness that non-professionals – including lay health workers, traditional birth attendants, family members and HIV-positive individuals themselves – may even be initiating treatment at home or outside clinics, with limited access to doctors or nurses. Ultimately, treatment is something that each individual has to take on and manage alone, every day, for life – albeit with support from others. None of this is easy; and it's a greater challenge in countries where so many people are dying, where so many people are terrified of the disease, where AIDS is highly stigmatized.

The challenge of treatment includes the urgent need to provide broad HIV education about the drugs and related issues such as side effects and drug resistance. But educating people about treatment isn't a simple matter of talking about the disease or even about drugs, but a complex matter of addressing people's attitudes toward health and illness, toward their own bodies. It requires providing that information in such a way that it is culturally sensitive and can be understood.

In much of the world, there is the basic challenge of literacy and poor education. People speak many languages and belong to different ethnic and social communities within one nation. They engage in myriad cultural practices and have different religious and spriritual beliefs. They use alternative medicines and healing practices. In Africa, for example, an estimated 80 percent of people rely on traditional medicines, in both urban and rural settings.[8]

Right now, the urgent focus on getting drugs into bodies has outstripped the ability of the international community to fill the gap of treatment literacy; training is only beginning for doctors and other health-care professionals. The job of accelerating access to treatment education has been left to NGOs and nascent activist groups at the grassroots level. In some ways that makes sense, because AIDS is still a local disease being fought and experienced at the local level. It has to be taken up by communities to work well – as seen in Cange. But right now, these groups and nascent programs are limited, and they lack funds and people to begin the job. Just look at the challenges facing groups like AFEW and Humanitarian Action in Russia.

Even when funding arrives, time is needed to get these programs off the ground. It took the better part of a decade for gay and AIDS activists in the US to move from protests in the streets to establish the myriad AIDS service organizations (ASOs) that now make up what some jokingly call "AIDS Inc." – the institutional infrastructure for fighting AIDS. And they weren't fighting an epidemic in which 10 percent or more of the population was directly affected. These ASOs are now ideally positioned to offer the benefit of their experience to other countries, and some are beginning to do that via "twinning" projects. But it's been slow.

Looking ahead, an important component of treatment preparedness and treatment literacy will be educating patients in developing countries about their rights, including their right to consent to or refuse participation in research and clinical studies. The global community needs to provide resources to help grassroots groups do this work now, not later.

Training

As the Mexico and Russia chapters show, there are few doctors experienced in using HIV drugs, and they lack diagnostic tools such as viral load and CD4 tests. Today, many health and academic groups around the world are responding by sending experts to help train doctors in developing countries. Academic and professional "twinning" programs offer an excellent mechanism for the exchange of skills and information between scientists, clinicians, laboratory technicians and others globally. But in some ways, sharing experiences between health professionals within regions may be more useful. Although Western specialists are quite experienced in treating HIV, and sometimes TB, they rarely cope with chronic malaria, sleeping sickness, or dengue fever. Field physicians in developing countries are the ones who have the expertise there, and are the experts in managing multiply co-infected patients.

Here, the efforts of medical groups like the International Association of Physicians for AIDS Care (IAPAC) are helpful. Working with the WHO, IAPAC has created training and education modules for health workers that are built on the continuing medical education (CME) models used in the US. But it relies on experts from the field, within developing countries – the pioneers of treatment – to train others. These lessons can be broadly applied to other sectors, be they NGOs, community-based programs, or activist campaigns. Instead of turning to the West for expertise, the West can help by turning to local experts and making their experience better known to the world.

Other medical and academic groups have also stepped forward to provide specialist training to health professionals in the field. The International HIV/AIDS Alliance, a leading NGO in the UK also worked with WHO officials to develop a useful new "Antiretroviral Toolkit for Programme Managers" – a "how-to" guide aimed at health officials in poor countries, and at ASOs who are heading treatment scale-up programs. It covers the basics of how to begin scaling up antiretroviral drug delivery and health services for HIV in poor settings.

Looking ahead, groups like IAPAC and other medical providers would do well to partner with local hospices, nursing organizations and frontline community players like W-TAG in Uganda or TAC in South Africa, in order to develop training models and materials that could teach individuals and communities to treat themselves, as Botswana's Darkoh stressed. Most importantly, alliances must be made with traditional healers and those who advocate alternative healing practices.

Hard-Learned Lessons

The WHO's public health approach to treatment reflects sobering lessons learned from a decade of antiretroviral use in industrialized countries, where patients have had to abandon antiretroviral treatment or switch regimens to overcome problems such as severe side-effects and drug resistance. The exact causal link between drugs and their side-effects isn't always clear, and may be an indirect result of therapy. Side-effects can also resemble symptoms related to HIV illness itself. What no one questions is the fact that while antiretroviral drugs are very potent against HIV, they cause a cumulative negative toll on the body. That's why many Western doctors and patients now delay starting patients on therapy, and reserve the use of protease inhibitors until patients require these more powerful but toxic drugs.

US federal treatment guidelines were modified in recent years to reflect that trend: they no longer advocate a "hit early, hit hard" approach to HIV treatment, and urge physicians and HIV-positive individuals to weigh the risks and benefits of therapy carefully with a given regimen. They stress paying close attention to one's initial, or "first-line" regimen, since this will dictate the course of treatment and what "second-line" or substitute (salvage) drugs may be used if a switch is needed. Many studies around the world show that HIV develops resistance after a period of time, a problem that develops more quickly if patients can't tolerate or adhere poorly to their regimens. WHO experts hope the global adoption of standard first-line "fixed-dose" regimens will reduce such problems.

Although the treatment guidelines for poor countries differ sharply from US guidelines, their end goal is the same: control of HIV using a three-drug antiretroviral cocktail that attacks the virus's ability to reproduce at different time points of its life cycle.

For many years HIV experts stressed that each individual is unique, with a distinct treatment and illness history. For that reason, US guidelines advocate an individually tailored approach to therapy that allows physicians to mix and match drugs freely to suit a patient's medical profile. That's a far cry from the WHO's new one-size-fits-all, standardized public health approach for poor countries.

Initially, protease inhibitors formed the backbone of three-drug regimens in the US, but later, alternative first-line non-protease regimens were approved. The US guidelines also recommended using laboratory blood tests to monitor immune T-cell levels (CD4 and CD8 T-cell tests) and viral activity in the blood (viral load tests), along with basic tests of liver function, and of glucose and lipid levels to monitor how the drugs may affect major organs like the heart, liver, pancreas, and kidneys.

In 1999 there were sixteen antiviral drugs and one anti-cancer drug, hydroxyurea, approved to treat HIV. New drugs and drug classes have been added to the list, which means many possible combinations. To boost potency in patients with advanced disease, some doctors have experimented with four- and five-drug regimens for patients. Other immune-boosting drugs, like interleukin-2, are being tried alongside antiretrovirals in clinical trials, as are therapeutic vaccines.

Many people use complementary and alternative medicines to boost immune strength as well, including traditional Chinese medicine, and ayurvedic medicine in India; both rely on roots, herbs and other natural compounds. HIV experts stress that drugs, herbs and natural supplements may interact with antiretrovirals, and this can affect HIV treatment. While more drugs represent more weapons to use against HIV, some Western experts feel it has led to their chaotic use, and the subsequent rise of drug resistance in industrialized countries. That concern is also behind the adoption of the WHO's "less is more" menu of drugs for poor countries.

Palliative Care

While millions wait to access antiretrovirals, there are other drugs that are lacking and could keep millions alive until they arrive. These include drugs for opportunistic infections like cotrimoxezole and fluconazole, which are used to treat HIV illnesses, and painkillers such as oral morphine and aspirin to alleviate suffering in patients dying of AIDS. Hospice workers estimate that a majority of their AIDS patients experience severe pain and need opioids, which are lacking in much of Africa. They advocate implementing the three-step ladder approach to pain management for AIDS that is used for cancer pain relief. It calls for using non-opioids like aspirin and paracetamol, then mild opioids, then stronger ones like morphine, until individuals are free of pain.[9]

Access to morphine is restricted because narcotics are strictly controlled; only physicians can use them in some countries, while in others they are outlawed. In 2002, for example, Tanzania did not permit distribution of oral morphine outside a few experimental sites, according to the Foundation for Hospices in Sub-Saharan Africa (FHSSA), an umbrella advocacy organization that is a leader in the field of AIDS hospice work. Governments fear that relaxing laws around such drugs will lead to narcotics abuse. That's the same reason Russian officials cited for the ban on methadone and buprinorphine to treat heroin users there. Given the scale of the epidemic facing Africans, health officials in a number of countries have now rightly moved forward to ease restrictions around access to oral morphine for dying AIDS patients.

In 1995 the self-funded FHSSA began focusing on the lack of drugs used to treat HIV-related illnesses, as well as of palliative care services and hospices in the region.[10] It's played a key role in pushing sub-Saharan governments to integrate palliative care programs and training for communities into new national treatment programs. As of September 2003, there were around 100 hospice programs in sub-Saharan Africa, with at least one formal hospice program in each of South Africa, Zimbabwe, Uganda, Botswana, Swaziland, Zambia, Malawi, Tanzania and Kenya.

Given the staggering number of people dying of AIDS now, many are dying alone, or perhaps with little help and no pain medicine at all. With few doctors or nurses, hospice groups in Africa are training community caregivers and volunteers to provide palliative care at home, under the supervision of nurses. They are also providing a range of services such as food distribution, income-generating projects, services for AIDS orphans such as bereavement and after-care planning, and collaboration with DOTS tuberculosis programs.

In August 2002 Peter Sarver, editor of the FHSSA hospice newsletter, summed up the situation facing the majority of those being targeted by the WHO's plan:

It does not appear that [antiretroviral therapy] will be able to address the widespread need for care any better than the jump to the use of cell phones in Africa can make up for the widespread lack of access to this new communications infrastructure . . . When it comes to AIDS, we must work against the denial and ignorance about the reality of the massive unnecessary suffering.

Quoting a fellow advocate, Jan Stjernsward, he added, "Before prevention takes effect and affordable curative therapies become available, the only realistic and humane thing to do is offer pain and symptom control."[11]

Advocates of palliative care are desperately hoping that the push to treat will accelerate their ability to provide enough care to keep millions from dying.

The Next Battle: Cheap Monitoring Tools

As AIDS drug prices began to drop in 2001, attention turned to the equally urgent need for low-cost diagnostic tools. Most tests considered routine for HIV management are out of reach for poor countries, and often cost more than the drugs themselves. They include T-cell and viral load tests.

In 2001, the cheapest viral load tests being marketed to African countries cost an average of $100, excluding equipment and laboratory facilities. Two years later, Roche had dropped the price of its popular viral load test to $19 for resource-poor countries. But that's still far too expensive for millions of people in poor countries, where the per capita health budget is typically under $5 dollars a year. The same is true of T-cell tests, which are run through flow cytometer machines that rely on immunofluorescent markers and other staining techniques to tag and distinguish CD4 and CD8 T-cells in a blood sample. More sophisticated tests, performed primarily in research laboratories, measure subsets of these two T-cell families to indicate where there may be a specific loss of immune T-cell function due to HIV.

In 2001, the cheapest flow cytometers for measuring CD4 T-cell counts cost $50,000 to $100,000, while other machines were for sale in the $40,000 to $80,000 range. These machines perform two tasks: identifying cell types (lymphocytes and leukocytes), and counting or measuring cell concentrations. Though the cheapest T-cell test may now cost less than $5 in some African countries, the prices of flow cytometers haven't fallen much. Beyond tests, there are other expenses, including the training and hiring of technical staff, maintenance and repair of broken equipment, and the shipping, storage and analysis of samples. "There's no question about our ability to afford it: we just can't," remarked Serge Diagbouga, an HIV doctor at the Centre Muraz in Burkina Faso, in the fall of 2001. "We need alternatives and, unfortunately, we need them soon."

HIV monitoring is used not only for disease management, but also in epidemiology, to screen blood, and for research purposes. These tools are needed in settings of abject poverty where there is frequently limited infrastructure. That means no running water, electricity or refrigerators; no good roads to transport tissue or blood samples across long distances; no doctors to administer tests; and no technicians trained to use diagnostic machines.

Reviewing the state of lab technology in most of Africa, Charlie Gilks, MD, a consultant to the WHO, spoke about the need for researchers and manufacturers to engage in innovative thinking when developing new testing methods. "Most of the discussion about these tools is skewed [by an assumption] that there will be laboratory technologies to do the testing," he said. "But there is a relative scarcity of trained cadres and technologists. Bear in mind that there are very fragile health systems that are being overwhelmed by the HIV epidemic."[12]

As Gilks noted, HIV has not spared health professionals in the worst-hit African countries. "In a country that has a 20 percent prevalence rate for the population, 20 percent of the medical and laboratory staff will be infected as well."

Emphasis on Clinical Management

Two years later, the demand for cheap tests remains pressing. What has changed – and radically – is the attitude of HIV experts in rich and poor countries regarding the necessity of having such diagnostic tests in order to put patients on therapy. A growing number of doctors working on the frontlines of global AIDS have successfully argued that such tests are very desirable, but are not required to start and even manage HAART patients. The lack of sophisticated monitoring tools presents a serious barrier, but it is one that may be overcome by well-trained doctors who rely on clinical criteria like weight-gain and resolution of symptoms to judge how well drugs are working.

That's the thinking behind the adoption of the WHO's new low-tech monitoring guidelines. Today, rapid HIV tests can provide accurate antibody results in minutes. Everything else – T-cell, viral load, resistance tests – is viewed as a step up the ladder, or as experts put it, icing on the cake. Others point out that a simplified approach to monitoring patients on therapy need not spell ineffective or inferior health-care. Some doctors have even argued that Western treatment guidelines for HIV rely too much on laboratory tests and give the body and the human patient short shrift. They've welcomed a greater focus on clinical skills for managing patients.

"Now that treatment is becoming available, the government is making a lot of effort to decrease the price of [anti-HIV drugs]," said Diagbouga.

> But we need to know the criteria before we put the patients on treatment. I don't think we can permit ourselves to distribute anti-HIV drugs to patients across Africa the way we give out aspirin. What we need is some kind of consensus for us in developing countries with limited money and resources, to get a panel of techniques that work not only for CD4 T-cell count, but also for viral load, that we can work to distribute and make accessible in our country, so that we can correctly follow our patients.

What Diagbouga and others want to know is how well clinical monitoring will match up to laboratory yardsticks, and that depends more on human skill than technology. No one can dispute that it takes more time and is more labor-intensive to use clinical or symptom-based management to follow HIV patients than doing a blood test. That skilled workforce is not something widely available yet in Africa, and it could take years to train enough people to do the job.

Developing New Tools

"I can design the best toys out there, but what's the point if no one can use them?" remarked Helen Lee, MD, a scientist at the University of Cambridge, at a 2001 meeting of experts in Bethesda, Maryland, to discuss cheaper HIV diagnostics. Lee is regarded by her peers as a master lab test designer. Surveying the super-high-tech tests now used in the West – such as phenotypic resistance testing – she challenged her peers to think innovatively, and focus on the actual field conditions in poor countries. "We've all got a million ideas and tricks up our sleeves that may not help anyone in Africa," she added. "The question is, what can we do that will actually make a difference?"

What's needed, say Diagbouga and others, are cheaper T-cell and viral load tests, and there are many in development (see Appendix B). Lee is particularly interested in developing a cheap dipstick or filter paper technology for T-cell and viral load testing, similar to those used to test for pregnancy or simple urine samples. She drew knowing laughs from colleagues by comparing the qualities of her ideal lab test for poor settings to a lover doing the Kama Sutra: it has to act quickly (results in thirty minutes); be simple (requiring ten minutes to train a nontechnician to use), cheap (costing 50 cents at most), stable (having a one-year shelf life), noninvasive (no syringes to draw fresh blood), and multiplex (capable of testing more than one sample at a time). Once the tool is ready, it typically takes years and a lot of money to test for efficacy in human trials, win FDA approval, and arrive on the open market. "Now," she grinned, "which one of you is ready to fund me to do that?"

In 2001 the answer wasn't clear. But since then the race has started among diagnostic test developers. Several clinical trials of promising tests have started. The Gates Foundation and other donors are backing a new diagnostic initiative that will be rolled out by the WHO, in conjunction with other agencies. Generic drug makers are pushing forward lower-cost generic HIV T-cell and viral load tests. These are likely to reduce the cost of patented products used in the US. Finally, treatment activists are making more noise about the lack of low-cost tests for the rest of the world.

For Africa and elsewhere, the next generation of laboratory tests will need to monitor the impact of multiple chronic infections and therapeutic regimens at the same time, as well as overlapping drug toxicities, side-effects, and drug resistance linked to these multiple pathogens. Several tests being developed use new technologies like gene chips that may fit the bill. The question remains: How quickly – and how cheaply? For now, the results are promising but slow.

Economic Pragmatism

The WHO's low-tech guidelines reflect a collective awareness that economics, not science, drive health policy in developing countries, and that this includes access to HIV care and medicine. But some critics have questioned the ethical reasons for adoption of a different therapeutic standard for poorer countries. The guideline authors defend their approach, noting that clinical guidelines for HIV therapy were developed for use in high- and middle-income countries. They are not meant to be a substitute for national AIDS treatment programs, but to facilitate the dramatic scale-up that is needed in countries with limited infrastructure and resources.

"I was part of the committee that came up with the guidelines," said Dr. Mark Wainberg, an HIV specialist at McGill University and former president of the International AIDS Society, who helped draft the WHO guidelines.

> I don't think they are perfect, but I doubt whether any similarly constituted group would improve significantly on the recommendations. In spite of my bias, I think that [the three-drug non-protease] concept is ethical as well as practical. Protease inhibitors were considered less reliable because of potentially non-monitored toxicities in resource-poor settings.

Dr. Sam Narasapa of Chennai, India, agreed. "I have no doubt that the regimen suggested will work," he said in 2001. "We need to be bold and ensure that this therapy will benefit individual patients. This will contribute to the reduction in viral transmission in the community. We must remember that these are guidelines and it is left to the individual physician as to how he will treat the patients. Training and hands-on experience are essential."

Treatment Hurdles

Assuming that low-cost drugs and tests become available, what are the barriers to global success with antiretroviral treatment? There are a number of known problems linked to either the drugs or to HIV's ability to evade them. If experts are right, then these problems may be diminished by relying on easier regimens and clinical monitoring. But it can also be argued that they will represent even more of a challenge for physicians and individuals coping with HIV and therapy.

Managing Side-Effects

Although protease inhibitors are linked to greater toxicity, all the anti-HIV drugs cause side-effects (see Appendix C). The greater the duration of therapy, the greater the risk of developing these problems.[13] Some are mild, or transient; some chronic. Some are very serious, disfiguring, or potentially fatal. Common and mild effects include fatigue, headache, nausea, fever, diar-rhea, and skin rashes, all of which may be manageable but affect one's quality of life. More serious problems include damage to the major organs that could lead to cancer, diabetes and heart disease in people on HIV treatment for life. Other serious side-effects include hepatitis (liver damage), kidney damage, high cholesterol, hair loss, nerve damage (neuropathy) and oral warts.

In recent years, one set of drug side-effects has generated great concern, as it poses a threat to long-term adherence. Lipodystrophy is a term used to describe a range of body fat changes and metabolic problems that were initially linked to use of protease inhibitors, but can also occur with non-protease drugs, notably d4T. It produces a gaunt look, with a loss of fat in the face, buttocks, arms and legs, but a fat gain in the stomach. It's not clear how much of a threat to health lipodystrophy poses, but it is worrying.

Lipodystrophy is linked to distinct problems such as high cholesterol levels and insulin resistance (which leads to diabetes); mitochondrial toxic-ity; lactic acidosis; and bone weakness.[14] What does all this mean for Africans or others who are about to embark on life-long therapy? Like US patients, they have little choice: treatment is a life or death matter. They need the drugs, and the drugs are potent but toxic. What will happen if and when millions in Africa begin experiencing serious side-effects? Experts are hoping that non-protease regimens will decrease the incidence of side-effects, but the data we have suggest they will occur. If anything, the reliance on nucleoside drugs as the anchor for first-line regimens sug-gests that some problems, like lactic acidosis and mitochondrial toxicity, could be a big threat.

The other challenge has to do with the existing baseline health in many of these countries, which is poor. Exposure to parasites and other illnesses causes problems like liver damage that may be exacerbated by anti-HIV drugs. With few resources to diagnose these problems, the task ahead is difficult.

The Global Threat: Resistance and MDR-HIV

Drug resistance is a common phenomenon that occurs with HIV. Resistance is a natural by-product of Darwinian evolution, but it is also the result of what's called drug selection pressure. HIV reproduces itself 10 million times a day, and each time it mutates. Some of these mutations help the virus survive and become resistant to a drug or drugs; other mutations cripple the virus. Multi-drug resistance to HIV occurs when the virus has mutated, or shifted its genes, in response to the presence of several drugs.[15]

In recent years, research teams in the US have argued that emerging multi-drug resistance (MDR) to HIV poses a growing threat to future control of AIDS in some patients.[16] In a much-cited study presented in December 2001 by Douglas Richman's group at the University of San Diego, over three-quarters of patients on HAART who were failing to suppress their HIV infections below detectable levels had resistance to at least one class of antiretroviral drug, and half had resistance to two or three classes.

Transmission of drug-resistant HIV is also on the rise. Investigators warn about rising MDR cases in newly infected individuals in big cities across America. Having MDR-HIV is making it harder to fight the virus in these newly exposed patients, too. Suppression of MDR-HIV is slower, and long-term success is less common than in those with drug-sensitive (or "wild-type") HIV. Barring development of an effective HIV vaccine or therapies to overcome resistance, a new wave of AIDS illness and deaths may occur in these individuals in the coming years, researchers warn.

"The fact that resistance is being transmitted in 20 percent of new infections is very significant," Richman said. "It means that a proportion of people practicing unsafe sex are people who already know they are infected and have been cared for and are taking medicines." Experts worry that transmitted MDR viruses could blunt the effectiveness of first-line regimens for some individuals.

The US studies reflect transmission rates in predominantly white, gay men living in urban settings where HAART has been used for some time. European studies are also troubling. In July 2003, a Dutch study showed that 10 percent of Europeans with HIV carry a virus with a resistant strain.[17] About 2 percent had an HIV infection that did not respond to two or more types of drug.[18] Other groups in Canada and Europe have also documented transmission of MDR-HIV.

The Global Picture

What does all this mean for the rest of the world? How big a threat is drug resistance – and MDR-HIV – for the millions who are just beginning to access antiretroviral treatment? Will we one day see a global epidemic of MDR-HIV, as we have seen with other diseases?

Many first-line TB and malaria drugs and regimens no longer work against resistant strains, making it harder to control these diseases. Second-line or salvage regimens are then used, that involve less powerful drugs. There is also multi-drug resistance to antibiotics across much of Africa and the developing world. Why should HIV be any different?

Many experts feel that drug resistance and MDR-HIV emerged in the US and Western Europe because people were initially treated for years with sequential and ineffective one- and two-drug nucleoside regimens like AZT and 3TC, before adding on protease inhibitors. The initial protease regimens were also hard to manage and toxic, leading to poor adherence in some people.

By comparison, individuals in developing countries are being offered once-daily, simplified but potent three-drug regimens. That could limit or delay the emergence of resistance to one or more drugs. But US studies also offer a global warning: they show that resistance to one or several nucleoside analogs marks the beginning of cross-resistance to all the drugs of this class.

"I think that even under optimal situations, currently available drugs are not sufficiently potent to inhibit all viral replication," stated Stephen Deeks, of the University of California at San Francisco, who treats a growing number of patients with MDR-HIV who now need salvage regimens. "Therefore the emergence of drug resistance is inevitable in most patients – it's just a matter of time."

The Great Debate

That view has led a minority of scientists and health officials in richer countries to warn against a rapid introduction of antiretroviral therapy in the poorest parts of the world. The critics include Robert Gallo, MD, and Luc Montagnier, MD, the co-discoverers of HIV. As news of the European studies made headlines, they warned that Africans could not do better than Americans, and instead, they predicted, a global roll-out of treatment will seed global resistance and limit our ability to control a worse epidemic in the future.[19]

Others disagree. They argue that withholding treatment from millions who will otherwise die soon is unacceptable. And the pattern of AIDS in Africa or Asia may not be the same as in the US or Europe, since we've learned a few things in the decade of using antiretroviral drugs in these countries. Partners In Health's medical director, Joia Mukherjee, M.D., treats MDR-TB and HIV among slum dwellers in Lima. While resistance complicates HIV treatment, she feels that ethics is the fundamental stumbling block: "We give our patients in the US HAART knowing full well they will develop resistance," she noted. "But somehow that additional 10-plus years of productive life is not considered cost-effective for Africans, Haitians, Cambodians in the world of public health." With 8,000 deaths a day from HIV and 5,000 from TB, she added, "[m]y view is that it's better to die in 10 years with resistant virus than to die now with drug-sensitive virus."

And, she notes, there's also reason to hope that death won't be the outcome for such patients in another decade, because new and different regimens are being used. Clearly, simpler daily regimens will help patients in Africa and elsewhere be more adherent to dosing schedules and give HIV less opportunity to evolve into resistant strains. That's an important reason the WHO is pushing drug manufacturers to coformulate more fixed-dose pills to boost adherence. "That is a safeguard against the chance of taking single or dual therapy," said Gilks of the WHO, in 2002. "I suspect – but have no data – that this is very important."

Future Unknowns

As my report from Brazil shows, there is some reason to be hopeful that the WHO's new guidelines will help keep resistance down in developing countries. In 2002 there were no reports of MDR-HIV in Brazil, though there were signs of some emerging resistance patterns.[20] In a mid-2003 update, Brazil reported a 6.6 percent rate of resistance among patients nationally – far lower than present rates in the US and Western Europe. How long will low resistance continue in Brazil? That's not clear either. In September, a team based at the University of Alabama at Birmingham found that the duration of initial regimens in 405 patients started on therapies between January 1996 – when protease drugs came on-stream – to October 2001 was 1.6 years. Half of the patients stopped therapy because of side-effects, many linked to use of toxic protease drugs. Two factors also shortened the duration of their first regimens: their use of injection drugs and their history of opportunistic infections.

The US experience suggests that Brazil and other developing countries may be enjoying a grace period. But HIV resistance has proved itself to be affected by the passage of time. We don't know what pattern of resistance to expect from the new fixed-dose pills, but we do know that once resistance develops to a single drug, cross-resistance can be a problem with other drugs of the same class. Since nonprotease regimens like Triomune are being introduced on a mass scale, the future risk for Africa is the loss of an entire class of drugs – nucleosides – or the loss of nukes and non-nukes too. Studies show that resistance to nukes can reduce the efficacy of non-nukes. Since protease drugs are so toxic and so expensive, there aren't many alternatives for Africans who develop drug resistance.

As in the US, some African patients have scrambled to access lifesaving medicines, and a small minority have taken one or two antiretroviral drugs before accessing three-drug regimens. For that minority, resistance may be a problem requiring alternative drugs.[21]

Similar patterns are seen in Asia, where AZT monotherapy and a few other drugs were available to a small minority of individuals.[22] But what about effective three-drug regimens that are introduced within largely treatment-naive populations? That's what we face today, globally. The vast majority of the 42 million people with HIV haven't taken any drugs so far.

Although resistance is certain to increase, Joep Lange, MD, president of the International AIDS Society, estimated in 2003 that the rate of resistance in developing countries will be only 2 percent if people start on effective three-drug regimens and adhere well to them. The use of new fixed-dose three-in-one pills will make adherence much easier, he predicts, though the issue of access to a consistent supply of drugs will be a factor that could affect resistance. And over the course of time, resistance to fixed-dose pills may occur.

If that happens, what substitute regimens will be available for individuals in these countries? How effective will a switch to other therapies be if broad cross-resistance has developed within one or another class of drugs? Protease drugs are expensive – will cheap generic alternatives be available? How will we monitor resistance? Few African laboratories offer resistance testing for individuals, because the tests are prohibitively expensive, even in the US. Instead, experts advocate using resistance tests for population-based epidemiological, or "sentinel surveillance" studies of resistant HIV variants.[23] That will tell them how prevalent resistant viruses are in a given population.

Unfortunately, the WHO's new low-tech guidelines won't be able to offer doctors much guidance. They rely on monitoring clinical symptoms. The only way doctors will be able to know whether patients may be developing resistance to treatment is if and when they get sick – a sign of drug failure. By then, it might be harder for salvage therapies to work.

Daniel Kuritzkes would go further to bridge the US–Africa monitoring gap. He would like to see a better correlation between symptoms of clinical failure and the laboratory standards adopted to report resistance test results. That kind of information would benefit doctors and patients everywhere. He would also like more clinical trials of promising experimental drugs in Africa, and other settings where less resistance now exists.

The burning issue, then, is not whether multi-drug resistance to HIV will emerge globally – the clear consensus is that it will, and there's evidence that it already has in a small minority of African patients who began therapy with suboptimal regimens years ago. The great unknowns are how much resistance will develop to the new, simple pills, how quickly or slowly this will happen, how hard it may be to control MDR-HIV disease medically, and how easily these viruses are transmitted.

From the HAART epicenter in San Francisco, Deeks urges us to learn from the recent past.

A few years from now, a lot of people are going to be doing very well and likely will always do well – we can't lose sight of that. And there will be people who are going to look like US HIV patients in the early nineties, with significant AIDS-related complications. There will probably be a lot more of them than we expect.

New but Costly Weapons

Fuzeon (T-20) is a new fusion inhibitor drug that works against resistant HIV strains and was recently approved in the US by the FDA. Unfortunately, the drug has to be injected under the skin twice a day, and can cause some sensitivity at the site of injection, so it's not convenient. It's also been priced at an astronomical $20,000 for a year's supply by drug manufacturers Roche and Trimeris.[24] They justify this exorbitant price by arguing that the drug is complex to make, requiring 106 manufacturing steps. In the US the drug is marketed to individuals failing on other regimens, but few can afford it there either. Tipranavir is another drug used against resistant viruses.

Then there's the recent news that Trizivir, the all-nuke pill that's gained popularity in the US, isn't as potent as other non-protease first-line regimens.[25] In Moldova, for example, 80 percent of patients being put on therapy are given Trizivir, a regimen known to be less effective than other combinations in patients with advanced disease. Activists have blamed the Global Fund for financing treatment programs that use either suboptimal (less effective) first-line regimens to treat AIDS. But Global Fund officials say that the Fund has no say about what drugs are bought or used by the government, since they are a financial lending body. Such decisions are the province of the WHO. It has backed Trizivir as a less effective first-line alternative to other efavirenz-based regimens.

Adherence: Cost is the Factor

Due to the barriers I've listed above, adherence is predicted to be the big challenge in resource-poor settings. Yet patients are managing very well in model projects like those of MSF and PIH in Haiti. Reports from the recent Paris IAS meeting in July 2003 showed that individuals in pilot treatment programs have statistically higher rates of adherence to HIV regimens – 90 percent and better – than patients in developed countries like the US with its 70 percent adherence rates.

Apart from side-effects, the real barrier to adherence is no surprise: cost. A study undertaken in 2002 in Botswana, prior to the government roll-out of treatment, found that when people had to pay for their own drugs, adherence fell and suboptimal regimens were used.[26] If cost were removed as an obstacle, adherence would climb to an estimated 74 percent. What actually happened was better: adherence was 83 percent in one study of 176 patients who received the drugs free at the Maun General Hospital, where adherence was strictly monitored. Once the issue of cost was removed, poor adherence was due to forgetfulness, side-effects, lack of access to the medical site, and lack of privacy. The last issue relates to stigma, which makes people on therapy afraid that others will discover they are HIV-positive.

Adherence increases when such barriers are lowered, through strategies such as peer support groups, DOT programs and the community-based *accompagnateur* model. DOT programs are thus gaining in popularity.[27] But DOT isn't for everyone, and as I mentioned earlier, there are ethical issues to consider. DOT programs also require a huge investment in training. "In order to do DOT in our program in Khayelitsha, we'd need to train thousands and thousands of *accompagnateurs*," pointed out MSF's Rachel Cohen. "That's simply not feasible."

One finding is that Africans are highly motivated to become healthy and stay healthy, because they have seen so many people die.[28] Since they begin taking the pills when they are very ill, their speedy recovery also provides powerful proof of the efficacy of therapy, compared to US patients who are often started on therapy when they are relatively healthy, and may not witness such dramatic results, producing in lower adherence over time.

Compared to the success stories, China provides a warning for those who are implementing treatment without preparing communities in advance for the challenge of adherence, or providing good medical support for those on therapy. In November 2003, a Chinese official reported that a fifth of HIV patients given free antiretroviral therapy in hard-hit areas – more than 1,040 out of 5,289 – had abandoned their treatment in the first seven months of the program.[29] Many were poor villagers or farmers who were exposed through a blood-bank scandal. The high drop-out rate was blamed on severe side-effects and a lack of alternative regimens, as well as a dearth of trained physicians to manage patients with side-effects.[30] China has fewer than 100 doctors with experience treating HIV-positive patients.

A Scary Surprise

In August 2003, researchers at the University of California at San Francisco, led by David R. Bansberg, MD, dropped a small bomb on the AIDS world. His group showed that resistance mutations occur more often in patients who adhere well to their regimens than poorly – the reverse of long-standing dogma.[31] "These findings will make us rethink the argument that life-saving drugs should be denied to some populations because poor pill-taking behavior might accelerate the creation of resistant mutations of the HIV virus," declared Bansberg. His group found that resistance mutations were twice as likely to develop in patients who took 80 percent or more of their antiretroviral medicines than in those who only adhered 40 percent of the time. "Ironically, it is the 'good adherers' who developed more resistance rather than the 'problem' patients," noted co-investigator Andrew Moss, PhD. (At the same time, other studies show resistance is low in individuals with very high adherence – above 90 percent.)

Why?, everybody wanted to know. The short answer lies in Darwin's findings about drug selection and drug pressure. By religiously taking their pills on time, "good" adherers maintain a constant pressure on HIV, forcing the virus to try to escape attack. Every time HIV copies itself, it mutates. In good "adherers," the virus may be copying itself faster in order to try to outwit the drugs. That could lead to the creation of a lot of drug mutations that spell resistance.

The implications of these findings are important, not only for AIDS therapy but for TB therapy, too. Many doctors assume that patients who fail TB therapy are simply non-adherent. But what if they're not? What it could mean for Africa is that, with 90 percent patient adherence rates, such religious pill-taking could theoretically speed up HIV's activity – and lead to more resistance. Either way, it seems, resistance is a threat, regardless of where patients live or how well they manage their pills. The UCSF group stressed that their findings should not encourage patients to take less of their drugs. After all, drug failure has been linked to drug resistance in many, many studies. And those with resistance still derive a clinical benefit from being on treatment. Still, the news is something that WHO experts and individuals on therapy will have to grapple with, given the lack of resistance tests in poor settings.[32]

The Impact of Nutrition

Poverty not only makes it hard to access treatment, but hard to adhere, as researcher Helen Ayles of the Zambart Project reported in 2002.[33] Simply put, it's hard to take pills without food. Food is an issue that continually cropped up during my country visits. I have no evidence, only my personal observation, of a link between the patients who develop resistance to therapies and their lack of food to swallow pills. The experience of Te Ofa in Haiti is a case in point: when he had no food to take his pills, he felt nauseous and threw up. That affects drug absorption, and the concentration of medicine that fights HIV. There's not much science to back this – yet. Studies are needed to investigate the relationship of nutrition to drug resistance, adherence and efficacy. Creative solutions are also needed to introduce nutrition and food packets into the WHO's simplified treatment formula to address this barrier.

The same is true for clean water. If there are organisms that cause diseases in untreated water, and HIV patients drink that water to swallow their pills, they risk exposure to leishmaniasis, for example, one of the new OI's cropping up in patients in developing countries. Delivering clean water and food to HIV patients should be regarded as an inherent part of AIDS treatment programs. In India, some doctors provide nutritional supplements for patients to take with their daily HIV pills, in an effort to increase absorption of these drugs. In Uganda, a number of NGOs have learned that providing seeds to grow food is more useful than food packets in ensuring sustained nutrition, for affected individuals and communities who are healthy enough to farm. (Of course, it may not be helpful if the seeds are "terminator" GM seeds from Monsanto, which won't grow for more than a season and may colonize existing plants.)

HIV and Viral Sex: New Threats

HIV (or HIV-1) is a human virus that evolved from primate, or simian viruses. It is steadily evolving into viral subtypes, or clades, that differ genetically from three main viral types called Group M, N and Group O (outlier viruses). Group M subtypes are lettered A through H. As HIV reproduces, some of these subtypes merge and create new, or hybrid mutants. These are called recombinant subtypes; examples are B/C, which is spreading in southwest China, and A/B, a subtype linked to HIV outbreaks in Russia. There are over fourteen hybrid strains that have been identified, and it seems new ones are reported at each new AIDS conference.

A recombinant virus carries the genes of each parent virus and can be a stronger, or more lethal, virus. As the virus evolves inside a person, recombinant viruses may become dominant. If the parent viruses carry mutations that make them resistant to drugs, the recombinant viruses inherit that resistance. Experts now worry about whether recombination on a global level will make it harder to treat and control HIV in the future. Recombination thus poses a challenge to prevention efforts. These viruses can not only be transmitted, but now require us to create an effective vaccine that can generate a broad range of immune responses to the many viral subtypes. Similarly, microbicides need to work against recombinant viruses.

Superinfection

The emergence of more powerful and more resistant viruses has also produced several cases of dual infection or co-infection, as well as superinfection.[34] Dual infection occurs in HIV-positive individuals who are exposed to a second distinct virus during the period of acute infection, before they have developed antibodies. Experts worry that these second viruses may be more powerful, and potentially lethal, than the initial strain. These viruses can later recombine to generate new hybrid viruses – something called superinfection. In August 2003, University of Cape Town researchers reported on four cases of dual infection that led to superinfection in a small study of sex workers. They concluded that dual infection and HIV recombination may occur frequently in such high-risk groups. What worried everyone was the discovery that these women also became sick much faster.

The Cape Town report is the second in 2003 that provides early clinical evidence of the threat of dual infection and superinfection to the control of HIV.[35] Last spring, a University of Washington team reported on four individuals with dual infection who progressed to AIDS or death within two years after initial exposure to HIV. "Detection of dual infection is becoming more common, especially in regions where multiple subtypes are circulating," declared Jandre Grobler, the lead researcher in the Cape Town study.[36]

Experts can't really say how *much* of a threat superinfection really is – or to whom. For example, they don't know if the South African sex workers had some genetic factor or immune defects that caused dual infection in the first place.[37]

What does this mean for people on HIV treatment now, or for prevention, or vaccines? What does it mean for HIV-positive partners who want to forgo condoms or for people on therapy who choose drug holidays? Luc Perrin is a Swiss researcher who is a leader in the field of superinfection. Looking at the big picture, he feels the data so far do suggest that superinfection causes more damage to the immune system. If he's right, it may also be harder to develop a vaccine to control more diverse hybrid viruses. But some experts also stress that the immune responses in people with HIV or AIDS are different from those of healthy HIV-negative individuals who will be getting preventive vaccines, making such comparisons difficult.

Paul Farmer is among those who urge caution in extrapolating from results from such small studies, and from data involving commercial sex workers who may be at a higher risk of exposure to unprotected sex and therefore also STDs than other groups. He isn't ready to conclude that we have clinical evidence of extra immune damage linked to superinfection either. "If we have evidence of this, it's awfully preliminary," he said in September 2003. But he does feel the growing caseload of superinfection deserves our attention, adding, "I think it's serious."[38]

The emergence of superinfection has important implications for HIV prevention, including vaccine and microbicide development. Until we know more, experts urge HIV-positive individuals to use condoms and avoid unprotected sex, even when having sex with another HIV-positive individual. They also urge HIV-negative individuals to use condoms and practise safer sex.

HIV's Shadow Epidemics

Across the developing world, HIV is linked to poverty and rides on the coat-tails of endemic co-diseases: tuberculosis, malaria, hepatitis, tropical diseases, fungal infections, and so on. Treating HIV means managing multiple infections, and requires using drugs that interact. These diseases may produce similar symptoms that complicate their diagnosis and treatment.

In the West and other rich countries, the use of antiretroviral drugs has sharply curtailed the incidence of HIV-related infections (opportunistic infections). OIs develop when HIV has caused a loss of immune function, as measured by T-cell levels. Often, underlying or dormant illnesses may arise. Globally, we may see new or different OIs crop up in HIV-positive individuals and those on therapy in developing countries. In the US, not all OIs have fallen in people on treatment: cancers like lymphoma and viruses like human papillomavirus, for example, remain a threat.

At the Paris IAS meeting in July, some studies showed that antiretroviral therapy reduced OIs in developing countries. But other reports suggested that a greater emphasis should be placed on the treatment of OIs that cause death in HIV patients.[39]

One emerging problem is "immune restoration syndrome" (IRS), a usually transient, but often acute illness that occurs two to three weeks after starting HIV therapy.[40] It develops when antiretroviral drugs cause the rebounding of dormant or undiagnosed infections in patients with AIDS or deep immunosuppression. In India, doctors found that a large proportion of Indian patients – 66 percent – developed immune restoration syndrome within two to twelve weeks of starting antiretroviral therapy.[41] The most frequent OI was extrapulmonary tuberculosis. The infection wasn't picked up with a chest X-ray, since it occurred outside the lungs. Many patients who developed extrapulmonary TB had low CD4 T-cell levels when they started HIV drugs.

Another problem is that the standard PPD skin tests used to detect exposure to TB don't work as well in AIDS patients.[42] And again, access to skin tests and chest X-rays is not readily available in the poorest settings. Other non-TB pulmonary infections were also reported at the Paris meeting in patients going on HIV therapy.[43]

These studies raise important questions: What kind of additional routine pre-screening of HIV patients should be done to detect undiagnosed infections prior to starting antiretroviral therapy? What is the role of OI prophylaxis therapy, given the large variety of endemic diseases in many regions? How does HIV therapy affect the control of these diseases?

Such studies from the West are now pushing doctors to consider the need for routine Pap (vaginal) and anal swabs to monitor human papilloma virus (HPV) in HIV patients on therapy. There is also a relatively cheap non-invasive tool, the Hybrid Capture 2, that can detect HPV in samples. These tools and screening guides need to be implemented in developing countries.

The Great Killer: Tuberculosis

According to the WHO, one-third of people with HIV globally also have tuberculosis, and 70 percent of them live in sub-Saharan Africa.[44] TB remains the most common OI, and is often the first sign of HIV infection. It is also the leading killer of people with HIV. The two illnesses are synergistic – meaning that HIV and TB act like engines to fuel each other's activity and impact on the body. Individuals with active TB and HIV may get sicker more quickly. TB causes anemia, and leaves the body vulnerable to other HIV-related infections as well. Individuals with HIV who develop TB may also have a harder time controlling their TB infections.

Like HIV, TB treatment is difficult and requires taking four drugs daily for a long period of time – typically eighteen months, though shorter courses are also advocated. One of the critical limiting factors is that some TB drugs can't be taken with potent protease inhibitor drugs, as they reduce their effectiveness to subtherapeutic levels. A recent report also warned about the potentially fatal use of TB drugs rifampicin and pyrazinamidine when taken together. Rifabutin is a substitute for rifampicin, and causes less negative interactions with protease inhibitors, but is not generally available in resource-limited settings. Two TB drugs, isoniazid and rifampin, also have complex interactions with anti-fungal drugs like ketaconazole and fluconazole – commonly used in HIV patients.[45] They render the antifungal therapy ineffective in some patients.[46]

Reports regarding the impact of antiretroviral therapy on TB in poor settings are mixed. A new study by reputed Ugandan researcher Peter Mugyeni, MD, of the Joint Research Clinical Centre in Kampala found that drugs for HIV reduced TB by 80 percent. At the JRCC, around 40 percent of deaths of patients with advanced HIV disease are caused by TB. Next come toxoplasmosis, PCP, cryptococcis – all fatal in AIDS patients. Ironically, the advent of generic HIV drug now means that it's cheaper – and more effective – to use these drugs to prevent TB and PCP in HIV patients than anti-TB or PCP drugs on the Ugandan market. It costs $12 for an anti-HIV regimen for two weeks, versus $100 for other prophylaxis regimens for the same period. Another Paris IAS study found that side-effects with TB drugs were not that much worse when antiretrovirals for HIV were added.

Unfortunately, the best regimen for use with TB drugs is the one that isn't as powerful as other HIV cocktails: Trizivir. AZT (or d4T) and drugs like 3TC and efavirenz can also be used with rifampicin, but here too there are concerns about drug interactions.[47] All these issues simply underscore the complexity of TB–HIV co-management.

Treatment Breakthrough for MDR-TB

In June 2003, a long-sought breakthrough occurred in the treatment of drug resistant TB when doctors from New York School of Medicine used a new antibiotic named linezolid (brand name Zyvox) to save the lives of five patients dying of MDR-TB at Bellevue Hospital in New York City.[48] The drug is FDA-approved for use against penicillin-, methicillin- and vancomycin-resistant bacteria. A twice-daily linezolid pill was effective against strains resistant to nearly all current TB treatments when used for between nine and thirty-three months. Four patients also received aerosolized interferon gamma thrice-weekly. After completing linezolid therapy, there was no trace of TB in the sputum of patients' lungs, nor did the drug cause many of the severe side-effects linked to other TB drugs. Because the drug is approved for other uses, it can be used off-label by physicians.

For developing countries, this news is fantastic. Larger clinical trials are needed to confirm linezolid's effectiveness, and to explore how the drug interacts with antiretrovirals and other TB drugs, issues regarding future linezolid-resistance, and how it might be combined with other TB drugs into new fixed-dose pills, and so on. It remains to be seen how quickly generic linezolid will become available. Several advocacy groups are working to push new TB treatments, including the Global Alliance for TB Drug Development, the WHO, MSF, and others.[49]

Malaria and Other Tropical Diseases

There is no doubt that, like TB, malaria is a disease of poverty. It is one of several diseases endemic in poor and tropical countries, others including yellow fever, sleeping sickness, filariasis, dengue fever, Chagas disease, Japanese B encephalitis, among others. Some are spread by insects, others by parasites that spawn in rivers and untreated waters. Many of these diseases produce similar symptoms: fevers, loss of weight, anemia. When they occur as co-infections in people with HIV, they may become harder to treat. Similarly, HIV can expose these underlying, often chronic infections. Without diagnostic tests, the task of managing co-infected patients on therapy is much harder.

Unfortunately, the widespread and erratic use of insecticides and drugs has also led to insecticide- and drug-resistant species, making it harder to control the spread of these endemic illnesses. Chloroquine resistance is widespread in Africa, and there are few alternative drugs to treat malaria. Gates Foundation money is being used to research and develop new treatments.

There is one powerful new drug: artemisinin. Early studies show it is very effective, even against chloroquine-resistant mosquitoes. But brand-name artemisinin is ten times more costly than chloroquine, and thus its use is limited globally. Clinical trials are underway to compare the efficacy of artemisinin alone and in combination with another TB drug, sulfadoxine-pyrimethamine.

In November 2003, AIDS activists from Health GAP warned that some African countries were using their Global Fund grant money for malaria to buy insecticide-treated bed nets and chloroquine, rather than the more effective, albeit pricier, artemisinin.[50] Experts argue that this strategy is a recipe for failure – and more malaria resistance. "There is almost no evidence that this strategy has ever succeeded or is actually of any biological or scientific sense," argued Professor Bob Snow of the Kenya Medical Research Institute. He added that Uganda was buying this failing combination at a time when it was associated with a clinical failure rate of 33 percent or more by day twenty-eight. One site in Uganda reported a failure rate of about 80 percent on day fourteen.[51] Snow criticized the Global Fund for doing a poor job at peer-reviewing proposals, he said, while "WHO is not providing the technical leadership countries deserve."

On the HIV front, co-infection with malaria makes it that much harder to treat. In the future, there's hope that generic manufacturers will package and develop new fixed-dose combination pills for malaria, as they have for HIV and TB. Activists are calling for a price battle to reduce the cost of brand-name artemisinin.

The same is true of other so-called "neglected diseases" – illnesses that kill millions in poor countries every year but for which new treatments are lacking. Since these diseases don't affect people as much in industrialized countries, multinational drug companies have abandoned their research and development; there's too little profit in this work. Groups like MSF have taken the lead in campaigning for new funding for neglected diseases.

Viral Hepatitis

Hepatitis is another common co-infection of HIV that leads to liver damage (hepatotoxicity). Around the world, exposure to hepatitis B and C has greatly increased. Injection drug users are especially at risk from hepatitis C, which can be transmitted in blood in shared syringes, or through unprotected sex. Hepatitis B is so prevalent among gay men that experts urge vaccination for hepatitis B for this population in particular. Sex workers are also at higher risk of exposure to hepatitis B; so are individuals with chronic exposure to parasites and pathogens that damage the liver. Since many of the antiviral drugs are processed by the liver, they also cause drug-related damage to it, increasing the risk of hepatitis. In the US, some co-infected patients on HIV therapy have died of liver failure, which experts link to the increased hepatotoxicity of therapy.

Three drugs – ddI, d4T and nevirapine – may increase liver damage in individuals with active hepatitis, and should be avoided. That rules out the WHO's first-line fixed-dose regimen for a lot of people; instead they have to use single drugs in other combinations. 3TC and tenofovir, a newer drug, are active against hepatitis B, but generic tenofovir is not yet widely available.

For those going on therapy who may have had prior exposure to hepatitis strains that lie dormant, there's also the risk of this infection becoming active if HIV is not controlled. And it may also emerge in individuals who harbor a dormant infection and develop immune restoration syndrome after starting therapy. These issues pose more challenges for doctors who need at least basic blood tests to monitor liver function. Many frontline doctors feel that liver tests are among the most essential laboratory tests, because of the impact of drugs on the liver.

HIV-2

HIV-2 is a sister virus to HIV-1 (usually known as "HIV") that is also transmitted by blood or sexual fluids, and causes a slower type of immune illness. It is endemic in Western Africa, where people may be co-infected with both HIV viruses. Unfortunately, non-nucleoside drugs, or NNRTIs, are inactive against HIV-2 (as well as Group O HIV-1 subtypes). That means people living in Senegal, Ivory Coast, Ghana and Sierra Leone, for example, may have a hard time with the WHO's new guidelines. They can't use first-line regimens that include non-nuke drugs; doing so can lead to drug resistance and drug failure. That leaves only nukes and protease inhibitors, and the latter are costly, although a generic version of indinavir is available as a single drug. There is Trizivir, a fixed-dose three-in-one, all-nuke pill, but it may not be as powerful for those with AIDS. It could eventually lead to nucleoside cross-resistance, which won't leave any drugs but protease inhibitors for affected patients. Other drugs are becoming available, but as single drugs they won't be as easy to manage as convenient daily pills.

Needs of Special Populations

Although public health officials advocate a standardized approach to HIV treatment, the reality is that treatment has to be modified for different populations, including women (pregnant and not-pregnant), children, those with co-infections, those dealing with substance abuse, and so on. Myriad social, economic, and cultural factors impact on the access to treatment of these different groups. There are also disproportionately affected groups in some countries, including, for example, prisoners and sex workers in Russia, soldiers, miners, and truckers in southern Africa, and men who have sex with men in Morocco and Cuba.

Women

Although antiretroviral therapy can be equally effective in women and men, studies in many countries show women often access therapy later. Around the world, women often have less access to health services in general, including HIV services. Recent data from the decade-old United States Women's Interagency HIV Study (WIHS), an ongoing longitudinal study of HIV, suggest that women may respond differently to treatment than men. Women also appear to develop some more severe side-effects than men do, including lipodystrophy and diabetes. These side-effects were worse in African-American women in their study, though there is considerable debate over whether these differences are related to gender, race, or other genetic factors. Such factors could influence women's immune response to vaccines and microbicides.

These observations raise the question of what drugs are best for use in women, including pregnant women, in developing countries. For example, the nucleoside drug d4T isn't recommended for pregnant women, and US studies link it to higher rates of lactic acidosis and lipid problems in some African-American women. Then there is nevirapine, a backbone of the new fixed-dose pills the WHO is advocating. In Uganda, a number of women I interviewed had to abandon nevirapine due to rashes and severe hypersensitivity. Will other drugs be available for them? Some doctors are also concerned about nevirapine's effects on the liver in patients in developing countries. In India, for example, doctors report a higher rate of hepatitis in HIV patients on therapy, which reflects a high rate of prior liver damage.

The concerns about nucleoside drugs also extend to girls. Unfortunately, there are no large-scale gender-based studies being rolled out in developing countries, though WIHS researchers in the US strongly advocate this idea.[52] Learning from the US experience, a global research priority should be to implement gender-based studies alongside new treatment programs in order to track the impact of new fixed-dose regimens on women and girls, and carefully monitor drug side-effects.

Other challenges are non-medical, and relate to social, emotional and cultural factors that impact on women's health and treatment for HIV. As the chapter on Uganda noted, a growing body of research shows that sexual trafficking, prostitution, violence, rape – including marital rape – and domestic abuse are contributing heavily to the spread of HIV in women and girls across the world, and to a high degree in parts of Africa.[53] So may customary laws and cultural traditions on inheritance, marriage, divorce, polygamy, virginity rites, ritual sex, male and female circumcision.

These factors affect women's and girls' ability to seek help, including information and services for testing and treatment of HIV. They highlight the urgent need for counseling and mental health services to be integrated into HIV programs. And they reveal the extent to which gender-based abuse and inequality are intrinsically linked to what advocates for women rightly call a global female AIDS epidemic.

Pregnant Women

The global focus on HIV prevention has led many countries to implement HIV screening of pregnant women, and to establish MTCT programs to prevent mother-to-child transmission. MTCT-Plus programs are also beginning. That means pregnant women who are also ill with HIV may be among the first to access treatment in some countries.[54] But there are problems associated with drugs such as AZT and nevirapine.

HIV can rapidly develop resistance to nevirapine when the drug is used alone to prevent maternal transmission of the virus in MTCT programs. There is growing worry that it may become harder to control HIV later in these women. It may not be. But it raises concerns about how well a fixed-dose combination pill containing nevirapine, a non-nuke, will work in women who took the drug during pregnancy who harbor NVP-resistant viral mutants. Some worry that the widespread use of the drug in MTCT programs may also seed resistance to nevirapine in wider populations and, down the line, blunt the efficacy of first-line combinations in developing countries.

But experts from MSF and other groups working in the field to roll out antiretroviral therapy back a first-line regimen of nevirapine, d4T and 3TC.[55] Resistance to 3TC also occurs quite quickly when the drug is used alone, while studies show that d4T causes neuropathy and is the biggest culprit in causing lipodystrophy, or lipid problems. It also interacts with rifaimpicine, a TB drug. Another non-nuke, efavirenz, can be substituted for nevirapine because it can be used with rifampicine – but not in pregnant women. Efavirenz has suspected teratogenic (cancer-causing) effects on the fetus, and therefore should not be given to pregnant women.

For those who can't take d4T, AZT is also a substitute, but it causes anemia, also a common side-effect of pregnancy, tuberculosis and malaria. So AZT isn't a great choice for pregnant women, especially if they have these co-infections. The bottom line is that there aren't many options that don't have downsides for pregnant women in developing countries.

There are other issues related to drug efficacy. There is substantial body of data showing that use of a single drug such as AZT or nevirapine, or dual AZT/3TC can prevent maternal HIV transmission in the majority of pregnant women who receive such MTCT regimens. But recently researchers have argued that such regimens are suboptimal: if they are ineffective as treatment to stop HIV, they shouldn't be advocated for prevention, either. Some advocates are pushing for use of three-drug MTCT regimens that, they believe, would increase the success of MTCT prevention regimens and reduce the risk of resistance to nevirapine or 3TC. That would call for a change of the present MTCT guidelines. Comparative MTCT studies are needed quickly to determine if they are right, and how this might reduce the risk of spreading nevirapine resistance on a global level.

Children

As in adults, the use of antiretroviral drugs has quickly benefited children, including infants, born with HIV or exposed after birth. But the crisis of access is very different globally, due to the high death rate of HIV-parents, which has led to an epidemic of HIV-positive orphans. Although MTCT programs are being initiated, millions of women have had no access to prophylactic AZT or nevirapine, and their children are born HIV-positive. Studies show infant mortality is higher in mothers with HIV or AIDS, who may not be able to nourish their newborns adequately due to illness.

HIV treatment in infants and young children is even more difficult than in adults. Many studies have documented the greater challenge of adherence for children. Although many of the antiretrovirals are available for children and infants in liquid formulations, access to pediatric drugs at all the necessary dosages doesn't exist.[56] The drugs taste bad and are hard to swallow, as well as causing side-effects. Some require mixing powders with clean water – something lacking in poor and remote settings.

As with adults, there are also concerns about side-effects and cumulative toxicities, and issues of resistance in children. These problems are even greater, since children face long lives on treatment – decades more than the current generation on therapy. HIV drug side-effects increase over time. What will this mean for infants starting on antiretrovirals at birth? Will the use of non-protease regimens decrease this risk to children slated to begin therapy in poorer countries, as is hoped?

Children also go to school, and must cope with incorporating treatment into their lives. It would be easier if they had pills or liquid drugs that they could manage on their own as they got older. As with adults, what are needed for infants are simplified three-in-one, fixed-dose capsules that can be broken and mixed with food, or made available in pre-packaged formulations in small volumes. But these aren't available yet.

As parents die of AIDS, young children often become care providers, breadwinners and then orphans – a scenario that's become common in sub-Saharan Africa. Many children are forced to survive on their own at a young age, and turn to sex work when they become old enough to do so, exposing them to HIV and other sexually transmitted diseases. Globally, the sexual vulnerability of children to HIV is a crisis of incredible significance. In his recent travels, UN AIDS ambassador to Africa Stephen Lewis has talked candidly and with horror about the epidemic of sexual violence and rape that is being directed at young children, especially orphans, across Africa.

The non-medical needs of HIV-positive children around the world are numerous, and impact on their ability to cope with HIV. They need emotional support and counseling to deal with HIV and their fear of illness and dying, as well the grief and loss associated with the death of parents and loved ones, with the trauma of rape and violence, and so on. They need food and housing, and as surviving breadwinners, money to care for and support young siblings. They need help dealing with the stigma of HIV in schools and in their lives, help in developing a positive attitude toward their bodies and sexuality. Most governments have so far given little consideration to the lifelong needs of this growing population.

Although orphans' services and homes exist in all countries, the AIDS crisis has long overwhelmed the existing resources of orphan care providers in the hardest-hit countries. The stigma of AIDS can make it harder for these children to get help and find new homes; instead, rejection by relatives and communities, and by orphanages that fear AIDS, is all too common. Over the past decade, many international and national relief organizations and agencies have started focusing on the crisis of orphans, but they are still afraid of HIV-positive children, as the reports from Haiti and Russia show. And as I keep stressing, the ban on travel for HIV-positive individuals limits the ability of outside adoption agencies to help these children.

Injection Drug Users

The increase of HIV among drug users has become a huge problem in Russia and other Eastern European countries, China and Southeast Asia, and India. Like TB and other diseases of the poor, drug addiction is a problem linked to poverty and economic crisis, and those who are engaged in active drug use find themselves on the margins of society. They are often in poor health and susceptible to diseases like tuberculosis, hepatitis and sepsis. In Russia, as in the US, prisons are full of people jailed for using or trafficking in narcotics.

For obvious reasons, it's much harder for someone who's heavily addicted to heroin to adhere to a daily HIV-drug regimen. The same is true for alcoholism, an often overlooked problem that is an especially serious problem in Russia. That's why few treatment programs offer HIV drugs to active drug users. Instead, drug addiction programs are promoting harm-reduction strategies and drug maintenance programs that substitute methadone or buprinorfine for heroin to help addicts get clean. Unfortunately, these drugs and programs aren't available in much of the developing world. Instead, drug users face arrest, and tend to avoid encounters with institutions.

The challenge of reaching out to drug users is significant when it comes to getting people into testing and treatment. It demands more than anti-HIV programs. It requires government to address complex socio-economic issues that fuel the rise of illegal drug use. Step one is to increase funding to drug addiction treatment programs. After that, they can get into HIV testing and treatment programs. But here too, there are other challenges. It's common to hear of people in recovery turning back to drugs after they've tested HIV-positive. Those in recovery need consistent support to stay clean or sober – an important aspect of adherence to HIV therapy. Studies from developed countries show that substance abuse and active depression are two predictors of poor adherence to HIV treatment.[57]

Highlighting the Military

Although many African and Asian governments have drafted broad prevention campaigns at the national level, leaders in both regions have failed to deal seriously with spiking infection rates within a key group: the military.

So have international health officials and political leaders. They have delivered speeches, but there has not been high-level attention to HIV in Africa's armies as a key focal point for urgent education and prevention campaigns. But the movements of armies and the sexual activity of soldiers are linked to the continued spread of HIV. Governments bear a direct responsibility to address this distinct crisis. While their leaders lobby for global help and money for prevention and treatment, these governments actively fund and fight simmering border wars that fuel HIV's spread, affecting civilian women and children disproportionately.

In South Africa, where there are more HIV-positive people than in any other country, over one-fifth of the military is estimated to be HIV-positive. Yet in October 2003, Defence Minister Mosiuoa Lekota was quoted as saying this high prevalence should cause "no alarm." His statement was met with just that – alarm bells of concern – expressed by TAC, who accused the minister of "misleading the country."[58] The situation is proportionally more grave in Angola, Congo and Malawi, where 50 percent of the military are HIV-positive. In Zambia, the rate is 60 percent, in Zimbabwe, 55 percent, and in Swaziland, 48 percent.[59]

Bridging the Treatment-Prevention Gap

One of the great promises of global AIDS treatment is that it will boost prevention efforts and build a stepping-stone for vaccine and microbicide programs. That's because HIV counseling and testing are the first steps for individuals seeking care and treatment. Treatment itself offers hope, and this is a great incentive for people to seek testing, as seen in Cange, Morocco and elsewhere.

The June 2001 UNGASS meeting helped start country discussions of AIDS and a broader debate within global civil society regarding the need to expand HIV education, prevention, and testing programs quickly, and link them to new treatment initiatives. Globally, world leaders signed a Declaration of Commitment there which requires them to draft the blueprints for comprehensive national programs. But these are still actions only on paper for many countries. Many governments are still unwilling to dedicate serious money to fight the epidemic, commit to treating those affected, or take many of the other concrete steps they must to mobilize civil society. Instead, too many political leaders across Africa, Asia and Eastern Europe continue to practice denialism. Their absence of leadership perpetuates social ignorance of the epidemic and stigmatization of those with HIV. On a broad, global level, many people still know very little about HIV and AIDS, and there are few targeted education efforts to reach them.

Although many countries have prevention programs in place, some are barely off the ground. Globally, fewer than one in four people at risk from HIV is able to access basic information about the disease, according to a rough UN estimate. Voluntary counseling and testing services are limited. In general, testing is available in major cities and in a few centers in many developing countries, but not in rural areas. In countries where innovative prevention programs are funded, they are usually small-scale, and target communities at high risk, such as sex workers, drug users, or men who have sex with men. But they fail to reach married women or street children – groups who are very vulnerable to HIV but may not be as visible. Social and cultural attitudes toward sexuality are often to blame for the lack of information and prevention materials on HIV. Discriminatory laws also interfere with the ability of vulnerable groups such as prostitutes, injection drug users, and sexual minorities to risk disclosure and access to HIV testing services. Meanwhile, prisoners have limited access to health-care, and this is true of access to HIV services.

Turning to the future, there are some who worry that an increased emphasis on treatment will harm prevention efforts. They point to US studies that suggest some individuals no longer worry as much about exposure to the virus because they have the option of treatment.[60] At UNGASS, the prevention versus treatment debate threatened to divide the global community, although in the end there was a broad consensus that they are integrally linked. The programs I looked at showed that treatment is introducing a badly-needed discussion of HIV and AIDS, as well as sexuality and social attitudes toward taboo subjects like homosexuality, prostitution and drug use. This broad civil discussion will go a long way toward educating people about how to avoid sexually-transmitted diseases. Because of the scale of death in hard-hit countries, the issue is not about people growing complacent about AIDS; it's still about denial and fear and stigma.

MTCT and MTCT-Plus

The adoption of MTCT prevention and MTCT-Plus treatment programs require that prenatal and obstetrical services be available to pregnant women with HIV. But studies from developing countries show that most poor women lack these services, particularly in rural areas.

In order to get into MTCT programs, women must be willing to be tested for HIV. This deters many women who fear being stigmatized. HIV-positive mothers also need alternatives to breast milk in order to avoid passing HIV on to their infants after delivery. In most of the world, women breast-feed their children by personal choice and out of economic necessity. Many can't afford infant formula, which also can't be used in settings where there is no clean water. Infant formula isn't as nutritious as breast milk, either. As I discussed in the Uganda chapter, there are also cultural and social challenges to women's adoption of formula; if they don't breast-feed, they risk disclosure of their HIV status to their families. That continues to be a real problem for HIV-positive mothers.

Despite these barriers, enrollment in MTCT programs has greatly increased, and does offer some women a stepping-stone to treatment. So far, the roll-out of the MTCT-Plus programs has been steady but too slow. In May, only 400 women had accessed therapy via the MTCT-Plus program of the Columbia Mailman School of Public Health team. That was almost twice the number they were treating in March.[61] Aside from the Columbia program, the Bush money and the CDC's GAP funding are backing myriad MTCT and MTCT-Plus programs. MSF also has MTCT programs, as do other smaller groups.

Post-Exposure Prophylaxis (PEP)

The efficacy of post-exposure prophylaxis, or PEP, programs remains controversial. PEP involves giving at least two antiretroviral drugs to an individual within seventy-two hours of their suspected exposure to the HIV virus. The drugs attack the virus immediately, preventing it from reproducing and establishing an infection. At least that's the theory. A growing number of countries offer PEP drugs to health professionals in cases of accidental exposure to the virus, and to victims of rape. These are mostly small scale programs, and due to the limited availability of antiretrovirals few health professionals have accessed PEP services. That's also true of women who have been raped. In the US, small-scale PEP programs offer drugs to individuals who suspect they've been exposed to HIV, and gay men in particular have made use of these services in major cities.

As with MTCT programs, there are also doubts about the efficacy of PEP regimens that rely on two drugs, as opposed to three. Again, if two-drug regimens are considered suboptimal for treatment, why should they be used in prevention, especially in cases of acute infection? It's well-known that HIV levels are high in the blood during the period shortly after exposure. That would call for potent regimens to block a rapidly spreading virus. Some experts have even questioned whether existing 28-day PEP regimens could foster drug resistance if they failed to prevent HIV exposure.

Microbicides

One area where the global gap in resources is felt most keenly is that of women-controlled methods of prevention. Although research into microbicides is increasing, too little money is being invested in this arena, given the potential impact of such a weapon. Today, male condoms are the main tools being delivered, but these too are being limited by the Bush agenda. The Female Condom works well to block sexual exposure to HIV, but it's more expensive than male condoms. Nor is it a tool that has been advocated strongly by public health officials. The average global citizen hasn't made the Female Condom a part of his or her safe sex life.

Funding is now increasing in the field and there has been recent progress. Six candidate microbicides are being considered for Phase 3 clinical trials of their efficacy. Experts are predicting one could even reach the market within five years. That would represent a major step forward in the battle.

Vaccine Dreams

Without a cure for HIV or AIDS, the world's hope lies in a preventive HIV vaccine. There's also hope that a therapeutic vaccine could be used to boost immune defenses in those on antiretroviral therapy. But for now these are pipe-dreams. Since the launch of the International AIDS Vaccine Initiative years back, the search for a vaccine has continued, but has produced no major breakthroughs. The biggest recent step forward has been in proving it is possible to mobilize people to participate in vaccine studies in countries like Haiti, Thailand and South Africa.

The challenge of developing a vaccine hinges on many of the issues I raised in the treatment section, from basic immunology and virology; from how HIV causes infection and harms the immune system, to drug resistance and superinfection, and to tantalizing questions about genetic resistance and the impact of co-infections and co-diseases on immune defenses. A key challenge is that of developing a vaccine in countries like South Africa, where HIV incidence is so high.

Today, dozens of candidate vaccines are in various stages of testing, but only a few have reached the stage of large-scale phase III efficacy trials. Several vaccines are now being tested in Africa, India and China. Most of the global vaccine trials involve viral subtypes found in Africa and Asia, such as subtypes A and C. Some are testing vaccines that induce cellular immunity to HIV – the primary arm of the immune response; others are studying antibody-based vaccines – the secondary arm of the immune response.[62]

Recent months have brought mixed news. First there were the disappointing results in the VaxGen efficacy trial, carried out jointly by the US, the Netherlands, Puerto Rico and Thailand.[63] The trial involved 2,545 HIV-negative individuals, many of them former injection drug users. Unfortunately, these studies failed to offer proof of efficacy. But they provided useful insights regarding community participation and attitudes towards vaccines. Some activists are critical of the large-scale trials being planned now, arguing that candidate vaccines being tested are too weak against HIV. A similar charge was leveled against the VaxGen product.

As with low-cost diagnostics, researchers have a vaccine wish list: they'd like a vaccine that can be administered orally, is stable in different temperatures, can be administered once and provide long-lasting immunity, and most importantly, that is very cheap and easy to manufacture on a mass scale. Other vaccine studies, including those for malaria, TB, dengue, and other tropical diseases, are also underway.

Spotlighting Blood Safety

In Africa, the spread of HIV through blood products and dirty needles has garnered recent media attention. Several researchers have proposed that this route is more important than was thought, including Dr. David Gisselquist, a US physician who thinks that a third of AIDS cases globally are linked to contaminated needles in medical treatment.[64] That assertion remains unproven, but has led to increased attention to this route of HIV transmission. Until recently, the WHO estimated that dirty needles caused 2.5 percent of African HIV cases, for example.

In May 2003, a research group from Germany argued that exposure to dirty needles, rather than sexual exposure, is a significant cause of HIV transmission among South African children. In June, UNAIDS issued a report suggesting that 80 percent of the blood transfused in the strife-torn Democratic Republic of Congo may not be clean. And of course, the world now knows about the HIV blood scandal in the central provinces of Anhui and Henan, China.[65] China just got a $98 million Global Fund grant, which will be used to help treat these citizens, and also to put a health prevention infrastructure in place, including the addressing of blood safety.[66]

Meanwhile, the spread of HIV through needles used in hospitals and by injection drug users is a big concern for health professionals. In Africa, many nurses and health workers lack gloves and sterile equipment to protect themselves from exposure to unsterilized equipment and needles.[67] They have demanded protection as have consumers who fear vaccination for other diseases, or giving or receiving blood transfusions in hospitals in Africa. A major investment is needed – and is included within the various national AIDS plans – to upgrade the ability of countries to assure blood safety.

Dirty syringes are also behind the fast-growing HIV and hepatitis caseloads in Asia, including Southeast Asia, and Eastern Europe. Access to disposable needles is needed in these regions. In Russia, the Soros Foundation and the Open Society Institute deserve great credit for pushing needle-exchange and support for drug users despite an intransigent and punitive Russian bureaucracy. So do activists in Thailand working to promote the civil rights of intravenous drug users. A number of international groups are working to develop safer syringes, which could reduce the risk of HIV infection through occupational exposure. But these programs have yet to be embraced for widespread use.

The various HIV blood safety reports prodded US Health and Human Services' Tommy Thompson, the US chair of the Global Fund for AIDS, TB and Malaria, to launch a review in June into links between AIDS, dirty needles and contaminated blood products. So far the bulk of the Bush $15 billion in global AIDS money has gone to prevent sexual exposure to HIV. But Senator Jeff Sessions (R-Ark), among others, feels Congress should allocate more money to needle education – and possibly a clean needle-exchange program, if the threat is more significant.

Research Challenges

The plethora of reports and news coming from developing countries regarding HIV treatment, different drug regimens, subtypes, strains, adherence, resistance and superinfection represents a wealth of knowledge about HIV disease in different populations. It also invites research in all these areas. Today, several groups are pushing for clinical trials of drugs and treatment studies to monitor closely the impact of treatment in target populations and settings. New research is focused on HIV and TB, rather than on HIV and malaria.

There's a long list of important studies, too many to list here. On the treatment front, my wish-list includes longitudinal and comparative efficacy and safety studies to judge the effectiveness and impact of the new generic fixed-dose pills on treatment-naïve populations. We need to look at how these nonprotease pills work in women's bodies as opposed to men's, and in infants, children and adolescents. We need to study the impact of HIV treatment on TB, malaria and hepatitis treatment – and vice versa. We urgently need to study the efficacy of new therapies like linezolid for resistant TB and artemisinin for resistant malaria in co-infected HIV patients. We need to study how poverty, hunger, and the range of socio-economic issues such as homelessness, joblessness, drug addiction, migration, violence, rape and domestic abuse affect access and adherence to treatment.

As treatment is rolled out, we also need to know more about the baseline health of groups being targeted.[68] We need to study the use of traditional medicine and alternative therapies.

Turning to emerging global and resistant viruses, we need to know how well existing and novel pills and tests work against hybrid viruses and different subtypes in different populations. We also need more research and testing of new drugs and vaccines for other neglected diseases, something that MSF is pushing. And we need to establish mechanisms that will ensure that new drugs and products that emerge will be affordable and available on a mass scale.

On the prevention front, we need studies that look closely at how STD screening and treatment of genital herpes impact on HIV acquisition, and at the possible impact of new vaccines for herpes. We need a lot more money for microbicides, and the kind of political focus that's been given to treatment. If the world wanted a good microbicide, we'd have one much sooner, and this would have an enormous impact on the epidemic.

Ethics of Clinical Research

It's also true that many communities may be wary of participating in such research programs. As South Africa's experience shows, informed consent is not the norm in the world. Instead, there's plenty of evidence to show that poor people are often used as guinea pigs by unscrupulous researchers and drug companies. In a blistering review in the *Nation*, investigative researcher Sonia Shah found that drug companies can achieve quick, positive results of their clinical trials in very poor countries where doctors are on the take, where regulatory standards are lax or unenforced, and where patient advocacy is limited. As she wrote, "Over the past decade, the drug industry has quietly exported its clinical testing overseas where oversight is slim and patients plentiful."[69]

The results of this unfettered access are good studies and unethical ones. What makes the difference are Institutional Review Boards (IRBs) and community watchdog groups who have a say in the design and conduct of trials. In the US and Western Europe, AIDS activists had to fight to get on the IRB's of some trials, and scrutinize the fine print that detailed inclusion or exclusion criteria. The same scrutiny is even more necessary on the global level.

The French agency, ANRS, has assigned itself the task of reviewing AIDS research in developing countries, and will be a source for communities to learn what is happening in their backyards. But even they require community oversight. In 1996, ANRS researchers doing clinical studies of treatment for cryptococcus in Burundi, and MTCT studies in Ivory Coast and Burkina Faso, were accused by ACT UP–Paris of carrying out non-ethical trials.[70] The trial in Ivory Coast was stopped as a result.

It is important for these studies to be organized and carried out in such a way that the data from different groups and countries can be evaluated and compared. All this requires a considerable investment in data management, in the design and funding of clinical studies and trials, and in the training of community educators to engage affected communities and individuals, including uninfected people. To guard against unethical trials or abuses in clinical research, a global ethical standard for conducting HIV and AIDS studies in developing countries could be adopted. Less may be more when it comes to implementing treatment and diagnostics, but not when it comes to ethics: more attention is needed to avoid future abuses.

That's just the beginning of a long list of future "to-do" studies that will help us determine how much benefit we may ultimately derive from the global treatment effort. The question is: Which studies will be funded? That depends on who controls the purse strings. Where will the demand for such studies come from? And the community oversight? Much will depend on the engagement of civil societies and on people with AIDS who join the ranks of activists to hold governments accountable to their citizens.

PART IV

From Durban to Bangkok

14

AIDS AND EMPIRE II:
THE COST OF DELAY

Throughout this book, I have looked at a number key challenges on the political, legal, medical, social and cultural level that will determine how quickly and effectively we can implement treatment in the world's poorest countries. What follows in this final section are some of my insights regarding the overall progress we have made – and the setbacks that still plague us. This provides a rough and admittedly subjective yardstick of our progress to date, which is what I set out to do when I began reporting for this book in 2000.

I'll begin with the issue that continues to dominate all discussions of treatment, past and future: drug access, and the politics behind that access. After that comes the financial cost, the groups involved, the treatment challenges, and the potential role and response of communities in meeting this historic demand. Each one of these subjects merits its own book, but I will simply try to touch on what I regard as some of the critical lessons and insights that I've drawn from these first steps.

Let me start on a positive note – the historic, revolutionary vision and commitment by grassroots activists who, rightly, cast the issue of access to lifesaving AIDS medicines in the language of human rights and justice. By focusing on the moral and humane requirement to treat, to care, and to act, they have done the world an enormous service, reconnecting us with one another – North and South – over the huge gap of historic inequity. Many lives have been transformed by their actions, as much for residents of rich nations as for the poorest. We have all benefited from the feverish public debate over AIDS drugs, because the global epidemic affects our collective future, while directly threatening the lives of now 46 million individuals – in Botswana, Haiti, Russia, and other countries reported on in these pages – who are now beginning to access lifesaving medicines.

One benefit for everyone is the shift in how we – people all over the world – now view AIDS and the treatment of the epidemic. It has become a global public health issue, not merely a private health matter affecting individuals with HIV. As such, it is engaging international agencies, humanitarian organizations and political leaders in a very different way than the epidemic has in Western countries. The key difference is how health-care and access to resources are regarded. The development of drugs, tests and treatment guidelines for AIDS in rich countries reflects a reliance on private and employee-based health schemes and third-party payers. It assumes that individuals, taxpayers and companies in these wealthy countries have a high degree of choice when it comes to spending their money on their health-care. That's why HIV treatment guidelines in the US and Europe stress individualized treatment, while those for poor countries advocate standard-ized regimens in public health programs where budgets are very limited.

There is an argument to be made that a higher standard of care is being advocated for the richer nations since individuals there have access to trained doctors, specialists and high-tech, state-of-the-art diagnostic tools that provide a more accurate means of treating and monitoring HIV disease. The WHO doesn't feel that way; it believes that a public health approach to HIV and AIDS that emphasizes clinical monitoring and patient education is equally or more effective than an over-reliance on mon-itoring tools without a similar investment in patient education.[1]

Fundamentally, the adoption of a different approach to HIV care for rich, as opposed to poorer patients reflects the degree to which the drugs and high-tech tools we consider so essential to managing HIV in the West may not be as critical as we thought. HIV treatment guidelines in industrial-ized countries reflect market-based medicine, where profits, not health needs, drive drug development. Drug companies want consumers to have unlimited treatment options because they want to sell their products. They do not support socialized medicine or universal health plans that may place limits on health spending. They continue to make more profits in the phar-maceutical arena than those enjoyed by almost any other industry. They are entirely invested in having drugs remain squarely within the US-based capitalist system, where the laws of supply and demand create an endless variety of medical drugs and products.

At a fundamental level, then, the ongoing battle over access to AIDS drugs is about economics and the location of essential drugs as commodities in that global market system. That's why the multinational drug companies have fought so hard to defend their patents and prevent generic competitors from providing cheap drugs for Africa. They wanted – and still aim – to prevent the open debates that took place in the media over AIDS drug pricing to spill over to other medicines.

That's exactly what's happened, of course, and that is why the battle for AIDS treatment remains revolutionary. Thanks to Cipla and the Indian upstarts, and the actions of consumer watchdog groups like Health GAP, the global public now knows what Wall Street drug industry analysts and insiders have always known: it costs far less to produce antiretrovirals and other drugs than we were told. Moreover, the multinationals don't always develop these drugs; in many cases, academic groups or small biotech companies do. The multinationals simply buy and market promising drugs, and reap huge profits.

The exposure of these long-hidden details is highly threatening to the drug industry, and is likely to lead to further challenges in the fields of cancer, heart disease and diabetes, where lifesaving drugs are priced so high. Whether US and European consumers decide to take on the patent holders or their governments to demand access to cheaper lifesaving drugs in these areas is the multibillion-dollar question that haunts big pharma companies. But at the very least, consumers worldwide are more aware that they are massively subsidizing multinational corporations in the arena of drug development and sales.

All of this is taking place at a critical time, when consumers in all countries are hotly debating the high cost of health-care to their economies, and the merits of universal health-care versus the US-style third-party-payer system.

Looking beyond AIDS or health, these developments do represent a sea change, a historic advance, because they've also thrown open many doors – in law, economics, human rights, politics, foreign aid and development – causing a ripple effect and broad change at the global level. The media debates over the role of foreign aid, foreign debt, globalization and privatization in relation to global AIDS and health, for example, have given leaders and grassroots groups in developing countries more information and new means to counter economic and political agendas imposed by outside governments and donors.

Within developing countries, the biggest and most important development, aside from actual access to medicine, is the urgent discussion of all aspects of AIDS that was not happening before 2000. It is causing a profound social change by altering attitudes around sexuality, gender, and the status of vulnerable groups. The arrival of treatment is not only helping to rebuild countries by strengthening health infrastructures and by bringing new money to focus on national and development issues, but also by engaging citizens in their own future. All of this is nation-building at its core, and all of it is helping to address the inequities of access and information now dividing rich nations from poor. That is the revolutionary promise of the global battle over AIDS drugs, and why it will continue to transform societies profoundly, even after the issue is no longer about AIDS or even disease.

Now comes the reality check, the actual situation as it remains for 6 million people who are now ill with AIDS-related diseases and need lifesaving drugs today. By the time you read this book, another million will be dead.

Given the fast-changing arena of global treatment, it's difficult to predict how many people will actually be on AIDS drug therapy by 2005 – the WHO's 3×5 deadline for treating 3 million people in poor countries. Unfortunately, the politics of profit continue to dominate – and seriously limit – the global treatment agenda. Given the current level of spending on AIDS and the opposition of key players, it's safe to say that in the coming year we will not treat the 6 million people in poor countries who we know need these drugs now, today, in the coming year.

Even if there were unrestricted global access to generic AIDS drugs, too few steps have been taken in the past two years, and especially in recent months, to establish mechanisms necessary to procure and deliver the drugs to meet current demand. Fundamentally, what was and is still required is far more political will, money, activity and commitment at all levels, within all governments. That is true even in Brazil, the model for the global prevention and treatment roll-out. As world leaders have grown fond of saying, we need many Brazils. That would call for a universal public health system, progressive leaders, generic production, defiance of the powers-that-be who are keeping expensive drugs and tests from the reach of millions – and all on a global scale. And that we'll never have.

What, then, have we got? And how far have we come? Let me start with the numbers, the broad estimates of access that exist today. And let me compare that with 2001, the year of the famous Declaration of Commitment at UNGASS. That is when I began my own investigations for this book, and it provides a useful point of departure, statistically speaking.

In May 2001, just prior to UNGASS, the WHO gathered HIV experts in Geneva for an international consultative meeting on the global AIDS pandemic. At that time, Dr. Bernhardt Schwartlander, then with UNAIDS and now with the Global Fund, estimated that approximately 3 million people could "reasonably be expected" to be on HIV therapies by 2005. The cost of this effort would be roughly $4.4 billion, of which almost half – 43 percent – could be used for AIDS medicines, and the remainder for laboratory capacity (12 percent), training, monitoring and health infrastructure development.

To succeed, global funding would have to increase thirty-fold to meet the *minimal* treatment needs of the then-36 million people living with HIV/AIDS. It was estimated that 150,000 to 175,000 people in developing countries had access to antiretrovirals then, but only 25,000 were in hardest-hit Africa. To meet the needs there, access would have to be scaled up 100-fold.[2] At that meeting, experts agreed to reserve treatment for those in later stages of HIV disease and AIDS. They also began drafting their simplified guidelines for HIV treatment and monitoring.

If the global scale-up occurred, 40 percent of those with AIDS or symptoms of HIV disease would get access to antiretroviral drugs, with a range of 30 percent for coverage in sub-Saharan Africa to over 50 percent for Latin America and the Caribbean. The estimates were not made for Eurasia, where the epidemic has further exploded.[3]

Thus the WHO's 3×5 plan was born – and quickly stalled.

Global Fund Woes

The engine for the 3×5 roll-out was and continues to be the Global Fund, which in some ways has proved to be a surprisingly nimble, effective funding mechanism for the disbursement of grants to countries. In other ways, it has capitulated to the Bush administration and the interests of big pharma companies. The result is that the Global Fund lacks money to do what it pledged to do. It remains a battleground where government leaders and civilians wrestle with each other as the accusations of foot-dragging pile up.

Below I'll review some of the political battles that have plagued the Global Fund, but I first want to note how the funding situation stood in July 2001. The request from UN head Kofi Annan was for $7 to $10 billion annually. The Bush administration initially pledged $200 million for the Fund's first year, the Bill and Melinda Gates Foundation another $100 million, and the G-8 countries began throwing in more. The Fund established its Secretariat in January 2002, and began disbursing grants – a total of $1.5 billion to 153 programs in ninety-two countries, with 65 percent of funds going to African programs. But little of that money actually flowed out to countries in 2002; instead, much of it started moving late that year or earlier this year.[4] The lack of funding delayed implemention of both the UNGASS and 3×5 goals.

In July 2003, activists were decrying the nearly empty coffers of the Global Fund, which had collected only $1.24 billion from the richest eight countries in the world.[5] That month, European Union members of the G-8 promised they would give $1 billion a year to the Global Fund, matching the Bush administration's May 2003 pledge of $1 billion (though in July the US House of Representatives allocated just $500 million for the program). As a key G-8 member, France tripled its donation from $58.7 million to $176.1 million. President Jacques Chirac called the European move "historic."[6]

But AIDS activists felt very differently. They denounced the US and European leaders for failing to live up to their pledges to the Global Fund and their public commitment to the Declaration of Action issued at the 2001 UN Special Summit on AIDS (UNGASS). Worried, ACT UP activists led a "die-in" protest at a Paris donor's meeting on July 16, carrying 16 body bags, representing the 16,000 people who die every day of AIDS. They continue to demand that the wealthiest countries increase their pledges to the Global Fund to meet current demand from countries.

Last year, the Global Fund hoped to grant around $4.9 billion for operations for 2002 to 2004, but by the time of the donor's meeting had secured total pledges of only $2.6 billion. An immediate infusion of $600 million is needed for the rest of 2003, said Global Fund officials. But US officials feel Uncle Sam's contribution is adequate. US Secretary of Health and

Human Services Tommy Thompson, who was appointed in 2002 to chair the Global Fund – a move sharply criticized by activists – continues to argue that the US has done enough for now, and expects European allies to step up their pledges to make up the difference.[7]

Soft Money, Tough Agendas

The battles over funding reflect the different agendas of various major donors and governments, and they remain highly political in nature. Since he took office, President Bush has led the United States in undertaking uni-lateral action in foreign policy.[8] The administration's go-it-alone policies are reflected in Bush's $15 billion PEPFAR plan. The initiative called ini-tially for Congress to commit that money over the next five years, and will include $10 billion in new money. (It also provided the $1 billion US dona-tion to the Global Fund). The goal of the initiative is to prevent 7 million new infections – or 60 percent of new infections in target countries – to offer antiretroviral treatment to 2 million people, and to care for 10 million, including support for AIDS orphans.

While many applauded Bush's move, it must be noted that funds are being disbursed through a bilateral agency, US AID, while the program falls under the control of the State Department – a political, not health body. By creating a parallel funding mechanism that sidesteps the multi-lateral Global Fund and other UN agencies, Bush has created a mecha-nism to use foreign aid dollars to control programs that reflect US interests and his conservative social agenda. It also reflects the degree to which AIDS is now viewed as a security issue for the US, one that must be addressed through foreign policy, including foreign aid. Bush created a new, high-level Special Coordinator for International HIV/AIDS Assistance at the State Department, appointing Randall Tobias, former CEO of Eli Lilly, the Indianapolis-based pharmaceutical giant, to the post. Tobias has an ambassador's rank and reports directly to the Secretary of State, now Colin Powell. Randall's appointment, given his ties to big pharma, indicate his likely position on access to generics. The State Department is not requiring Tobias to sever his industry ties; instead, he told reporters he hoped his insider status would help him secure better deals on drugs.[9]

Controlling the Agenda

Bush modeled the prevention aspects of his global AIDS initiative on Uganda's national AIDS program. It is based on a "network" model of central and satellite clinics, complemented by mobile units. While that looks good on paper, it reflects a basic health-care structure whose base is US-controlled, as clinics, sites and programs are run through USAID, the US Department of Health and Social Services, NGOs, faith-based groups and willing governments – in that order, as laid out in an official press release from the White House. It deliberately avoids working with the multilateral UN agencies like the WHO, which are responsible for responding to global public health emergencies, and for control of infectious diseases like malaria and TB. The Bush initiative essentially privatizes AIDS treatment in developing countries, and gives NGOs more power than national governments. The danger is that this will not strengthen the existing public health systems, and will instead uselessly duplicate infrastructures. That spells less access for the poor, who rely most on public health systems.

Controlling Global Funds

Behind the scenes, the US has done a number of other things to sabotage the effectiveness of the Global Fund. Officials from bilateral agencies like USAID are persuading poor countries to reduce the amounts of their Global Fund applications. Jeffrey Sachs, the Harvard golden boy who offered up his dream of an AIDS war chest at the Durban meeting,[10] complained in January 2003 that USAID officials had helped downsize Malawi's application. It first requested $1.6 billion over four years, then settled for $197 million over five. By pressuring applicants to limit their grant proposals, donor nations are keeping the Global Fund afloat – barely – and avoiding a public relations disaster, charge critics.[11] They also put the screws to Richard Feacham, the Global Fund's pragmatic director.[12]

The current funding shortages are so severe that the Global Fund recently made a move that surprised even its supporters. Amid intense internal debate, its board members ruled that only the least developed countries can submit funding proposals for the next two rounds of Global

Fund grants, rounds four and five. That move is being contested by various groups within and outside the Global Fund.[13]

One of the very positive developments of the Global Fund is the creation of the CCMs – Country Coordinating Mechanisms. The CCMs represent an attempt to create a level of transparency in the grant-giving process, an important step that has indeed given a rare view of the global flow of money.[14] But in many countries, activists complain the CCMs are top-heavy, bureaucratic and dominated by government officials and a coterie of established NGOs, who are determined to control the AIDS effort – and the AIDS purse-strings.

Agency Turf Wars

As the lead UN agency responsible for accelerating treatment, the WHO in 2001 was crippled by a lack of leadership at the top, by staff shortages, and by a lack of human and material resources. Some of the money and talent had been shifted over to UNAIDS earlier, when the global effort was focused on prevention. Until July 2003, when Dr. Jong-Wook Lee took over as the WHO's new Director General, the agency was quietly struggling through a bureaucratic fight marked by internecine turf wars between UN agencies vying for control of purse-strings and programs.[15] These agencies ultimately want institutional power in the emerging global treatment agenda.

To its credit, the WHO did move on a number of important tasks required to scale up antiretroviral treatment. It established several working groups that began developing pooled procurement and delivery models; it began inspection of generic companies and products, and approved several for use; it gathered experts together and oversaw the drafting of its radical low-tech treatment and monitoring guidelines for resource-poor settings; it promoted "best-practice" models of care, treatment and prevention and the successes of pilot and model programs. It also recast the global AIDS battle as a public health issue, and focused on applying the lessons of AIDS to TB and malaria, and vice-versa. It established a global surveillance system to track the threat of HIV resistance and has worked with a number of governments, including Brazil, to push the treatment envelope further.

At the same time, the WHO is also a political institution, and agency officials are rightly accused of dragging their feet in inspecting and approving generic products by Indian suppliers, particularly the new fixed-dose combination pills not available in the US.[16] Activist groups like Health GAP accused the agency of caving in to pressure by the multinational drug companies, who strongly oppose generic competition.[17]

Had more inspections and approval of new fixed-dose pills occurred then, developing countries would now have access to these important medicines. This is something even top health officials like Dr. Schwartlander concede, though he defends the WHO's actions, given its limited financial and human resources at the time.[18] The result is that, two years after Cipla's revolutionary step, only four generic suppliers have had their products approved by the WHO.[19] Two years after UNGASS, WHO officials in July renewed their commitment to the 3×5 plan. They openly acknowledged that a critical year was lost following UNGASS, for a number of reasons: the failure of donor countries to make funds available; the US government's veto on generic medicine at the World Trade Organization; pressure from big pharma; lack of leadership from some political leaders in developing countries, such as Thabo Mbeki; and, yes, their own institutional failure to be more politically brave – to take charge of the global AIDS epidemic as the public health agency responsible for doing so.[20]

The Missing Link: Political Will

It is important to consider what could be achieved if true political will for treatment was forthcoming. For example, on September 11, 2001, when the US was attacked by al-Qaeda terrorists, the Bush administration responded by declaring a war, and it dedicated resources to that war: billions and billions of dollars. That war was partly in response to a threat of exposure to anthrax. Overnight, the Bush administration decided that this national emergency required extraordinary steps and demanded access to low-cost Ciprofloxin, made by Bayer. It then threatened to ignore Bayer's patents to import generic Cipro from Canada and – of all places – India, from Ranbaxy and other generic manufacturers of AIDS drugs.[21]

Another example: the Iraq War. Although we don't know the actual price tag of Bush's daily War on Terror, the initial amount approved by Congress was $79 billion to pay for the first phase of the war on Iraq alone.

That breaks down to $763,000 *per minute* of war. Contrast this $79 billion in start-up funds to the paltry $200 million in start-up funds given by the US to the Global Fund. Or to the $1 billion the US recently allocated to the Global Fund from the $15 billion Bush global AIDS effort. It now appears that less than $2 billion of the Bush money will be spent next year.[22] As the year comes to a close, and the drum-roll of national elections begins, Bush appears to be backpedaling on his fiscal commitment to global AIDS.

By comparison, Bush recently made a follow-up request for another $87 billion to maintain the effort to rebuild Iraq – a move that critics says will plunge the US further into the red. On a political level, then, the US has made its lack of commitment to global AIDS perfectly clear.

AIDS vs SARS

The recent epidemic of SARS offers an interesting comparison. In China, health ministry officials initially ignored the first reports in 2002 of a new, highly infectious, very rapidly spreading, apparently airborne pathogen. But when news of it leaked out, political leaders and global health agency officials intervened, forcing the Chinese to address their denial. Global health authorities eventually took many emergency steps to respond to the crisis, arguably because the SARS virus is a killer disease spread by coughing and sneezing that was fast traveling around the globe.[23] Why the difference?

The economic impact of SARS was quickly felt, compared with that of AIDS, which has been felt more gradually. The Asian markets began to unravel – including, most importantly, the global airline and travel industries, which were already suffering from the fallout of 9/11 terror attacks. SARS hit Wall Street where it feels the impact: in the stock market.

Within weeks, a coronavirus linked to SARS was isolated, and a variety of treatments tried. The WHO played a major role in fighting SARS. It worked with the Chinese, the US and other governments to dispatch rapid response teams to track the epidemic and halt its spread. Countries issued alerts and engaged and trained civil society to respond to the threat. Customs officials stopped travelers in airports, train stations, and border crossings everywhere. Health officials in local hospitals quickly reported any suspicious cases and quarantined them for short periods. At every level, from local to national government, citizens went on alert and instituted policies and programs to limit the spread of SARS.

Canada, particularly hard-hit Toronto, responded with war-like efficiency to the SARS threat. There, as in China, citizens quickly denounced attempts to segregate or discriminate against those with the virus (though, as I note in the chapter on Cuba, many blatant cases of discrimination have occurred in China related to its SARS quarantine). Meanwhile, Asian designers responded with notable aplomb to the regional threat by manufacturing fashionable facemasks that became an overnight cultural phenomenon. By comparison, worried Americans stopped traveling and trawled the internet to buy thick 3M face masks that filter out most infectious organisms – a throwback to the days of 1950s A-bomb shelters.

There were quick steps taken on the treatment front, too. Notably, several AIDS drugs were tried, including one that has had some impact. Top AIDS researchers like David Ho, MD, of the Aaron Diamond AIDS Research Center, and vaccine researchers, shifted their attention from HIV to SARS. At the CDC and National Institutes of Health, agency directors shifted scientists and resources to tackle the scientific challenges of SARS. After weeks, the global headlines began to fade. SARS fell off the radar, but the world is now better prepared for a new epidemic or a second wave.

All of this required a high degree of political commitment: to action, money, communication, and cooperation at many levels. It revealed how easily – and quickly – the world can respond to a life-threatening epidemic that it considers a global priority.

The US anthrax scare of 2001 is another case in point. So is the West Nile Virus scare. All were threats to which governments quickly responded with action. Global AIDS, for all its pandemic devastation, is still not being treated as a serious threat that deserves America's – or the world's – urgent attention, not compared to Ebola, anthrax or terrorism. SARS made that very clear.

Debt Relief

Given the current picture, new sources of funding are needed by governments to pay for their national scale-up efforts around AIDS. Debt relief has been proposed, and could have a major impact, but has made little progress on the global agenda. Along with Africa Action and Jubilee 2000, rock singer Bono is providing a strong voice in favour of a debt-swap for AIDS drugs. His Washington, DC-based organization, Debt AIDS Trade Advocacy (DATA) lobbies Congress and works closely with grassroots groups who back the cause, particularly African-American communities and church groups. Debt activists continue to point out that countries like Nigeria – part of the so-called next wave of AIDS – could do an enormous amount with the $32 billion it now spends on debt repayments to foreign banks and donors. So could South Africa, with its $18 billion foreign debt accrued largely by the former apartheid regime.

It's amazing to consider that Haiti, which is battling endemic hunger and raging HIV and TB epidemics, must pay back interest on new loans, even as funds are blocked by the US-led aid embargo that has crippled the government's ability to fight AIDS. It's a vicious cycle, and keeps poor countries tethered to a yoke of dependence on foreign aid. As I mentioned early on, the global AIDS fight is one of development. That's another reason the debt issue deserves serious attention.

Once again, the War on Terror provides a pointed comparison. In December, as Bush officials began cutting back on funding for global AIDS, Bush suggested that France, Germany and other countries who strongly opposed the US war in Iraq consider dropping the debt Iraq owed them in order to help rebuild the country. So debt-swap is an idea that Bush himself advocates – when it serves his political agenda.

To date, a few countries have swapped debt for resources to fight AIDS, namely Mozambique, Senegal and Mali. Brazil recently proposed to drop Guyana's foreign debt to its larger former colonizer, and to use some of that money to help set up a national generic industry to produce AIDS drugs. As the pioneer, it is again showing leadership.

But the reality is that heavily indebted countries like Haiti and Russia are taking on more foreign debt in order to invest national resources to fight AIDS and rebuild infrastructure. These high-interest debt repayments further impoverish them.

The debt battle won't be easy. The US government and lending institutions like the IMF and World Bank have shown little inclination to back what could be an easy mechanism for freeing up billions without investing new money. Instead, Robert Zoellick, Bush's point man on the WTO and trade, has a mandate to lock in as many bilateral and regional trade deals like the FTAA as he can while he's got the job.

Another alternative to freeing up global funds is an international tax on citizens of developed countries. For a few dollars a year, the global effort could be funded by splitting the bill in this way, something that would appear to have only a small impact on US consumers. But who will lead that fight? Not US presidential hopefuls and political parties who are shy of increasing taxes during a pivotal campaign period. Still, the model exists. Zimbabwe recently introduced a surtax on corporate and personal income, devoting the proceeds to AIDS programs.

Shifting National Priorities

While so much attention focuses on the US and G-8 leaders, it's important to consider the money that does exist in the national budgets of developing countries. If African nations devoted a fraction of their national defense budgets to AIDS, for example, a lot of money could be redirected. It's easy enough to argue that AIDS presents a great security issue not only to African and Asian countries, but to their armies. Why not shift military spending and manpower to help roll out AIDS treatment, provide education, guard drugs warehouses, and fund other services? It would be a peacetime act that could go a long way to strengthen the power and long-term security of these nations.

The Role of Private Money

Given the political realities of the Bush agenda and the limited commitment of the G-8 countries to funding the global AIDS program seriously, advocates have put forward a number of proposals for new funding streams. More private money is trickling in from donors and foundations. On the prevention side, the Bill and Melinda Gates Foundation is in a class by itself. Along with HIV prevention and vaccines, MTCT, TB and malaria programs, there is money going to dengue fever research and the WHO's new HIV Diagnostic initiative. Gates has increased funding for countries like Botswana, and most recently, India. Gates Foundation money has mostly gone to prevention, with the exception of Botswana's treatment program. Some activists criticized it and the International AIDS Vaccine Initiative during the UNGASS meeting for arguing against shifting resources to treatment, a debate that pitted prevention and treatment activists against one another and nearly derailed the UN summit.

The Rockefeller foundation has also focused on prevention, and pushed MTCT and now MTCT-Plus programs such as the one being rolled out by Columbia University's Mailman School of Public Health. As I pointed out in Chapter 12, the Soros Foundation has greatly expanded harm-reduction programs and TB programs, and has helped nascent advocacy groups like AFEW to get started. The foundation has focused its support on the most vulnerable populations: drug users, sex workers and prisoners. It is now eyeing Africa.

Smaller groups have made other important contributions. The Population Council, for example, has funded key research into microbicides, paving the way for others. Today, the US government has increased its budget for HIV microbicide research, though it is still a fraction of the budget for HIV vaccine research. Other donors, like the Ford and Henry Kaiser Foundations, have provided an array of grant money for projects around global AIDS. The Pediatric AIDS Foundation backs research and programs for children with HIV, and has helped highlight the needs of orphans.

The Clinton Foundation

On the treatment front, the William Jefferson Clinton Foundation has emerged as the big surprise player, and has secured several key victories. Clinton's team, led by his former right-hand man in the White House, Ira Magaziner, moved forward with a clear role: to help nations draft sound and comprehensive AIDS plans, secure additional funding, and identify gaps in their infrastructure and capacity to deliver on national goals. The Clinton model promotes a public–private multisector response in which private groups and NGOs work closely together to boost the public and private infrastructure for health-care delivery. As promised, Clinton has tapped new donors like Canada, Ireland and other European countries, and was lobbying Japan in November 2003 to offer more support to African countries.

AIDS activists were initially wary of Clinton's foray into global AIDS work because of his failure to confront AIDS when president, including his role in pushing globalization, structural reform, and trade deals like

NAFTA and the Global Agreement on Tariffs and Trade (GATT). After all, it was Vice-President Al Gore, representing the Clinton administration, who first went to bat for big pharma companies back in 1998, when AIDS activists began pushing for access to cheaper drugs. Such is the irony of Clinton, now leading the charge to rebuild Rwanda, when his administration stands accused of failing to prevent the 1994 Rwandan genocide that fueled the AIDS epidemic there.

Clinton's turnaround on AIDS, however belated, has made a dramatic impact, and he is providing political leadership that is badly needed to counter Bush's policies around prevention. A major victory came in September, when the Clinton Foundation announced it had brokered a deal with four generic producers – Cipla, Ranbaxy and Matrix of India, and Aspen Pharmcare of South Africa – to purchase the most popular first-line three-drug cocktail for just 38 cents a day per person – down from an already slashed generic best price of 55 cents. That reflects a sharp drop from the $1.54 price-tag for a comparable brand-name regimen. The deal will benefit a number of African and Caribbean countries, including Haiti, Rwanda, Mozambique and South Africa. The Clinton group is negotiating to achieve a similar deal for India and other regions.

With this generics deal in hand, Clinton was able to persuade a wavering Thabo Mbeki to move forward on treatment. The Clinton team worked closely with HIV experts in South Africa to draft a national treatment plan, which was launched in November. At that time, the sixteen Clinton Foundation countries were expected to put 2 million more people on treatment, including 1 million in South Africa.[24]

Politicizing NGOs

Of all the NGOs, Médecins Sans Frontières has provided key leadership, advocacy and frontline experience in the sphere of global AIDS. It is the most political of all the NGOs and has spurred other groups like Oxfam to take very bold position on issues ranging from access to generics to criticism of Bush's trade policies. On the medical front, MSF's pilot efforts have provided "proof of concept" models for the larger roll-outs that have begun. They have used Brazil's generic drugs in their South Africa program and pushed for a greater focus on the need for research and new therapies for neglected and tropical diseases. Their teams have pushed governments and health ministers to move faster, and they have supported local physicians in their efforts. These groups are continuing to raise the bar for other NGOs, encouraging them to focus more on their commitment to the communities they serve than to the donors who support their activities or the governments who receive their help.

The downside of having so many players enter the field is the lack of coordination, and the competition for funds that inevitably arises when new sources of funding are created. In my visits to countries, I was kept abreast of turf-wars between government agencies, established and newcomer traditional NGOs. The result was a fragmented response in places like Russia, where a number of NGOs operate with scarce communication, each engaged in rolling out small-scale programs.[25]

The Role of Corporations

While governments struggle to respond to AIDS, the private sector lags far behind. The cost of doing business has gone up due to AIDS, and the loss of so many workers has forced companies in many countries, especially in southern Africa, to pay attention. They don't want to pay, but they've being forced to the table by the scale of their own losses. They are working with insurance companies and other third-party groups who are being asked to cover the health costs of millions of employees. Like government officials, corporate leaders have taken an ostrich-like attitude toward the overwhelming epidemic. As my report from Carletonville illustrates, the situation is changing in southern Africa, due partly to the activities of the Global Business Council. Richard Holbrooke continues to be an active cheerleader, pushing business leaders to commit themselves to the cause. The GBC's next targets are Asia and Eastern Europe, where businesses have yet to do very much.[26]

Reducing Drug Prices

There is no doubt that the fall of drug prices is directly equated with increased access to AIDS drugs in poor countries. Since 2001, drug prices have fallen more than 85 percent, and after the latest WTO negotiations some predicted they would drop lower.[27]

There are other ways to bring down cost. One is by scaling up production runs in drug factories – something that may now be possible if the orders for products are followed through with funding promises. Another is in the form of the pooled procurement models being advanced by agencies like the WHO, the Pan American Health Organization (PAHO), UNICEF and the International Dispensary Association (IDA). A key goal of pooled procurement is to assure a steady supply of drugs, and to make sure second-line or alternative drugs are available for patients who may develop resistance to initial regimens – something that happens often with AIDS drugs, as with TB and malaria drugs. Pooled procurement works best when there is a broad range of drug suppliers.

At the WHO, Dr. Lee has brought on a coterie of experts who have applied the Global Drug Facility (GDF) model used to procure and distribute TB drugs to the coordination of AIDS drugs. The health analyst group McKinsey & Company backed the GDF model for antiretroviral drugs as one that promotes "rational" drug use.[28] Rational drug use reduces the chance of chaotic prescriptions and shortages by ensuring the steady production and supply of high quality drugs. The downside may be that drugs are selected that may not be the most ideal for a given patient (see Chapter 13). Through competitive bidding, the GDF model has brought TB drug prices down to below $10 per patient – a fall of 30 percent for a standard six-month course of treatment.[29]

Looking ahead, the WHO and other agencies have a challenging job on their hands to inspect and approve new generic suppliers and products in order to achieve two of their critical goals: first, promoting the use of standardized first-line fixed-dose generic regimens, and second, achieving low drug prices through maximum competitive bidding. With the new WTO ruling on generics, there's still debate over how intellectual property laws governing patents will affect the use of new Indian and Thai fixed-dose pills not yet used in the West.

On December 1, 2003, the WHO announced the creation of the AIDS Medicines Diagnostics Facility, which will provide direct support to countries on procurement and management of health-care-related commodities. The WHO plans to establish a number of "buyers' clubs" – pooled procurement bodies – for antiretroviral drugs and low-cost tests.

But it will not procure the drugs directly, other than in exceptional circumstances.[30]

The Role of Watchdog Groups

The up-side of the pricing war is the greater scrutiny that has been applied to the overall field of medical and drug research and development. In the US, the role of consumer watchdog groups has been critical. The Washington-based Consumer Project on Technology, led by James Love, deserves a lot of credit for its prescient focus on the field of patents and intellectual property. Other groups are now emerging to provide in-depth analyses of the economic structures that control access to other commodities, such as food and clean water, and other essential resources that are critical to public health. The San Francisco-based International Forum on Globalization (IFG), a think tank addressing the impact of globalization, is now turning to look at essential medicines in developing countries as they relate to contested arenas like the WTO, and the looming Free Trade of the Americas Agreement.

The result of this activity is the occasional merging of two political movements: AIDS and access to drugs, and the anti-globalization camp. They came together to target the main lending and trade bodies, starting with fiery protests at the Seattle WTO ministerial meeting in 1999, and followed by small-scale actions at the World Bank headquarters in Washington, D.C., in 2000 (and again in 2002); the African Union Summit in Abuja, Nigeria in 2001 (where African activists led the battle); the G-8 meetings in Okinawa in 2000; Genoa in 2002 – another heated street battle; and the WTO ministerial meeting in Cancún in September 2003.

Unfortunately, these two protesting camps haven't found common cause beyond their opposition to the corporate agendas of these large global bodies. Few anti-globalization protesters were at the UNGASS meeting, for example. Nor does ACT UP take on environmental issues. While intellectual property issues affect access to medicines, as well as clean water and food, groups working in these movements continue to focus on single issues. That is both their strength and their weakness, and activists on both sides admire and criticize each other for this. The education of AIDS activists about the impact of structural violence in other arenas – the other ongoing wars against the poor – is gradually taking place, and leading to a deeper understanding of the impact of global economic policies on other arenas that also affect public health.

Money Talks

Where do things really stand with the Bush administration and other G-8 leaders, and their political commitment to access to treatment?

In September and October 2003, key events occurred that once again transformed the landscape of our expectations regarding access to anti-retroviral drugs. They reveal how little has really changed in the fundamental attitude of the US government and its allies in the pharmaceutical industry to the value of a human life, as opposed to profits. Bush and the G-8 leaders are continuing their solid embrace of the present market-based economic system for health, and of the patent system as the key weapon to defend the investments and profits of drug companies.

As AIDS and anti-globalization activists began plotting how to derail trade talks at the WTO ministerial meeting in Cancún, rumors began circulating out of Geneva about a potential compromise deal on the famous TRIPs agreement that still blocked global access to generic drugs. On September 25, frontline NGOs such as MSF, Oxfam, Health Action International, Third World Network, and the watchdog group Consumer Project on Technology issued an e-mail alert warning global activists of an impending "drastic sellout" on AIDS generics. The US government was seeking further restrictions on exports of generic medicines by adding provisions to the famous Paragraph 6 or "Motta Text" of the 2002 Doha Declaration.

Under the US-brokered deal, only the least developed countries could import generic AIDS drugs – regardless of their domestic ability to manufacture them. Other countries could import generic AIDS drugs only if they could prove that there was insufficient domestic manufacturing capacity to make them. To do so, they had to declare a national emergency or crisis and issue a compulsory license to import outside generics. Of course, countries who depend on tourism dollars and direct foreign investment try to avoid declaring national emergencies, so that still represents a de facto barrier. The deal would also allow Eastern European countries to import generics, but not after they joined the European Union; after that the same restrictions would apply to them as to richer countries.

"The proposed deal poses so many hurdles and hoops to jump through, we are worried it may not work at all," declared MSF spokesperson Ellen 't Hoen before the deal was passed. "By continually demanding more restrictions, the US seems to be pushing for a watertight system so that no generic drugs ever get through to the patients in developing countries who desperately need them."

The next day produced a shocking development: not only was the US pushing for countries to "opt out" of any generics deal, it had already secured that agreement from G-8 countries, from middle-tier nations like Brazil and India, and even from the Asian "Tigers" – Malaysia, Indonesia, South Korea, China. In other words, the leading producers of raw materials and finished products for AIDS drugs had agreed only to export, not import for their own populations. Under the agreement, these countries can only seek to import if they can prove they lack domestic manufacturing capacity to produce the drugs for their own market.

There was also a reference to a WTO review process for countries hoping to issue compulsory licenses to import on this basis. Both potential exporters and importers would have to issue compulsory licenses under the new, onerous, deal. Never mind that China and Russia – two very populous nations – have an exploding Eurasian epidemic, and that their political leaders are dragging their feet in responding to the crisis. Calling the US deal "an unmitigated disaster," Health GAP and its NGO allies promised to derail it, and began intensive lobbying to prevent its passage.

Their efforts were largely in vain. The next day, a *New York Times* front-page story hailed the US deal as a good thing for Africa.[31] It quoted Peter Allgeier, the deputy US trade representative, saying he was hopeful it would be made policy even before Cancún. Although the Gray Lady of Journalism has been consistent in its coverage of global AIDS issues, the *Times* story read like it had been penned by a Bush speechwriter.

As tensions mounted, some twenty developing countries expressed their reservations about any revision to the Motta text, calling it a flawed agreement that left out too many people. For their part, AIDS activists were urging WTO members to scrap the Doha Declaration and start again from scratch. On the eve of the WTO's final agreement on a revision of the Motta text, worried African leaders faced a critical ethical challenge: if the deal fell through, and nothing was resolved, further delay could lead to another 2 million dead by 2004. Reluctantly – bitterly in some cases – these leaders went along. On September 2, the US-penned deal became official WTO policy.

The outcome allows the poorest nations of Africa to import generics quickly from Ranbaxy, Cipla and other private suppliers – but only if such exports do not involve an industrial or commercial goal. In other words, the Ciplas of the world can't make any money selling their drugs to the poorest countries. Analysts wondered if private generic suppliers would feel there was enough incentive to manufacture cocktails costing 50 cents a day, or a dollar a day, given these market limitations. As they pointed out, many generic companies fail to sustain their businesses when markets are not well developed.[32]

On the positive side, the deal also means that the majority of people with AIDS in the worst-affected zones can legally access generic AIDS drugs via Global Fund and Bush administration money. They can do so without this threatening the patent system, or the monopoly on AIDS drugs, which continue to be priced at $10,000 per person per year in the United States. But that limited victory comes at the human cost of many lives in other developing countries, whose governments cannot easily import generics. The language of the new deal, which is subject to interpretation, is being viewed by AIDS activists as one that gives the WTO new powers to review – and challenge – any attempts by countries to import drugs using compulsory licenses. It also leaves a barrier in place. In order to access outside generics, the exporter must also secure a compulsory license.

The Collapse of Cancún

The US chess moves around Doha provided the Bush administration with a small victory in the war against generics, but it lost a big battle when WTO trade talks completely collapsed in Cancún. Thousands of anti-globalization protesters converged on the tropical resort city, including many workers and farmers from Central America and other developing countries. Behind the police barricades, talks were bogged down over issues related to agriculture and protests over protectionist US farm and steel subsidies. Brazil and Argentina led a bloc of twenty-two developing countries to protest against the US position, displaying new regional muscle. As street protests increased, a despairing Korean farmer who blamed WTO trade laws on the loss of his livelihood, committed suicide. This shocking event drew more headlines and also contributed to the chaotic breakdown of the Cancún talks – a blow for the US.

Furious, Bush officials warned Latin American leaders against a repeat performance at the upcoming FTAA talks in November in Miami. They singled out Brazil as a "won't do" country versus other "can do" countries, and threatened to make bilateral agreements with the latter if the regional accord did not materialize. Without missing a beat, the activist camps vowed to derail the FTAA accord and set their sights on Miami.

The New Battle Zone: FTAA and Free Trade

Activists dub the proposed Free Trade Area of the Americas (FTAA) agreement "NAFTA on acid," a bitter reference to the North American Free Trade Agreement that was implemented under the Clinton administration. Critics feel that NAFTA has drastically harmed developing countries, instead of helping them develop. A recent Carnegie Endowment report issued in time for the FTAA talks shares that view, offering Mexico as an example of a country that has economically declined due to NAFTA, defying pro-growth forecasts from a decade ago.[33]

As I discussed in Chapter 4, the FTAA rules on intellectual property that the US has proposed could threaten future access to essential and generic medicines. They go beyond the restrictions on intellectual property rights and related matters that were established in the WTO Doha declaration, and are referred to as "TRIPS-Plus" rules. Among the hightlights, the new rules would: extend existing drug patents beyond the current 20 years; block the use of compulsory licenses for five years when a patent exists on a drug; give five years of patent protection to pharmaceutical test data on drug safety and efficacy (submitted by a company in order to get a drug approved), thus preventing generic competitors from getting the critical information they need to copy these drugs. Finally, FTAA rules might allow the US to pressure governments to change national laws on intellectual property rights. Instead of the pro-public health language of Doha, the new ceiling would be firmly pro-patent and anti generics.

MSF recently profiled the case of Guatemala, where AIDS drugs are not covered by patents, allowing MSF to use generics in its small program there. In April 2003, the Guatemalan government changed its national laws to give big pharma companies five years of exclusivity on test data. "This means an automatic five-year delay in the availability of generic drugs, even if they are not under patent," says MSF. Although Guatemala is the only country that's changed its laws this way, "the FTAA threatens to extend such a provision to all countries of the Americas," concludes MSF.

Activists from MSF and Health GAP, among others, are now campaigning hard to persuade countries not to approve an FTAA accord. They argue that the Doha declaration should remain the international gold standard of intellectual property laws. In a letter to US trade representatives, Health GAP activists reminded them that both the WTO and the WHO had urged member states to avoid seeking greater intellectual property requirements on countries with significant public health needs.[34]

NAFTA to CAFTA

Undeterred, the US has moved to craft a smaller regional version of the FTAA agreement, called CAFTA: the Central American Free Trade Agreement. It too is a TRIPS-Plus initiative that supports greater patent protection on products. If the US can't get hemispheric agreement to free trade, it will start smaller, vowed US negotiators.

Given the difficult economic picture in much of the world, and especially in Latin America, countries in this region do want access to US markets for their products. Pro-business groups and trade ministers have actively pushed for such accords, while other government sectors and civil groups oppose the potentially negative impact of unfettered globalization on their local economies as a whole. The conflict pits economic development against public health – a no-win situation for all parties.

In the wake of the failed Cancún talks, US hopes for quick passage of regional trade plans like the FTAA, and even CAFTA, were dimmed – but not for long. Just two days into the FTAA meeting in Miami, the US surprised critics by announcing that, as promised, it had moved to sign bilateral free-trade deals with several "can do" nations in South and Central America and the Caribbean – Columbia, Peru, Ecuador and Bolivia. Talks are also scheduled to begin with the Dominican Republic in early 2004.[35] Regardless of whether FTAA or CAFTA pass or fail, the terms of such bilateral agreements may trump accords such as TRIPs in the area of patent protection.

Regional AIDS activists attending a Global Fund meeting in Panama drafted a petition that warned of the potential drastic public health consequences of such accords for the region. "It is unbelievable that, just as poor countries are beginning to get access to the cheaper generic medicine for AIDS, the US government is trying a new way to close the door," said Ruben Mayorga, a Costa Rican AIDS activist with OASIS, an NGO in Guatemala. He was equally angry at his own leaders. "We are vulnerable because of our economic problems, but it doesn't help that people in our own governments are helping them to do it."

The Religion Card

Bush's new AIDS initiative also gives outside groups with specific religious agendas greater leverage to determine the social, economic and health agendas of developing countries. He did a similar thing in the US, creating new drug treatment and AIDS initiatives so that faith-based groups could qualify for federal funding. These groups, of course, oppose condoms and innovative safer sex programs aimed at sex workers and gay men. The administration did this by rewriting regulations to relax rules that have prevented the government from funding such groups. They've also gone after AIDS groups, in San Francisco and elsewhere, who run explicit safer sex campaigns aimed at gay men, pulling federal funding from such programs.

Globally and domestically, this is not a benign agenda. It leads to discrimination and, ironically, could harm AIDS prevention efforts. Across the world, religious groups are responsible for providing many health and humanitarian services. But they are varied in their programs. Those that Bush supports tend to have a very conservative "family values" agenda. And conservatives take a dim view of homosexuality, and of outreach to such vulnerable communities.

Targeting Abortion

As I mentioned in the introduction, one of Bush's first acts as president was to make good on a campaign pledge to reinstate the Mexico City Gag policy first passed by Ronald Reagan, then cast aside by Clinton, which bans federal funding for any programs working abroad that support abortion. Bush officials immediately targeted Planned Parenthood, a major provider of women's and reproductive health services internationally. In a more recent move, the administration pulled funding for a small but well-regarded AIDS program for African and Asian refugees, Marie Stopes International. It did so on the same day Bush trade officials moved to block generic access for all but the poorest countries – a double blow.

Marie Stopes provides AIDS counseling and health-care services for thousands of people in Angola, Congo, Rwanda and Eritrea. Its activities have been praised in the past by State Department officials as "very useful" and "good work" – but that is not the point. Under Bush, the State Department went even further to try to push the anti-abortion agenda into the AIDS arena: it offered six other relief organizations money if they would sever their partnerships with Marie Stopes International.

One of its partners in China is the United Nations Population Fund (UNFPA), an agency accused by the Bush administration in 2002 of cooperating with the Chinese government to support abortions. According to a *New York Times* story, state department officials admit they have no evidence to suggest that Marie Stopes International is or was involved in forced abortions or involuntary sterilization. These now-banned practices still occur in China, where a one-child-per-family rule has long been in effect.[36]

The pulling of the Marie Stopes funding sent a chill through the NGO community, but is squarely in line with Bush policy. The groups, organized into the Reproductive Health for Refugees Consortium, declined the Bush administration's offer, calling the accusations "baseless."[37] It's worth noting that one of these groups is CARE, a major food donor in Africa, and in poor countries elsewhere, like Haiti.

Bush's ABCs

A key tenet of the Bush initiative is its focus on a Ugandan model that stresses prevention ABCs: abstinence, betrothal and, only when necessary, condoms. The latter are viewed as a last resort, according to Bush officials.[38]

The ABC plan in Uganda is credited with falling HIV rates, and with the adoption of monogamy among more young couples. That may well be, but epidemiologists have also noted that the high death rate in Uganda, as in other hard-hit countries like Haiti, played a role in the stabilization or plateauing of what they term "mature" epidemics. In other words, many of the people who passed along the virus in the early years are now dead.

My own experience is that the ABC model has failed many of the HIV-positive women and mothers I interviewed in Kampala, because they were virgins who got married and were infected by their often older husbands. They had practiced the ABCs until marriage, but were not tested before having sex with their husbands, and they did not use condoms because they wanted children. They were diagnosed in prenatal clinics – not because they showed signs of infection or illness. The ABC model may fit Bush's born-again Christian moral agenda, but not Uganda's social and cultural reality. There, women are expected to marry young and bear children. There are double standards regarding female and male sexual monogamy, and polygamy is practised by some groups. Many HIV-positive husbands had clearly had sexual relations before their marriages. Some were HIV-positive widowers who had buried wives who had died of AIDS. They had moved to new cities to remarry without disclosing their HIV status to their new spouses and, in some cases, had knowingly exposed these women to infection. Some women knew their polygamous HIV-positive husbands had not told their second wives about their HIV status; these first wives felt it was not their role to inform the other woman. In other cases, men had no idea they were themselves HIV-positive and possibly exposing their new brides to infection. But no matter: the ABCs fit Bush's "compassionate conservatism."

Reversing Gains

Further, the ABCs as promoted by Bush officials are not only a serious threat to the control of HIV in Africa; they may even increase the spread of the epidemic. They limit proven prevention weapons: education and discussions of sexuality and safer sex, aimed at young men and women; condoms; family planning services for women; targeted outreach to sexually vulnerable groups such as gay and bisexual men and sex workers. With 10 to 20 percent of Africans in some countries already exposed to this virus, withdrawing access to condoms seriously limits the ability of sexually active adults to avoid exposure to a lethal virus. This policy targets women especially, because they are socially disempowered in issues of sexual decision-making, and already lack access to women-controlled means of prevention, including female condoms. By increasing women's vulnerability to HIV exposure, the ABCs risk exposing future generations of now unborn children as well.

When safer sex and condoms are removed from the prevention menu, women and men who engage in commercial sex have no means of protecting themselves either. In all countries, prostitution is often a last resort for individuals with limited means of supporting themselves. Removing condoms will also greatly impact on gay and bisexual men, and on transgendered individuals who are at statistically higher risk of contracting HIV. Here again, homophobia raises its ugly head.

Looking ahead, it's important for health officials in Uganda and civic organizations everywhere to look closely at the repercussions of adopting models that may seem morally appealing to some, but fail to address the needs and vulnerabilities of the people, including young married women. It's one thing to argue against promiscuity and sex before marriage, but at the end of the day the US favoring of sexual abstinence over C may be tantamount to a death sentence for many if it becomes national AIDS policy.

Financial Stakes

It's important to understand that the Bush global AIDS plan was financially supported by big pharma companies, who paid up to $25,000 each to help win passage of the bill.[39] They wanted to make sure that they get a share of any new markets for AIDS drugs created by the program. Even they admit it: "Yes, it makes the companies look good," said John Vandenheuvel, a GOP strategist working for the Coalition for AIDS Relief in Africa, a lobbying group that supported the bill. "Yes, it helps them with the president. But there really is a practical matter for all of these companies doing business in Africa. All the major multinational pharmaceuticals have some type of [AIDS] program they are already using and would like to have it utilized as part of the [Bush] plan."

So the issues underlying the Bush global AIDS initiative are hardly limited to religious opposition to abortion, or condoms, or sex outside of marriage, or prostitution, or homosexuality. It's about profit. Bush officials continue to insist that Africa isn't ready for the millions it has to offer, which is why it pulled back $1 billion of the initial $3 billion authorized by Congress for the first year of the program. While US trade officials were working at the WTO to block access to generics, a group of GOP leaders toured Africa, including Senate Majority Leader Bill Frist (R-Tenn), a physician and conservative politician, and Senator Lamar Alexander (R-Tenn). Lamar told reporters: "My sense of things is that the African system can't absorb too much money too quickly."

In his view, Congress should put its money first into ensuring safe blood transfusions, use of clean needles and – no surprises here – establishing a private US agency to send volunteers to Africa to work with existing organizations. Hence, the famous Volunteers for Prosperity – Americans with good jobs, degrees and enough money to be able to volunteer to work in Africa – would actually benefit from the money earmarked for the poorest countries.[40]

Biotech Buy-In?

A telling aspect of the myriad agendas that underlie Bush's global AIDS bill is the last-minute inclusion of a clause, slipped in by Frist, that calls for the use of genetically modified foods in any food aid given to recipient countries. These GM foods, are largely produced by five US biotech companies: Monsanto, AstraZeneca, Novartis, Dupont/Pioneer and Avantis. As with AIDS drugs, the GM issue involves patent and profit battles within global trade bodies like the WTO.

The Bush administration has made it a priority to push GM foods and support big biotech companies. It has also used UN programs to "dump" surplus GM food, according to Greenpeace and Actionaid.[41] In recent years, several African governments have refused US food aid because it consisted of GM maize and GM seeds, and they fear these will cross-pollinate with local plant varieties and destroy local agriculture.[42] European countries have also rejected US GM food and demanded strict labeling of such products, to the anger of US agribusiness.

Within the WTO, the battle between US trade officials and those of very poor African countries has been fierce around this issue. One question to ask is: Now that the US has allowed generic AIDS drugs for the least-developed countries, will it win concessions on GM food? Will the global AIDS bill provide a neat entry not only for big pharma companies, but big biotech companies as well?

Privatizing Health

In a September–October 2003 issue of *Foreign Affairs*, political analyst Steven Radelet noted that Bush has backed the biggest increase in US foreign aid in decades. In his view, Bush is using foreign aid as a "soft" power that balances his use of "hard" power, like the war in Iraq or the War on Terror. In addition to his global AIDS program, Bush has allocated $300 billion to fight famine, and for "complex emergencies."

Several other foreign aid initiatives were launched by Bush in May 2003, along with his global AIDS bill, which, taken together, reflect an overall vision of private–public partnerships designed to promote his conservative religious agenda, as well as the economic ideals of free trade.

Similarly, Bush's new Millennium Challenge Account (MCA) is a fund that will provide $5 billion a year to selected countries "ruling justly, investing in their people, and establishing economic freedom." The emphasis here is on rewarding countries that adopt US economic reforms along with democratic political models. This is partly a response to the threat of terrorism, claim Bush officials.

The MCA will be run by a newly created government corporation, the Millennium Challenge Corporation, with oversight by a board of directors chaired by the Secretary of State. It will reward countries based on indicators of success that include factors like budget deficits, trade policy, immunization rates, primary school completion rates, control of corruption, and protection of civil liberties.

How will countries receiving MCA dollars feel about challenging the US on generic drugs? In 2006, the MCA may expand to cover middle-income countries, including, Radelet says, "several countries of strategic interest to the United States – such as Russia, Columbia, Egypt, Jordan and Turkey – raising the possibility that MCA funds would be diverted for political purposes."

Prevention: Losing Ground

The politicizing of HIV prevention is a dangerous trend. Even as prevention efforts begin to pay off in some countries, like Cuba, Uganda, Thailand and Haiti, the epidemic is fast developing in Russia and China, part of the runaway nexus of "next wave" countries hit by HIV. It is also rising again in the United States, particularly among certain groups, including young gay men, after having leveled off.

I wasn't able to visit China because, on the eve of my planned trip, the SARS epidemic broke out. But there, too, the numbers keep being revised upward. In November 2003, global health officials warned that more than 1 million might already be exposed in China, more than projected just a few months before. By 2010, there may be 10 million Chinese exposed to HIV – an unbelievable statistic. Chinese officials admit to 840,000 HIV/AIDS cases, and 150,000 deaths since 1985.[43] The WHO recently warned that more drug users were engaged in commercial sex, increasing the spread of HIV there and in Malaysia and Vietnam. With 1.2 million people in the Western Pacific region, 55,000 new cases are reported each year. By 2005, if the current rate of increase continues, 120,000 new infections will occur there annually.

What will happen if the Bush pro-abstinence, no-condom agenda is allowed to dominate prevention efforts? These numbers could get worse. That means governments need other sources of funding for targeted prevention efforts that will reach out to the heroin addicts in Russia, the young sex workers in India, the closeted gay men in Haiti, the unwed teenage girls in Mexico – instead of punishing them.

Revising the Future

In September 2003, world leaders met again at the UN to review progress since UNGASS. They declared that, without more funding, we will fall short of the prevention and treatment goals set forth at UNGASS in 2001. The Global Fund grants to date, if disbursed according to plan, will provide antiretroviral drugs for 500,000 people – a tripling of the coverage in poor countries and a six-fold increase in Africa. The drop in drug costs will change that number. Current AIDS-related funding for developing countries is expected to reach $5 billion by the end of this year, a 20 percent increase over last year and a 500 percent increase since 1996. But twice that amount – $10 billion – is needed by 2005 to achieve the goals laid out at UNGASS.

By the WHO's calculation in July 2003, the global treatment roll-out will increase slowly at first, extending treatment to thousands of people in countries in 2004 as national programs are put in place and training is extended to health professionals. But from 2005 on, it will rise exponentially. These calculations were also made before the events of September at the WTO, and others that have increased the odds of a faster roll-out. As more money comes, and new players jump in, these numbers are being constantly revised.

Another important step was made in October 2003 by Canada, which is considering revising national patent laws to make generics available to governments. That would make Canada the first country to export generic AIDS drugs legally, and to do so within the legal framework of the recent WTO – TRIPS agreement hammered out in the week before Cancún. But as I write, Canada has hit a number of stumbling blocks as it tries to amend complex laws on intellectual property, and make them fit with other accords.

This move, coupled with the drop in generic prices reached by the Clinton group, has caused the WHO to revise its projections beyond 2005. Now the new catchword is 4×6, or 7×10, depending on how optimistic activists and policymakers feel. In November, as it was putting the final touches to its revised 3×5 plan, the WHO estimated that 935,000 people would be on antiretroviral therapy in developing countries by 2005 under all existing programs, including those using Global Fund money and the World Bank's MAP money, among other sources. That left a gap of 2,065,000 for 2005.[44]

The Global Fund has also increased its estimates of the money needed. In July 2003, when Dr. Lee announced his plan to make good on the 3×5 plan, the Global Fund was expected to cover treatment for 400,000 people by 2008. The money would also provide voluntary HIV counseling and testing services to 31 million people. Funds for malaria would provide insecticide-treated nets to 51 million people and artemisinin-based treatment for resistant malaria for 3.6 million. It would provide short-course DOT treatment for TB to 2.9 million, and second-line therapy for drug resistant TB to 11,000 people.[45]

Now these figures will have to be revised. The drop in generic drug prices for HIV drugs means Global Fund money that's already been disbursed will cover many more people. The WHO plan does not cover TB or malaria, so these statistics remain the same, but they too are merely projections based on variables that are also likely to change as Gates money provides new insights into these diseases, as generic manufacturers produce fixed-dose pills for TB, and as other innovative strategies are applied to these concurrent diseases. It's important not to overlook the global hepatitis picture, which isn't covered by the Global Fund, but will be affected by the global focus on HIV.

The Emerging Picture

What does this all this mean with respect to people actually accessing therapy? Will there be more Brazils or not? Again, comparisons are useful. In 2001 a WHO survey showed that half of the seventy poorest countries had virtually no access to antiretroviral therapy, and no drugs to prevent mother-to-child transmission. In two-thirds of these countries, less than a quarter of the population had been tested for HIV. A year later, forty countries in sub-Saharan Africa had developed national AIDS strategies and a number were providing treatment through pilot and small-scale public-sector programs.[46] In addition to Brazil, some governments were providing free drugs to a small number of citizens: Botswana, Cuba, Costa Rica, Thailand, Nigeria and Senegal. After the first round of grants by the Global Fund, the number of people on therapy in developing countries doubled.

In 2002, 300,000 people were on drugs, with half in Brazil alone. The WHO's figures showed that only 1 percent of people in sub-Saharan Africa who needed therapy had it – some 50,000 people out of an estimated 4,100,000 who were ill and required the drugs immediately. In Asia, the figure was 4 percent – some 43,000 people on therapy out of 1,000,000; in Eastern Europe, 9 percent: just 7,000 people on therapy out of 80,000 needing drugs. But as my report from Russia shows, these numbers are low estimates of the true need. In Latin America, coverage was 53 percent, with 196,000 people on therapy out of 370,000. Again, testimony by those in Mexico shows that these official numbers must be treated with caution.

By the end of 2002 the WHO's estimate had increased the number of people on therapy in Africa to 70,000 outside Brazil. And round two funding commitments for 2002 from the Global Fund will provide treatment for almost a half-million more people. Beyond these numbers are ambitious plans for putting more people on treatment. The Economic Community of West African States (ECOWAS), for example, has committed itself to providing treatment for 400,000 people, which covers a third of those needing treatment in the region. Other countries have started making the drugs available both in the private sector and through small-scale private programs. Today, as the door to generics opens for the poorest countries, but not to those with a little more money, more than ninety developing countries have incorporated HIV treatment into their national programs – at least on paper.

Here are some updated country figures that show what the two-year push had achieved by July 2003. They are based largely on results from the initial phases of various national scale-up programs. In Botswana, 6,100 were on AIDS therapy, up from 4,500; in Burundi, 1,000, up from 600 a few months earlier; in Cameroon, 7,000, up from 6,000; in Thailand, 10,000; in Uganda, 10,000; in Togo, 450; in Senegal 1,500, with a goal of 7,000 by 2005. The situation in Latin America was also improving.[47]

From the perspective of doctors who had no drugs a few years ago, these numbers reflect considerable progress. "If you compare the situation in 1998 to 2003, it has dramatically turned in a good way," said Papa Salif Sow, MD, of Senegal in July.

Still, it's very uneven, and some major countries have had trouble. According to analysts on the ground in Kenya, there wasn't a single person getting drugs from the public sector there at the end of 2002. Now treatment is beginning, but there are delays associated with procurement and delivery. Countries like Angola and Sierra Leone are struggling with the aftermath of civil wars, while the Congo is still locked in internecine battles involving armies from neighboring countries. Even as governments commit to treatment, their soldiers are raping women and spreading HIV, and little action has been taken to stop them. That makes it hard to tally real progress when, for every step forward, more steps are taken to increase HIV's prevalence. Political will cannot be confined to an AIDS plan, but needs to include government commitment to address HIV in the army, as well as rape and war, and other regional engines of the epidemic.

Congo is a good example. In December, World Bank officials said they were prepared to give $1 million to the country to battle AIDS, while women continued to stream in to clinics reporting rape linked to the still-simmering civil war.[48] Half of all people in the country's hospitals were AIDS cases, and the epidemic may threaten half the country's population of 50 million within a decade, according to the national AIDS program (PNLS). HIV prevalence is now 12 to 15 percent in four of the country's eleven provinces – twice that of the provinces that were spared the worst of the five-year war. Over 80 percent of cases were linked to sexual transmission, in a country where many youths begin sexual activity at as young as twelve, and half of young people by sixteen. "If this trend continues, it will not be an exaggeration to say that in 10 years time there won't be a future generation," predicted PNLS director Jack Kokolomani.

This is also true of South Africa. But the political picture there and the global focus on its epidemic have radically improved – after years of what many consider criminal inaction by the Thabo Mbeki government. Given South Africa's regional power and its resources, its actions have had a severe effect on the whole region. It will take years to undo the damage Mbeki's policies have caused. A generation of Africans, including young people, are now suspicious of HIV and the agenda of doctors and treatment advocates, due to his misguided views on AIDS.

Mbeki's stranglehold on AIDS was broken by TAC and its allies by the National Association of People living With AIDS in South Africa (NAPWA), union activists from COSATU, frontline doctors like James McIntyre and Glenda Grey of the Soweto clinic, political figures like Bishop Desmond Tutu, openly gay judge Edward Cameron, Patricia Delille, an outspoken member of Parliament, Nelson Mandela and his wife, Graca Machel, and his ex-wife, Winnie Mandela, as well as many others across civil society, particularly student and youth groups. They formed a broad coalition with former anti-apartheid groups and mobilized what has become the biggest grassroots AIDS movement in a developing world. TAC's defiance and civil disobedience campaigns, its many fights with drug companies, its illegal importation of generic fluconazole, its national rallies – all were pivotal steps in the larger global movement.

It was TAC's re-launching of a civil disobedience campaign that tipped the balance toward victory in South Africa. November 19, 2003 will go down in history as the day South Africa regained hope. The government's national plan of free antiretroviral treatment has begun right away in two provinces, Gauteng and Western Cape. The goal is to treat 1.2 million citizens by 2008 – a quarter of the current HIV-positive population.[49] The cost of the plan could be close to $680 million dollars a year, with $45 million to be spent by the end of 2003. Over half the plan will focus on implementing treatment and building up the infrastructure.

A jubilant TAC cheered in the streets following the announcement. "We think that, with the best political will, we can bring 150,000 people into treatment in 18 months," Zackie Achmat told reporters. "If they do this, it will be the largest antiretroviral drug program in the world."[50]

Grassroots Activism

The political movement to demand access to AIDS treatment for poor countries remains a grassroots effort, led by small groups of activists, including many who represent people living with HIV and AIDS. Compared with 2001, there are more fledgling AIDS groups across Africa, Asia, Eastern Europe and elsewhere who have taken up the banner of treatment and prevention.

In South Africa, the TAC has provided a much-needed public face for people with HIV, one that is bold, smart and unafraid of the government or world opinion. It found powerful allies in COSATU and NAPWA. In Thailand, activists from NAPWA took to the courts in October 2002 to invalidate a patent claim by the US giant Bristol-Myers Squibb on a powder form of didanosine, or ddI, a nucleoside drug. They won, and Thailand produced generic ddI. Injection drug users formed a network that gave rise to the fledging Thai Treatment Action Campaign. T-TAC is also playing a regional role, networking with less established groups and individuals in Burma, Laos and Cambodia. They are now getting ready for the 2004 global AIDS conference in Bangkok, determined to gain universal access to AIDS drugs as TAC did in South Africa.

In Latin America, networks of activists have worked hard and cooperatively.[51] Some helped to import recycled drugs from donor groups in the US and Europe. Others have become experts, creating new NGOs that are now rolling out treatment education programs at the grassroots level. They are also watching the WTO and FTAA, and forging alliances with anti-globalization activists.

In Eastern Europe, activists are also networking, finding common cause after years of struggling in relative isolation. The grassroots movement is likely to have a major impact on the other regional drug war – against narcotics. Globally, the growing ties between activists in developing and developed countries have also provided a vital channel for sharing experiences of treatment and education, and to help activists influence national agendas for HIV.

The Human Tally

Global progress in treatment and prevention is unlikely to overshadow the deaths of the 3 to 4 million people who will not get drugs by the time of the Bangkok AIDS conference in 2004 – the next global landmark. Remember that 6 million need drugs *now*. If 1 or 2 million get them next year, 4 or 5 million don't. Given that the estimates of need are being made based on criteria of AIDS, i.e., very advanced illness, that mean many of them will die in the coming months. Each of these deaths is an indictment of our failure to do what we could in fact do, which is to treat them now. Globally, we have the money, and we have the drugs. We simply don't have the political will.

The human cost of our recent failure and delay in responding to this crisis is the deaths of 2.4 million Africans in 2002 – out of 3.1 million deaths globally. There were 3.5 million new HIV infections in Africa out of 5 million globally. Staggeringly, those between fifteen and twenty-four represented almost half (42 percent) of those new infections. The responsibility for that failure lies with each country and every government, with each political leader who did not act. It lies with George Bush, dubbed the greatest menace to democracy by George Soros, the man pushing democracy and harm-reduction in Russia.

Despite this failure, I want to close with a tribute to the pioneers, the physicians and the activists, those in the trenches who refused to accept the deaths of the tens of thousands of people who have now been saved due to the delivery of antiretroviral therapy since 2001. Against the highest odds, they have provided the world with a global response to AIDS and a blueprint for action.

AFTERWORD

Truth is a powerful weapon. Wherever it is lacking, it is essential that it should be provided. The identities of victims and perpetrators, the crimes committed, and the attempts made to explain them away or cover them up should all be revealed. Following a period of massive abuses, an essential part of the process of assessing responsibility and of demonstrating respect for those who suffered is the official disclosure of truth and acknowledgement of culpability.

Aryeh Neier, *War Crimes*, 1998.

Having summarized my thoughts on the global effort to scale up treatment for AIDS, I feel it is important to celebrate the critical steps that have been taken since the Durban conference in 2000. Has it been revolutionary? Yes, in some ways it has. The focus on drug prices and the war over patents has changed the landscape of access to medicine for people in poor countries. It has refocused global attention on the link of both economics and politics to global public health. The fight has taken place in the arena of AIDS, but it is already affecting other illnesses such as TB, malaria, and tropical diseases that also require urgent attention. The infrastructure being developed to deliver health-care is also a kind of nation-building, or development. Public health is becoming more of an issue of equity and human rights. We should celebrate every life that has been saved and every adult, child and infant who has been protected from exposure.

As I look to the future, at the forefront of my mind, however, is the continued human cost of delay. At the time of the Durban conference, 40 million people had HIV; in 2002 there were 42 million. The UNAIDS estimate on World AIDS Day, 2003, cited as many as 46 million – representing ten new HIV infections every minute. In 2000, the issue that dominated global headlines was drug prices. Once Cipla entered the arena, and the world learned about the true costs of manufacturing, the debate veered over to the cost-effectiveness of treatment, and whether saving those who were ill would somehow *harm* prevention efforts directed toward those as yet untouched by the disease.

When the opposite was shown to be true, as is documented in this book, and testing was seen as the first step to getting people into treatment, then the debate shifted to concerns about infrastructure and doubts about the ability of poor Africans to use drugs properly. Here, too, these last obstacles have proved to be decoys that have allowed political leaders and global health officials to put off for as long as possible their responsibility to provide access to treatment rapidly, and to care for citizens in the poorest countries.

Throughout this tumultuous period, it has still been considered acceptable for political leaders to debate openly who will live and who will die, in pragmatic and economic terms; to debate the merits of saving the uninfected versus the infected person; to weigh these human lives on a scale of human productivity and lost human capital. It has come down to dollars and cents: to how much treatment costs per person per year for each given country or municipality, versus the potential lost profits of the wealthiest multinational corporations in the most profitable industrial sector – pharmaceuticals. Although ethical, moral and humanitarian issues drive the activist movement for access to AIDS drugs, individuals at the highest echelons of government are displaying a rather easy acceptance of the idea of another 2 or 3 million dead as the details of treatment, or profit and losses, are worked out.

That still remains true, after all the early debates have given way to the simple fact that what pioneering groups first claimed is true: it is possible to treat the poorest people effectively with AIDS drugs, and it costs less to do so than we projected. The barrier to access is not poverty, or illiteracy, or the inability of Africans to take their drugs consistently, or any other indices of national development or capacity; it is a lack of political commitment, pure and simple. That is what essentially fills the global gap in treatment access. That is what seals the fate of those who lie in their village clinics, hospice or hospital beds right now, suffering with little relief, and with limited access to palliative care.

As with falling drug prices, the main shift in the arena of global AIDS has been our collective expectation of what is possible. Once drug companies decided to package three drugs in one, once Cipla decided to make a low-cost generic copy, once health leaders decided to adopt simpler guidelines for using and monitoring people on therapy, barriers fell away. The disease did not change – people simply changed what they thought about the problem.

Whether we decide the lives of poor people with AIDS around the world are worth saving, then, is really the fundamental ethical question that we face. It is essentially the same question we faced in 2000, and before that, in 1998, 1997 and 1996, when we began offering treatment to people in rich countries. The difference now is that we lack the comfort of false arguments that allowed many people to keep these central moral issues at arm's length. The main actors who have blocked access to treatment have hardly changed their stripes, only their tactics and reactions to developments in this field. But so have those pushing for access. Low-cost treatment is becoming more available, but it is not universal. There is money, but not enough of it, and it comes with many strings attached. Nor will it be made available without continued, intensive political fights.

I have singled out the Bush administration in this book as the greatest barrier to access to cheap AIDS medicines for the world. If Bush wanted to save the world from global AIDS, overnight, he could, in fact, move some mountains. But his administration – ultra-conservative, far-right Christians and their allies – have decided to erect new ones instead. The price of their policies will be paid dearly in continued death and suffering. We should hold them accountable for their actions.

Before antiretroviral drugs were available, and arguably before it was known that these drugs could be made so cheaply as generics; before the pioneering groups who are profiled in this book presented evidence of their ability to treat people in the poorest settings of Africa with minimal resources, perhaps the failure to do better, or at least to try, was something many people in the world could justify.

But that day has passed. There are really no good reasons, no matter how sophisticated or crude. There is only the continued complicity of those who act to block access to treatment, and the complicity of the rest of us who are aware of their actions and fail to stop them.

There are, however, sharp differences between these two groups, as Aryeh Neier points out in his 1998 book, *War Crimes*.[1] In it, he tackles the murky waters that separate individual from collective responsibility and guilt in the arena of crimes against humanity, when the subject is genocide.

Does the global treatment gap for AIDS drugs constitute genocide? Consider the first textbook definition of the word, put forward just before the Nuremberg trials by Raphael Lemkin, a Polish–Jewish scholar, working for the United States War Department. He defined the crime as "a coordinated plan of different actions aimed at the destruction of essential foundations of life of different groups." A more modern definition is "a variety of acts that in combination were carried out for the purpose of ending, or ending in significant part, a distinct group's continued existence."[2]

Who is being killed by this gap in AIDS treatment? The poor, regardless of nation. The most disenfranchised, regardless of nation. That the majority are not white in Africa, Asia and Latin America bears stressing again, in order to make it absolutely clear that racism is a major part of this crime.

The question of intent is the one that makes it so hard for human rights advocates to agree on cases of genocide. But think of it: we do know that withholding medicine, delaying money, blocking access to drugs, and otherwise failing to treat will cause 2 or 3 million people to die in the next twelve months. We also know that withholding condoms in African populations where HIV awareness is low and 10 to 40 percent of citizens are already HIV-positive is a recipe for spreading HIV. That's a core part of Bush's ABC prevention policy. Don't forget – almost half of new infections globally are in young people, who will then face a life with HIV and, without treatment, the threat of a painful death. Given the scale of the epidemic, and the characteristics of those who are suffering and vulnerable, then the term genocide is relevant. US officials and those in other governments who, at the WTO and in other forums, agree to economic deals that effectively block access to generic AIDS therapies for people in all but the least developed countries, knowing many people will die without them, are more than implicated.

"The very phrase 'crimes against humanity' connotes that it is not only a particular group that has been injured but the entire human race," writes Neier. "Accordingly, all have a responsibility to see that justice is done."[3]

I've introduced this weighty and difficult concept – genocide – with its historical gravitas and ability to make us wince, because I think it fits, for me, as the rare word I can find that matches the breadth and impact of the AIDS pandemic. And because, unlike the Holocaust, where some could claim ignorance of the fate of the Jews, we are collectively, in this world of instantaneous communications, fully aware of the consequences that a lack of HIV treatment will cause for some 6 million of the now 46 million people who need drugs today. It is going to cause them to die agonizing deaths, without even the benefit of medicines to relieve their suffering.

How many of those 46 million will die? It's impossible to estimate. But we can take a few rough measures from some of the countries I visited and extrapolate. In Carletonville, over 70 percent of young women are already HIV-positive. That's astonishing. So are the high HIV rates in the mining workforce and military of several of the African countries. If the South African government comes through, a sizeable percentage of those young women may access free generic pills made by Aspencare, possibly via an extension one of the mining companies' workplace treatment programs into the local community. But the Mbeki government is still dragging its feet in delivering on the plan, and stigma is preventing workers from taking advantage of the offer of treatment. I predict a lot of those young girls are going to get sick before they get to swallow a once-a-day pill, unless something radically changes in the present equation.

South Africa is at one extreme end of the spectrum, with such high prevalence rates. But look at China. One million people are already exposed, and the number is multiplying faster than officials can keep track. The dire forecast is 10 million Chinese with HIV by 2010. Will that spell 4 or 5 million more infections in China alone by 2005? That would outstrip the entire number of people the WHO is hoping to save by putting them on treatment. If treatment fails, we lose on the prevention front, too.

Lest we get overwhelmed, think of the alternative. With treatment, the majority of 46 million people could survive – and even thrive. It costs 38 cents a day per person. That price might go down to a quarter, who knows? We – the world – can afford this. It takes only a few weeks for a once-a-day pill to work, even in severe AIDS cases, as you've read. My point is: there is a solution here, and it's clearly visible to us now. What we need to see is how and why and by whom it is being blocked.

I also think it's important, as Neier argues, to stop promoting abstract notions of collective guilt that prevent individuals from confronting their own, often lesser, and largely passive complicity in such crimes. Too often, he writes, this leads to the absolution "of those who actually create great crimes on the grounds that if all are guilty, no one is guilty."

Considering the current state of global AIDS treatment, who is responsible? The actions of the CEOs of Merck and Pfizer and other drug giants are different from those of laboratory scientists who may have public health interests in mind when they create new compounds, or the average American shareholder in these large companies. Their actions are also different from those of the WHO and other humanitarian agency officials who lacked courage and leadership, or bowed to political pressure as they delayed in acting decisively to scale up treatment last year. They are also different from the actions of a George Bush or a Thabo Mbeki – elected leaders who are accountable to their citizens.

Yet we are all members of this global body politic. We are all threatened by AIDS. Even when we remain passive in the face of the blocking of AIDS treatment for the world, we bear a responsibility. Our knowledge of the crime makes us complicit. Our inaction thus speaks as loudly as our actions. As you read this book, you too have become complicit in the knowledge that it is still possible to prevent these crimes against humanity. Whether you accept it or not, you have a global citizen's responsibility to respond.

When I drove up the Haitian mountains by Jeep to visit the Cange clinic, I was thinking about the practical and logistical challenges to treatment, not politics per se. I was thinking about what was needed, what was being debated, and what was being provided to villagers in remote, rural Haiti: the concrete evidence – the proof of the concept – that AIDS treatment can work in the poorest settings. That's what I went searching for and, as this book documents, I found plenty of it.

But I also encountered what I started to call, to myself, privately and then more publicly, crimes against humanity – only a few of which I document here. The more countries I visited, the more I made the connections that link the issue of lack of access to AIDS drugs and health-care to specific economic policies.

The gap in treatment is not a historic given; it's been created and is actively maintained. Not by faceless corporations, but by key individuals within those commercial entities who use soft-money contributions to political leaders to promote pro-business policies that may run counter to global health needs. These people have names, they have e-mail addresses, they often have very conservative political agendas. They are united by their stakes in businesses that are part of the global economic system, one that views new forums like the WTO and the FTAA as tools for enrichment. They tacitly accept global inequity and feel little responsibility for how their actions affect citizens everywhere. These individuals, through their institutions and corporations, have gone to great lengths, often far away from the sphere of HIV and AIDS, to prevent 40, then 42, now 46 million people from accessing lifesaving drugs to treat AIDS and other diseases.

In his recent book, *Pathologies of Power*, Paul Farmer referred to this politico-economic matrix as structural violence. He called it "a set of historically given . . . and often enough, economically driven conditions" that impact negatively on health access for the poor.[4] Systemic structural violence, he found, is "a broad rubric that includes a host of offenses against human dignity: extreme and relative power, social inequalities ranging from racism to gender inequality, and the more spectacular forms of violence that are uncontestedly human rights abuses, some of them punishment for efforts to escape structural violence." Structural violence, not drug prices, is the root cause of the global gap in AIDS treatment. That is as true today as it was twenty years ago, when AIDS first appeared on the shores of Lake Victoria in Uganda, or the villages surrounding Cange in Haiti.

I'd like to close *Moving Mountains* with a quote from a statement made in the fall of 2003 by a group of Zambians living with HIV and AIDS in Lusaka, where a few thousand people have started treatment. They presented their global plea to Stephen Lewis, the UN Secretary General's Special Envoy for HIV/AIDS in Africa. Lewis is among the people I most admire in the global AIDS arena, because he has refused to give in to his growing despair, and has remained a remarkable and passionately humane emissary – a one-man Cassandra of sorts – warning political leaders of the price we are paying for their denial and complacency in the face of our century's greatest global threat.

"For each day that passes without people accessing treatment we attend funerals," said the Zambians.

> People die. We hear a hundred reasons for not providing people with treatment. For each reason given, lives are lost. The government must realize that it has a responsibility to provide health-care for its people. Any government

that fails to put in place measures to ensure the health of its citizens is not a government worth its name. Such governments should resign. If it does not do so, then people are justified to remove it by any means necessary.

The right to life and dignity should not be a preserve of the rich and powerful. What we are seeing in Zambia is a microcosm of what is happening globally. The HIV/AIDS crisis is not a crisis of lack of resources. It is a crisis of lack of conscience. It is the obscene gap between the haves and the have-nots that is driving this holocaust.

Let me end with the old Haitian proverb: *Deye mon, genyen mon*. Beyond the mountains, more mountains.

And behind more mountains, more people – our collective future.

World AIDS Day – December 1, 2003
San Francisco, California

Appendix A

LOW-TECH TREATMENT GUIDELINES

The main topics covered in the WHO treatment guidelines for resource-limited settings concern the initiation of antiretroviral therapy: when to start, what drugs to use, when to switch, how to monitor treatment, problems of toxicity and resistance, and specific treatment issues concerning women (including pregnant women), children, drug users and other special groups. These also cover potency, dosing, drug interactions, managing HIV-TB co-infections, and the difficulties of distinguishing symptoms of HIV drug failure from immune restoration syndrome.

The guidelines limit antiretroviral therapy to patients who have AIDS or are sick, using WHO staging criteria for HIV disease. This covers individuals with WHO Stage IV disease (clinical AIDS), those with WHO Stage I, II and III HIV disease and CD4 T-cell counts below 200, and those with WHO Stage II and III HIV disease with a total lymphocyte count (TLC) of below 1,200. They recommend a dual nucleoside analog regimen of AZT/3TC combined with a non-nuke like nevirapine (NVP) or abacavir (ABC) for first- and second-line therapy, or substitution of compatible combinations like d4T/3TC, d4T/ddI and AZT/ddI. Other combinations are toxic and should never be used together, for example AZT with d4T. The guidelines duly note that cross-resistance to nukes can develop, making adherence important. Side-effects such as lactic acidosis and mitochondrial toxicity are of particular concern to pregnant women and children.

In terms of monitoring, the guidelines suggest that any doctor can offer HIV therapy if HIV antibody testing is available to a patient and the doctor is trained to do syndromic management. The first step involves basic clinical monitoring: obtaining a patient's past medical history; identifying current or past opportunistic infections (OIs); screening for co-infections such as tuberculosis; and for women, testing for pregnancy. Details of these guidelines are outlined in Appendix B.

The guidelines offer a tiered scale for laboratory testing, starting with "absolute minimum tests," which include an HIV antibody test and a blood test for hemoglobin (a protein that enables red blood cells to carry oxygen from the lungs to the rest of the body) and hematocrit levels. "Basic" testing includes a white blood cell count and differential that can pick up common antiretroviral side-effects such as neutropenia, and provides a total lymphocyte count, or TLC (a measure of the total number of immune system cells, including CD4 and CD8 T-cells). In studies to date, the authors note that TLC correlates poorly with CD4 T-cell levels, but provides a good marker for prognosis and survival when used with WHO clinical disease staging criteria. Other "basic" tests include blood sugar, liver and kidney function, and pregnancy tests. "Desirable" tests include bilirubin (a liver test), amylase (a pancreatic test) and serum lipids; these are particularly useful to monitor antiretroviral toxicities as well. CD4 T-cell tests are also "desirable," but a viral load test is merely optional.

Drug resistance tests don't make the cut at all, being too costly. But resistance testing for sentinel purposes is needed to identify resistant viral strains in a given population. The WHO is now setting up a Global HIV Drug Resistance Network to assist member states in this task. To help individuals adhere, the guidelines recommend a low-cost formula used in the US: patient education, continued counseling and, when possible, involvement and support by the family and community. They also suggest a strategy of Directly Observed Therapy (DOT) for antiretroviral therapy, borrowed from TB management. What isn't adequately addressed is the issue of public stigma, which makes people reluctant to get tested for HIV – a critical step in accessing antiretrovirals – and reluctant to seek care until they are quite sick. That includes discrimination by health professionals who fear exposure to HIV.

Risks for Women and Children

The guidelines highlight the risks of using standardized regimens and specific drugs in some groups. Women who plan to have children, or who are at risk of unplanned pregnancies, should stay clear of Sustiva (efavirenz) which carries the potential risk of causing birth defects. Since resistance to nevirapine can develop quickly, women might want to save that drug for prophylactic use when pregnant. A small minority of patients are hypersensitive to nevirapine, which can cause a rash; if undetected, this can lead to fatal Stevens-Johnson syndrome. But the downside of a substitute regimen like AZT/3TC/abacavir is that its efficacy is not known in patients with advanced AIDS or very high viral loads. There's also a risk of hypersensitivity to abacavir in children. Finally, lactic acidosis and mitochondrial toxicity pose special risks for women and children, but the long-term consequences are impossible to gauge. Longitudinal studies and national toxicity databases could help assess this risk.

People living in West Africa may also find that the WHO's suggestions won't work as well, because they carry a viral strain of HIV called Group O, and a sister-virus called HIV-2. These viruses are endemic in the region, and naturally resistant to non-nukes. Unfortunately, the guidelines don't spell out where they are now most prevalent. Looking ahead, sentinel monitoring for Group O and HIV-2 viruses is needed.

Could a three-nuke substitute work for these patients? Generic all-nuke combination pills are gaining popularity in places like India and sub-Saharan Africa. But the WHO authors hold back on recommending them as a first-line regimen, based on limited efficacy data. There is also greater concern about increased toxicity and cross-resistance to the entire class. How well will non-nukes work as an alternative salvage regimen for such patients? That's another open, but burning, question.

What about double nukes? Avoid them if possible, say the experts. Such regimens are known to be less potent and to lead to resistance. But what if there's no money for three drugs? Case studies show patients can still benefit from suboptimal therapy. Ethically, many doctors choose to treat sick or dying patients with two drugs, and to grapple with resistance later. To their credit, the WHO guidelines support this choice. If a two-drug regimen appears to be working, they suggest keeping a patient on the regimen and switching over to three drugs when possible. "The concession regarding two drugs reflects reality and represents a dilemma since individuals have a right to benefit from such therapy, notwithstanding the problem of drug resistance," acknowledges McGill University's Mark Wainberg, MD.

Where does that leave protease inhibitors (PIs)? The advantage of these drugs is their potency; their drawback is toxicity, higher pill counts, and their potential interactions with drugs used to treat TB. Due to their cost, PIs offer a good switch or salvage regimen when combined with two nukes. Generic companies are moving forward to market fixed-dose pills, including PIs.

Field Application

How useful are these guidelines for doctors and patients? That depends on who's treating and who's being treated – and for how long. What's good in theory can be hard in practice. It's also important to consider what is missing from the guidelines. There is not much attention paid to food and nutrition for patients on antiretrovirals, but field doctors say this is a critical aspect of managing malnourished patients with HIV. STD screening and treatment, and prophylactic treatment for OIs, are also given comparatively little attention. There's passing mention of complementary herbal therapies and traditional medicines used in different countries. Non-medical and social issues that impact on access to care also fall outside the scope of the guidelines.

The guidelines note that co-infections like TB impact on HIV and vice-versa, and that HIV drugs interact negatively with TB drugs. They suggest treating active TB cases first, to avoid stressing the liver and causing drug interactions, but that's often hard to do. The phenomenon of immune restoration syndrome poses another challenge to syndromic management. Some US patients have experienced serious flare-ups of hepatitis after the initiation of antiretroviral therapy, due to the emergence of latent infections. This issue is likely to be more of a problem in developing countries, where hepatitis is widespread.

Appendix B

LOW-COST MONITORING TOOLS

The WHO's low-tech treatment guidelines include a simplified approach to monitoring patients on HIV therapy in resource-poor settings. They rely on CDC clinical staging criteria to monitor symptoms of HIV and the response to therapy. CD4 T-cell counts are used only to assess how well therapy is working. Viral load tests are not used at all (see Appendix A).

Under the new "no-to-low"-tech guidelines, HIV patients are screened and treated for TB before starting HAART, to avoid negative drug interactions between drugs that affect the liver. At that time, hemoglobin, liver and renal tests are also done. Based on CDC staging criteria, those with AIDS or clinical symptoms of HIV disease, or with no symptoms but with CD4 T-cell counts below 200, are qualified to begin HAART. Clinical evaluation of patients would take place at month one, with basic biochemistry and CD4 T-cell counts at month four and, when possible, a viral load test at month six. Others advocate a similar model, with slight variations in the schedule of follow-up tests.

In 2001 there was little solid information on how well clinical monitoring stacked up to the laboratory gold standard of the West – viral load and T-cell tests. Today there's quite a bit more evidence, but much of this comes from well-trained experts in pilot treatment studies. It remains to be seen how other doctors across Africa cope with this challenge.

A New Tool: Total Lymphocyte Count (TLC)

Experts are advocating the use of TLC as an alternative to a CD4 T-cell count, to assess the impact of therapy on survival. The TLC measures non-T-cell lymphocytes (B-cells and natural killer cells) as well as T-cells, with the latter making up the biggest portion of the TLC (though not necessarily in HIV-infected individuals). This approach requires only a light microscope, whereas CD4 T-cell tests require expensive flow cytometry. Although major hospitals in Africa have flow cytometers, the technology is relatively expensive and requires a trained operator.

How good is TLC? "Although total lymphocyte count doesn't predict who does badly [on treatment], it did reflect on survival," said Charlie Gilks of the WHO in 2001, referring to his own studies. "It is a pretty good prognostic that also correlates with CD4 T-cell count." In a presentation on surrogate markers at a 2001 Bethesda meeting on low-cost diagnostics, Victor De Gruttola of the Harvard University School of Public Health also weighed in on the adjunctive value of TLC: "Longitudinal monitoring of lymphocytes could have value for disease progression," he remarked. In small studies of people with HIV, De Gruttola found that "the mean value of TLC drops 12 percent a year, so it is meaningful in people after they develop AIDS." Once they're on therapy, TLC may not be as useful.

That's George Janossy's criticism of TLC. A top researcher from Royal Free and University College Hospitals in London, he dismisses TLC as an alternative to CD4 T-cell tests for long-term monitoring. "My opinion is that using lymphocyte counts is useless for those who need to live," he stated. "It picks up disease only at late stage." Once patients begin recovering on therapy, that strategy won't work as well, he argued.

Adapting Tests to Africa's Needs

In Senegal and Ivory Coast, clinical staging has been used successfully in small pilot projects, along with other alternative tests, to measure T-cell counts. But some African researchers worry about accepting guidance from clinical markers and lab tests whose standards derive from the blood or immune profiles of non-Africans. Little is known about what constitutes "normal" blood, lymphocyte or T cell levels among different African populations, including those with HIV. Chronic endemic diseases like TB, malaria and parasites can suppress immune function on their own, to a certain extent. TB, for example, can cause a 20 percent drop in total lymphocyte count that does not rise fully to baseline levels after successful TB treatment. Similarly, parasites can lower hemoglobin levels.

In Senegal, Serge Diabouga and colleagues, in collaboration with French researchers, have used a new low-cost system to monitor T-cell counts: "Dynabeads." This technology uses magnetic beads or particles that are coated with antibodies to T-cells' CD4 receptor. The results can be read by standard light microscopy. In a study done in seven African laboratories, Dynabead results correlated well with those from CD4 T-cell tests performed by flow cytometry. Like TLC, Dynabeads represent a labor-intensive technology that requires time-consuming manual counting; but it beats having a more sophisticated machine that requires steady electricity and someone to operate and maintain it. The Dynabead system is far cheaper than flow cytometry – only $2,000 for the equipment and $5 per test. It takes only three days to train a technician to use it. Today, the system is available at a 30 percent discount from the WHO, through a procurement plan the agency oversees. Given the constraints of manual labor and the need for highly trained technicians, it's not likely to be a long-term solution for Africa's needs, but it is filling the gap for now. Several Latin American governments are starting to use Dynabeads in their HIV treatment scale-up programs.

Testing New Products

In April 2002, a follow-up forum on low-cost diagnostics was held in Washington, DC, sponsored by the Forum for Collaborative Research, which later held a follow-up workshop at the July 2002 World AIDS Conference in Barcelona, followed by another in February 2003 in Boston. These meetings have allowed key players to share updates on the development of an array of alternative approaches to monitoring CD4 T-cell counts and viral load, as well HIV drug resistance and state-of-the-art technologies that can test for multiple infections at the same time. At the April meeting, participants formed working groups to fast-track progress on viral load and T-cell tests.

"The goal of the meeting was to map out the process of validation for alternative technologies," said Veronica Miller, MD, of the Forum. "One of the problems that we have come across in this work is the lack of leadership from organizations that should be taking that role. Development from industry and academia has been slow." Others have criticized the WHO and its representatives for failing to be better team players when it comes to sharing information and pushing forward on a unified, low-cost diagnostics agenda. "It's a turf war," said one critic, requesting anonymity. "The WHO wants this to be their baby."

One reason for this may be a new influx of funding from several foundations. In spring 2003, the Bill and Melinda Gates Foundation gave $30 million to help set up a new diagnostic initiative under the WHO's auspices. As part of the WHO's 3×5 program, it is setting up an AIDS Medicines Diagnostics (AMD) facility that will coordinate efforts to develop, test and procure low-cost monitoring tests and other tools.

The Gates Foundation funds were originally going to be handled by the Foundation for Innovative New Diagnostics (FIND) in Geneva, under the leadership of Giorgio Roscigno, former development director of the Global Alliance for TB Drug Development in New York. FIND's first target is an alternative TB test to replace time-consuming, often inaccurate sputum tests.

Gregg Gonsalves of Gay Men's Health Crisis, who co-organized the initial Bethesda meeting along with Ben Cheng, then at Project Inform, a San Francisco AIDS organization, is among those who pushed for an HIV diagnostics initiative along the lines of the International AIDS Vaccine Initiative. The IAVI program includes a pricing plan to ensure that any vaccine products it helps to develop will be affordable and distributed to poor countries. That thinking is behind the WHO's model diagnostics plan, and will help ensure that the products will be cheap when they finally reach markets. Gonsalves also worked with the Doris Duke Charitable Foundation on a grant program for research on new diagnostic tests. Recently, the European Commission has also indicated that it plans to fund this now-hot field, and will probably support the WHO's new diagnostic facility.

"I would say I'm incredibly encouraged by how collaborative everyone has been, as well as willing to share new data," said Cheng, now at the Forum.

In June 2003, Gonsalves was busy planning a meeting of big and small companies that currently manufacture HIV diagnostic tests. "We really need to start pressuring these companies to make cheaper tests available to meet the demand that's out there," he said. "As a community, we've kind of dropped the ball." He's hoping for a commitment to a tiered pricing model similar to what now exists for patented drugs, with an offer of tests at cost, or steeply discounted, for the poorest countries – a step that parallels what's occurred with HIV drugs.

Going with the Flow

In the West, flow cytometry is used for two kinds of analysis: large-scale, sophisticated scientific analysis, and more practical clinical analysis. Research laboratories use instruments equipped with multiple laser light sources that can distinguish between various sub-subsets of T-cells, dividing CD4+ and CD8+ cells into different functional categories. The second use is for medium to large-scale clinical analysis of patient samples by labs. Clinical laboratories use simpler instruments for such purposes as CD4 T-cell counts. About half the laboratories in the US use "double-platform" methods; these combine results from flow cytometers and hematology analyzers to arrive at a T-cell count. Others use "single-platform" methods, in which all the information can be collected by the flow cytometer alone. The cost of flow cytometers depends in part on how many tasks the machines are designed to carry out. The number and cost of different reagents used also affects test prices. Experts have determined that using two or three reagents produces the best results. In general, they agree, it's easier to count CD4 cells accurately than CD8 cells.

If test designers like Howard Shapiro, MD, have their way, however, existing CD4 T-cell count and viral load tests will soon seem as bulky and outdated as an LP compared with a CD. Cytometers will become smaller and simpler, and incorporate cheap, mass-produced parts. Boston-based immunologist Shapiro advocates combining inexpensive light-emitting diodes, plastics, digital technology and new antibodies to create immuno-fluorescent equipment that's cheaper to use and easier to maintain than flow cytometers. In 2002, at the Bethesda meeting, he predicted that a prototype could be built in less than a year. That hasn't quite happened, but he's not far off track.

Shapiro recently reviewed data emerging from initial studies of a half-dozen prototype flow cytometers (*Practical Flow Cytometry*, fourth edition, Wiley-Liss Publishers, 2003). These experimental approaches use different staining and "gating" methods to capture and sort cells in order to count them.

New Approaches to T-cell Analysis

The FACsCount (BD Bioscience) is a small, inexpensive machine that uses a green He-Ne laser source and prepackaged reagents to do T-cell subset analysis. It is being used in Brazil, India and Thailand. Another instrument, Luminex's Model 100 flow cytometer, has also been adapted for this task. In London, Janossy has pioneered the use of low-cost flow cytometers using cheap red diode lasers. When "Panleucogating" (a simplified fluorescent staining technique) is used with a primary CD4 gating in a double-plat-form system, "the red diode laser instruments yielded absolute CD4 T-cell counts that were closely correlated to those generated by a state-of-the-art 'full technology,'" said Janossy in a recent technical review.

Red diode lasers are also used in Partec GmbH's new CyFlow flow cytometer, which can be applied to create a mobile laboratory in an SUV with off-road capability to do CD4 T-cell counting, say company experts. But according to Janossy, the CyFlow system is being promoted for use in the field although it hasn't been tested in multi-center trials – an important step, he felt.

Earlier I mentioned the Dynabeads system, which has been field tested in Senegal and elsewhere. It is being used increasingly in Africa and in Latin America.

A Promising Candidate: Easy Count

In Shapiro's view, one of the most exciting new T cell technologies involves Easy Count, a prototype instrument being developed by the Immunicon Corporation in the US, and the University of Twente in the Netherlands. Easy Count is essentially a low-power fluorescent microscope that uses a digital imaging chip, like those used in inexpensive cameras, plus software, to provide a T-cell count in about a minute. It's the size of a toaster, runs on long-lasting battery power, has no moving parts, and doesn't require a trained operator. In other words, it's as close to the Holy Grail as we've gotten so far. Results of the Easy Count system should be comparable to those of existing flow cytometers, say experts. Based on early results, the

WHO planned to build several Easy Count systems for clinical field testing. Then came news that the current models don't differentiate well enough between monocyte and CD4 T-cells, and that the reagents that were initially used were no long available. The WHO has put its field tests aside while Immunicon goes back to the drawing-board and new reagents are sought.

Another newcomer is Beckman Coulter's Cytosphere kit, a bead-based kit for light microscopic counting of CD4 absolute count (total lymphocyte count). It's relatively cheap – $8 in poor countries – very simple, and requires no instruments, and can be used in remote sites. But it is labor-intensive, requiring trained technicians to use it. The kit has received early evaluation by the FDA, said Cheng, who added that Beckman Coulter is trying to come up with a pricing strategy for the developing world.

Another newcomer is the SemiBio Ligand Catcher, a biochip for CD4 cell counting that uses an antibody-coated glass slide to obtain fast, rapid absolute CD4 counts using a light microscope. In a recent progress report, SemiBio reported a close correlation (0.95 correlation coefficient) between its test and flow cytometry. It must be noted that only four of thirty-three blood samples tested came from HIV patients; the others had other diseases, and one control was a healthy volunteer. But the company repeated their test results, which have yet to be validated by independent testing. "Our results encourage the use of this alternative technique in developing countries with limited economic means," SemiBio concluded.

Alternative Viral Load Tests

What about alternatives to a PCR viral load test? This virologic tool is currently used to evaluate the success of antiretroviral therapy. Insufficient suppression of HIV indicates the appearance of drug resistance, or some other problem reducing treatment effectiveness. Even at $19, for some developing countries Roche's PCR viral test is too pricey to be used routinely in patients. A cheaper choice may be the Retina HIV-1 Rainbow "real-time" NASBA test, which uses a different technology than PCR and can detect all HIV-1 subtypes. It yields results in just two hours, and in early studies it was comparable to the standard but more expensive NASBA – the NucliSens HIV-1 test, by Organon Teknika, which delivers results within sixty minutes and is FDA-approved. The Retina test is now offered at $20 to $25 outside the US market – unfortunately, too expensive for many countries.

The TaqMan PCR test is another, cheaper option that involves a simple, one-step test similar to standard HIV-PCR tests. Its advantage is that it can measure ninety specimens at once, with results in two to three hours. The main drawback is the large initial investment needed to buy the system. Another is the lack of standardized reagents. "Basically everyone makes their own primers and probes, typically under research lab conditions and not under GMP [Good Manufacturing Practice]," explained Susan Fiscus of the University of North Carolina, a highly respected diagnostic researcher. "Thus there can be a lot of variation from lot to lot, which might lead to erroneous results."

Some experts are more excited by the heat-denatured p24 antigen test, in which HIV levels are inferred from the detected amount of free HIV core protein. This test costs $6 to $8 in Africa. Jörg Schüpbach of the University of Zurich found that the sensitivity and specificity of the heat-treated p24 antigen test is comparable to existing PCR viral load tests. In a study of nine adults on HAART, the p24 antigen disappeared as quickly as viral RNA. In a larger comparative study of 155 patients on HAART who were followed for 154 days, the p24 antigen test was better at predicting survival than HIV PCR, and is a good predictor of subsequent disease progression.

Unfortunately, it's been hard for others to duplicate Schüpbach's promising results in testing in multiple labs. "The assay works, but the results obtained do not seem to be quite as sensitive as the results obtained in Zurich," stated Fiscus, who's been testing the p24 antigen test.

An additional test that's generated excitement is the Cavidi ExaCir reverse transcriptase test. Recent data from several groups around the world suggest that it is more sensitive than the heat-disassociated p24 antigen test, and just a little more expensive – around $10 to $15 per test, said Fiscus, who's also testing this technology and says there's a bonus to this test: "The reverse transcriptase that is isolated can also be used to assess phenotypic drug sensitivity [see glossary]." For now, no one's putting a future price-tag on this potential resistance test. "I guess it would depend on the number of drugs being evaluated," added Fiscus.

The Future: Dipsticks and Heel Sticks

Many HIV experts are excited about using dried blood spots (DBS) and heel sticks (a pinprick to the heel to get a drop of blood) rather than larger syringes, which require refrigeration. This well-established, simple technology is routine in pediatric care, and uses a dipstick. Specimens can be put into a sealed plastic bag and shipped, and remain stable at room temperature for up to a year. Heel-stick methods are less invasive, and may be especially useful for monitoring pediatric HAART patients.

According to Fiscus, the DBS technique is also applicable for HIV antibody measurements, as well as those of actual virus levels. It is applicable for both gene sequencing and resistance testing, too. But Fiscus explained that

> [t]he only thing that is less difficult about the dried blood spot is the collection and storage. There's no need for trained phlebotomists or freezers. In order to do a viral load, you still have to do a commercial viral load test, so it gets to be $50 to $100. The best thing would be to elute the p24 from the dried blood spot and use it in Schüpbach's enhanced p24 antigen test. We are still trying to get this to work – so far no luck. The DBS do apparently work in the Primagen test.

Testing Many Diseases at Once

An exciting new option is a multiplex microgene chip technology. It is behind new products like the HIV diagnostic "Taste Chip," under development by John McDevitt at the University of Texas at Austin, and Bill Rodriguez at Harvard. They began developing their system for detection of rapid and chronic HIV in 2001. Their new rapid, portable gene chip test contains multiple plastic wells, each containing a microbead coupled with a reagent (such as antibodies, antigens and oligonucleotides). A single blood sample will allow for simultaneous detection of multiple infectious micro-organisms – for example, hepatitis B and C, HIV, CMV, and mumps.

The multichip technology can be used to measure HIV antibody, p24 antigen, HIV RNA (viral load), CD4 and CD8 T-cell levels, as well as drug resistance, using a single drop of blood. Best of all, the tests will be dirt cheap, costing a few cents, not dollars. An HIV Elisa antibody test that now costs $25 to $80 will costs ten cents; a CD4 or viral load microchip test only $1.50. The equipment consists of a hand-held microchip reader that runs on a simple battery, not mains electricity, making it ideal for developing countries. In February 2003, Rodriguez said progress was going so well that field tests of an alternative CD4 T-cell test would soon begin in Haiti,

Botswana and South Africa. He was applying to the Gates Foundation, the National Institutes of Health and other donors for $5 million to bring the product to market within a year.

In the Forum's working group, there's fresh enthusiasm for the multi-chip concept, but also for the Cavidi and Primagen tests. "I am not sure there is a single technology that excites me most," said Cheng. "They all have their pros and cons. I think if we really can develop a dipstick for viral load and CD4 that would be a major advance." Looking ahead, he added, "I think there is a need for other diagnostic tests, including hepatitis, TB, resistance, etc. But also easy, cheap and reliable assays [laboratory tests] to monitor for side-effects."

George Janossy is also excited, but more about what he calls "simple flow" cytometry, and far less about other approaches. As for the other toys, they might work, but would they be better than "simple flow," as he calls flow cytometry?

> People are admirable for trying to reinvent the wheel and suggest the use of frequently very impractical non-flow cytometric methods, because theirs is a hopeless task. Flow cytometry is simple. It discriminates between the CD4+ T cells (small cells) and CD4+ monocytes (large cells) which other methods cannot do easily. So you will face an untold number of dreadful problems with other methods (dipstick, magnetic field counts, etc.). The reality is that the current acceptable cost of flow cytometry is already down at $2 to $3. That is the price to beat.

Without missing a beat, Janossy also noted that costs could be reduced by using no more than two reagents, and cutting their price. That would make "simple flow" a "winner over other cumbersome methods."

Low-Cost Resistance Tests

What about tools to monitor potential resistance to antiretrovirals? Due to the currently very high cost of resistance tests used in the West – between $400 and $1,000 – most clinicians in poor countries advocate their use only for population-wide surveillance of emerging drug-resistance patterns. For most individual patients, doctors stress adherence to dosing schedules, so as to maintain optimum drug levels in the body. Adherence can be improved by prescribing simplified regimens and following the Directly

Observed Therapy (DOT) model used in TB control (see Chapter 6). Nor is adherence solely to blame for the problem, as I discussed in the section on resistance in Chapter 13. Even people who strictly adhere to their regimens may see resistant strains emerge over time. Without cheap tools to monitor resistance, how can we directly assess the scale of this threat? "We need to look at the failure of TB control," said Salif Sow, MD, an HIV expert in Senegal, who attended the Bethesda meeting. "We're going to need tests to follow this in HIV."

Resistance tests also require trained doctors to understand the results. Here, there's also some good news about emerging low-cost resistance tests. A Swedish team led by Anders Malmsten recently reported on a simple test that combines viral load and phenotypic drug susceptibility testing by measuring virus-associated reverse transcriptase activity.

A New Optimism

Despite the current lack of tools for most patients, the prevailing attitude among frontline doctors and testing experts has shifted to open optimism. Today, it appears that India, Thailand, Senegal, Burkina Faso, Nigeria, Uganda and South Africa are the most active countries in the area of developing monitoring technologies, said Cheng in mid 2003. He added that the twenty-one nations of the Caribbean are about to get involved in this arena. Elsewhere, many governments that are rolling out national treatment programs are also involved in training doctors and technicians to use diagnostic tests. For now, the major hurdle still remains cost. After that, said Cheng, the list includes: "Ease of use, throughput of the assay, reliability, how it compares to the gold standard, physical requirements and training requirements."

For now, a number of immediate hurdles are blocking more rapid access to low-cost tests. On a technical level, aside from low-cost flow cytometers, there's too much variability and possibility for error among the standardized blood samples and reagents used today. That makes it hard to compare the quality of various new products and approaches. Another problem is the lack of communication between industry and bench researchers, which has slowed progress, according to Janossy. Some companies are reluctant to allow independent testing of their products by outside groups. Then there's the overall lack of interest in low-cost diagnostic technologies by the industry as a whole. That's the main reason Gates money is being used to jump-start a diagnostic initiative through grants to researchers.

Several years ago, for example, Avant Immunotherapeutics produced the TRAX CD4 enzyme immunoassay as a cheaper, proven alternative to flow cytometry for CD4 T-cell counts. Avant sold the product to Immunogenetics. Today it is off the market – an abandoned but still promising technology.

"Clearly, these instruments do not need to be more complicated than a compact disc player equipped with a fluid cell and a microsyringe, and supported by fast, user-friendly software," said Janossy of the goal of low-cost flow cytometry. "The simple reagents provided in bulk at low costs should not be a problem either. The problem with this proposition, however, is that currently industry is singularly uninterested to either produce such simple instruments, or, once made, to submit these to multi-centre analysis."

Generics may represent another future avenue. In the past two years, private Indian generic companies have started developing generic T-cell and viral load tests, as well as looking at tests and kits for diseases like TB and hepatitis. But many questions remain here too, regarding quality control and the capacity of generic companies to mass-produce new products on a global scale.

Doubts about Tests

There's also a serious concern that's recently cropped up: doubts about the usefulness of Western-based antibody tests for some non-Western patients. HIV-1 subtype B viruses prevalent in the US and Western Europe were used to develop diagnostic antibody tests in the West. But in Africa and parts of Asia, subtype C and A viruses are more common, and many hybrid viruses exist globally. A recent Nigerian study by leading author G.M. Odaibo looked at blood tests in 85 patients and found most Elisa and rapid test results did not accurately detect HIV infection. "The implications for prevention and therapy are enormous," concluded the Nigerian researchers.[1]

Another new study from Argentina found that false-positive test results occurred with several commercial rapid HIV tests, when used with blood samples that lacked antibodies to gp41, an HIV surface protein. "For this reason, we consider that HIV screening assays must be evaluated with all specimen types in the settings of their intended use," concluded M. Vingnoles and colleagues at the University of Buenos Aires School of

Medicine.[2] A group in Cameroon found a different result: four rapid tests and two antibody tests worked well in terms of sensitivity and specificity to detect HIV in non-B HIV subtypes taken from fresh, routine blood samples.[3]

What all this points to is an urgent need to determine and compare how well existing tests being used globally to detect HIV really work in non-US, non-European individuals, and whether new tests are needed based on various HIV subtypes that exist elsewhere. Without an accurate antibody test, even syndromic management can't be initiated. From a global point of view, experts should act quickly to review existing prevention studies, to determine whether current epidemiological forecasts are accurate, in light of these new findings.

Research Wish-List

Looking ahead, developers and activists agree that the biggest hurdle in the way of obtaining these tools is a weakness of political will. The shortlist of what's needed is easy to see: to begin with, there's an immediate need for government leaders and activists of all stripes to push diagnostic manufacturers to lower their product prices drastically for poor countries. More funding and donors are needed to train technicians and establish diagnostic laboratories in developing countries.

Here, the concern raised about the validity of antibody and rapid tests now being used in Africa needs to be immediately addressed: if they don't work as well in individuals with other subtype viruses, we need alternative antibody tests. The global roll-out of prevention and treatment relies on the success of HIV screening as the first step toward identifying those needing care. Across Africa, most programs use Western Blot tests to confirm antibody test results.

To get the ball rolling, the WHO's new AIDS Medicines Diagnostics facility needs funding and the full support of the political and scientific community, as well as from industry. The WHO immediately needs to procure and deliver high-quality, uniform reagents in order to field-test promising new technologies accurately. And they need to provide independent comparative information quickly on the current studies involving Dynabeads to interested governments and projects hoping to use this new system.

The last word goes to George Janossy in London, a can-do guy like Shapiro, who wants everyone – including his peers – to simplify the task at hand. On the issue of quality reagents, he noted that the Thailand Government Pharmaceutical Organization is now bulk-distributing inexpensive CD4/CD45 reagents to hospitals in the country, and providing an assurance of their quality. That's a useful model for others to follow. He also feels that flow cytometry manufacturers should be compelled to submit their new tests and equipment for independent international evaluation of their quality – before marketing them to African countries. "If these steps are known to the world, then it becomes obvious that inexpensive CD4 testing is currently a reality. Do not believe a word if they say to you that monitoring is difficult," he urged. "It is just a question of will and collaboration between those who wish the field moving."

Appendix C

HIV-RELATED METABOLIC SIDE-EFFECTS

Resources

For easy-to-read information on side-effects and other aspects of HIV therapy, check out community Internet resources such as the New Mexico AIDS InfoNet <www.aidsinfonet.org>, AIDS Meds.com <www.AIDSmeds.com> and review articles by John James in AIDS Treatment News <www.atn.org>. For more technical material, see Project Inform's site <www.projectin-form.org>, the Treatment Action Group's site <www.tagline.org>, the National AIDS Treatment Access Project (NATAP) <www.natap.org> and The Body <www.thebody.com>.

There are also sites for information on alternative and complementary therapies to counter the deleterious effects of antiretroviral therapy. Check out Immunet <www.immunet.org>, DAAIR <www.daair.org> and the Canadian AIDS Treatment Information Exchange <www.catie.ca/network.html>.

For HIV professionals, comprehensive and academically oriented reviews can be found at HIV Insite <www.hivinsite.org>, which is affili-ated with the University of California at San Francisco. Other universities and academic medical centers with excellent Internet resources regarding treatment of HIV/AIDS include Johns Hopkins, New York University Medical Center, the University of Alabama at Birmingham, and Harvard University. See also the Centers for Disease Control <www.cdc.gov>, the World Health Organization <www.who.int> and the Kaiser Foundation's website <www.kaisernetwork.org>.

Selected Glossary

Lipodystrophy is a broad term used to describe a range of body fat changes and metabolic problems that are linked to use of anti-HIV drugs, especially protease inhibitors. Experts distinguish fat gain (lipohypertrophy) from fat loss (lipoatrophy), since both can occur in the same person at once, and affect different parts of the body, including under the skin (subcutaneous), in the face, neck, arms and legs (peripheral) and stomach (called central or truncal adiposity). Lipodystrophy is also linked to distinct side-effects such as high cholesterol levels and insulin resistance (which lead to diabetes); mitochondrial toxicity; lactic acidosis; and bone weakness.

Cause: The exact cause of lipodystryphy is unclear, but the processing (metabolism) of anti-HIV drugs affects fat cells, including those in the liver. A 2002 report on children suggested a link to impaired growth hormone (GH) secretion. Some experts suggest monitoring for GH secretion in children, and the use of recombinant GH therapy for those with excessive intra-abdominal fat loss. The strategies are being evaluated for adults.

Diagnosis: There are several diagnostic tests used that measure body fat and tissue, and evaluate levels of cholesterol, insulin, and certain body enzymes. A DEXA scan uses imaging technology to measure whole body composition.

Mitochondrial Toxicity refers to damage to the body's mitochondria, which are the energy producing units of cells. Studies show that anti-HIV drugs, especially nucleoside analog drugs, or 'nukes', lead to a loss of mitochondrial DNA and cell damage.

Lactic Acidosis is a rare, potentially fatal and rapidly progressing illness caused by an abnormal increase of lactic acid (or lactate) in the blood. The most common side-effects of lactic acidosis are sore muscles; nausea; vomiting; severe fatigue; rapid, deep breathing; abdominal pain; cramping; numbness or tingling; and muscle weakness (myopathy), which quickly gets worse. Doctors are careful to distinguish lactic acidosis, an extreme condition, from elevated lactate levels (hyperlactemia), which is a common condition in people taking antiretroviral drugs.

Cause: There is a relationship between mitochondrial toxicity and lactic acidosis. When damage occurs to mitochondria, and muscle cells are forced to get their energy without oxygen (anerobically), they produce lactic acid as a waste product. This causes the soreness in muscles, and cramping in marathon runners, for example. It has been reported in people on anti-HIV therapy who develop lipodystrophy and get fatty livers. Lactic acidosis can also cause kidney damage and hearing loss.

Diagnosis: A blood test exists to measure lactate levels, but experts are divided about the usefulness of test results, since doing exercise (climbing stairs, walking quickly) before taking the test can increase lactic acid levels. Lactate levels over 5 mmol/L in the presence of symptoms can indicate progressive lactic acidosis.

Bone cell loss is measured on a scale ranging from mild (osteopenia) to more severe (osteoporosis), which indicates the risk of fracture. Based on reported cases to date, avascular necrosis appears to target the joints of the hips and shoulders. Experts say there may be little clinical evidence of bone loss, and it is can easily be missed by an X-ray, and even with more sophisticated imaging equipment like a Dexa-Scan. The main symptom is acute pain that is not alleviated with anti-inflammatory drugs or painkillers. By the time clinical symptoms appear on a Dexa-Scan, people may require hip replacement surgery.

Diagnosis: A BMD (bone mineral density) test measures bone strength, based on the density of bone cells. A BMC (bone mineral content) test measures which bones cells are affected. For an overview of the emerging problem of HIV-related bone loss and disease, see my April 2002 article in *POZ* magazine (Anne-christine d'Adesky, "Hip to the Future," *POZ*, April 2002).

Appendix D

FACTORS AFFECTING ADHERENCE

A recent African study of factors that affect adherence to treatment showed that the cost of care in Botswana was the primary barrier to adherence in Africa. AIDS community advocate Lance Sheriff provided this summary of the study:

> Financial constraints, including though not limited to the cost of anti-retrovirals, were reported to be the most significant barrier to antiretroviral adherence in patients living with HIV infection and AIDS in Botswana prior to the introduction of free treatment. The study, published in the November 1 (2003) issue of the *Journal of Acquired Immune Deficiency Syndromes* reported that though 54 percent of the patients reported that they took their drugs as prescribed, if cost were removed as a barrier, 74 percent would have been adherent, which is comparable to rates of adherence in the developed world.[1]
>
> The study highlights several problems that will affect decision making by governments, donors and public health officials throughout the developing world as antiretroviral treatment is introduced. Decisions about the balance of free treatment provision and cost recovery will need to be taken in the light of evidence suggesting that cost of treatment is the biggest single determinant of non-adherence in all studies so far carried out in Africa.
>
> The findings also suggest that other economic issues apart from the cost of medication have an influence on adherence in resource-limited settings, and that these need to be taken into account when planning treatment pro grammes.

Lack of strict adherence to highly active antiretroviral (ARV) therapy is one of the key challenges to AIDS care worldwide. Treatment adherence has been closely correlated with viral suppression, while non-adherence has contributed to progression to AIDS, the development of multi-drug resistance and death. Adherence is often perceived to be a significant barrier to the delivery of ARV therapy in sub-Saharan Africa.

Currently Botswana has the highest estimated prevalence of HIV infection in the world. More than 330,000 people of a population of 1.5 million have been infected with HIV, and there were 26,000 estimated deaths due to AIDS in 2001 alone. Statistics from 2002 indicate that 38.8 percent of economically productive and sexually active adults (aged 15 to 49 years) have HIV/AIDS.

To evaluate the possible social, cultural, and structural barriers for adherence in the Botswana population, researchers conducted a cross-sectional study involving 109 adult patients (over 18 years) receiving at least three months of ARV therapy in three private clinics in Botswana (two in Gaborone and one in Francistown), between January and July 2000. Patients' reports of their own adherence and their care providers' estimates of adherence (taking at least 95 percent of their doses correctly) were the primary outcomes of the study.

Although the percentage of patients who were adherent 95 percent of the time was roughly the same by patient (54 percent) and doctor assessment (56 percent), these assessments were only in concurrence 68 percent of the time. According to the patients, the principal barriers to adherence included financial constraints (48 percent, including the cost of antiretrovirals 44 percent of the time), stigma (15 percent), travel/migration (10 percent), and side-effects (9 percent). Even though natural resources make Botswana one of the wealthiest countries in Africa, the cost of triple combination antiretroviral therapy remains far beyond what its citizens can afford on their own. At the time this study was conducted, the vast majority of patients on antiretroviral therapy were buying their own drugs with the help of medical insurance, but less than 1 percent of the HIV-infected patients in Botswana had such insurance. To make matters worse, medical insurance typically covers only one quarter or one third of the entire cost of triple-drug therapy. Consequently, most patients using antiretroviral therapy in this study were receiving suboptimal regimens with only 43 of the patients receiving triple-drug therapy. Sub-standard regimens are less effective and that, in and of itself, could have been expected to dampen the rates of adherence. But the study authors also reported that patients in this study often had no choice but to interrupt treatment, because they could not afford to renew their prescriptions. Limited finances also made it difficult to travel to the clinic site, sometimes more than 1,000 kilometres away, to renew their prescriptions; in addition, some simply couldn't afford to take time off work to travel to the clinic site.

Logistic regression analysis showed that if cost were removed as a variable, the expected rate of adherence to therapy would be 74 percent. The proof of this came shortly after this study was conducted, when Botswana began to supply free antiretroviral therapy to several thousand patients through a network of district hospitals and smaller sites throughout the country.

As the authors of the study had predicted, adherence levels were substantially better in patients receiving free medication. Preliminary data to this effect were presented at the Second International AIDS Society Conference in Paris in July. A study in a subset of patients in the programme receiving treatment at Maun General Hospital used a very strict definition of adherence in this study (100 percent).[2] Even dosing late was treated as non-adherence.

Using this strict definition, the 176 patients were adherent 83.16 percent of the time (on average, patients took their medication in exactly the way prescribed on 24.9 days of each month). Once cost was removed, the leading barriers to adherence became forgetfulness (26.92 percent); access to the site/drug, 37 (20.33 percent); and lack of privacy, 33 (18.13 percent).

During a plenary during the same conference, Dr. Ernest Darkoh, the Operations Manager of the Botswana National Antiretroviral Programme spoke about the challenges and lessons learned while implementing the programme. One of the challenges is "maintaining adherence. We've managed to maintain 90 percent rates, or levels of adherence."

He noted that there were other initiatives planned by the Botswana government to further improve adherence, including improvements in the distribution of antiretrovirals, increased availability of clinical and laboratory monitoring, and strengthened health infrastructures for delivering care.

As shown in the study in the *Journal of Acquired Immune Deficiency Syndromes*, the remainder of patients in Botswana and other resource-limited settings who are forced to pay for the medicines themselves will be at much greater risk of poor adherence and most will be on sub-optimal therapy.

Similar findings have been produced from an analysis of 159 adults who received antiretrovirals through the Senegalese government's national treatment programme between 1999 and 2002. This study found that the probability of 95 percent adherence declined if individuals were required to contribute more than 15 euros per month towards the cost of treatment.[3]

Appendix E

RESISTANCE AND MDR-HIV

HIV drug resistance can be detected using one of two types of tests. Genotypic tests detect specific mutations in the HIV gene that are linked with resistance; phenotypic tests measure how well HIV grows in the presence of drugs – a more sensitive and direct measurement. (The Virco company also produces a "Virtual Phenotype" test, which predicts phenotypic resistance from genotypic results.)

The evidence of rising MDR-HIV transmission in acutely infected individuals in the US comes from a ten-city survey conducted by Douglas Richman of the University of California at San Diego, and colleagues including Susan Little. Their survey was part of a National Institutes of Health project focused on early HIV disease, and covers the period from May 1995 to early 2000. It reflects sexually transmitted early HIV infection among mostly white gay men in major US cities with high HIV rates.

In 2002, Little said that her studies found that 23 percent of newly acquired HIV has some detectable drug resistance based on tests of its genetic makeup (genotyping). MDR-HIV stood at 10 percent according to genotypic tests, and 6 percent according to phenotypic ones. "There is a significant increase, by genotype by phenotype, any way you look at it," Little remarked. "One-drug and multi-drug . . . resistance has gone up substantially." By comparing these results with data from the 1995 to 1998 era, when protease inhibitors were widely introduced, the UCSD team noted a fourfold increase in resistance to anti-HIV drugs.

To Little, the intriguing finding is the apparent persistence of MDR mutations for well over a year. "We and a couple of groups have looked at [MDR] persistence in newly infected persons, and they are, to the best of our knowledge, infected with a single strain of virus," she stated. Given this finding,

> as the prevalence of drug resistance in new infections goes up in those people who transmit HIV secondarily [via unsafe sex], they're only going to transmit — we think — resistant virus. I would expect that resistance in the population would go up, and a major dependent variable will be the prevalence of patients with new HIV infections and drug resistance.

Little's new data suggest that, perhaps in places like San Francisco where there is maximum access to antiretrovirals, the balance is tipping in favor of resistant viruses.

Not so fast, says Sally Blower.

Blower is a biomathematician at the University of California at Los Angeles who has spent the past ten years forecasting epidemiological trends like MDR-TB and antibiotic resistance. Using a different mathematical model and a technique she called "uncertainty analysis," Blower predicted a different, less scary MDR future for the world in the September 2002 issue of *Nature Medicine*.

"This type of modeling is much more like physics or hydrology or climatology where you actually learn the system and write down equations that describe that process," Blower explained. Since no one really knows the viral fitness of MDR-HIV viruses, nor how easily they are transmitted, she decided to model 1,000 different HIV drug-resistant viruses taken from San Francisco patients. She varied the estimate of their potential fitness, or ability to replicate, and determined how well they might be transmitted at different fitness levels.

"We showed by actually modeling the problem that you can have a high prevalence or drug resistance, but a low transmission," Blower summarized. Although people on antiretroviral therapy have a greater risk acquiring resistance the longer they're on therapy, she thinks that they are likely to pass a mixture of wild-type and drug-resistant viruses to other people. If wild-type viruses prove more fit, as many studies indicate, then resistant viruses will lose the Darwinian war on the population level. The spread of drug-resistant HIV into new, untreated bodies will be low. Based on the current numbers, her model predicts that between 3.88 percent to 20.8 percent of new HIV infections each year in the US will be resistant.

Who's right? Maybe both groups. Many factors can affect viral dynamics and transmission, including which populations are surveyed and when, the types of drugs used, the duration of therapy, virus subtypes, the presence of co-infections like TB or STDs, immune control, the ratio of wildtype to resistant variants, and, importantly, if and when individuals engage in risky sexual behavior. "It's difficult to estimate the infectivity of resistant [HIV] virus," agreed Daniel Kuritzkes of the University of Colorado Health Sciences Center, another pioneer in the field. He is nonetheless worried: "It's clear that nucleoside resistance has little difficulty being transmitted because we see it, and Susan Little's is the most comprehensive survey in the US." Despite different forecasts, Blower added, "I do not see any disagreement between what the UCSD group is saying and what we have published: we are all in agreement that there is and will continue to be transmitted resistance."

Little pointed out that current US treatment guidelines assume that newly infected individuals have no past exposure to HIV drugs. "Somehow the additional ten-plus years of productive life is not considered cost-effective for Africans, Haitians, Cambodians in the world of public health." These guidelines will need modification. "In order to adequately assess our strategy, we ought to know how common the problem of MDR is," Little contended. "I would argue it's time to start strongly considering routine resistance testing for chronically infected people, at least at the research level." She also favors extending resistance tests to acutely infected individuals prior to beginning HAART.

In Europe, treatment guidelines already do that. Swiss researcher Luc Perrin feels that resistance screening in persons with acute HIV represents "one of the best ways to follow the progression of resistance in the general population." He recently found a 10 percent rate of drug-resistant HIV among a group of 325 newly infected Swiss patients, but only four had MDR-HIV that resisted all three classes of antiretroviral drugs.

The emerging consensus is that antiretroviral therapy will have clear benefits for individuals by reducing suffering and saving lives. By lowering viral load in individuals, treatment also impacts positively on public health by decreasing the risk of HIV transmission, based on studies from Africa and elsewhere. On a population level, though, the global introduction of therapy is likely to lead to a gradual increase in MDR-HIV, and there will be consequences.

"It's the old risk–benefit argument," said Little. "The short-term risk of drug resistance when treating people is very small compared to the huge personal benefit for the patient, but the long-term consequences for the population are significant if you don't intervene with more potent drugs or a vaccine before the resistance gets out of hand." Blower called for all parties to abandon what she called "a *National Enquirer* view of resistance," and instead to clarify goals. She said, "People in Africa are infected and dying. We need to be clear: Are we trying to treat people? If we are treating, then let's treat as many as possible as well as possible – that's the only strategy. But if we want to have an epidemic control strategy, then what is it? Is it to have as little drug resistance as possible? Or to decrease transmission rates? Or decrease AIDS death rates? We can decide a treatment strategy, but at this point, it's so vague and woolly that nobody articulates what they want."

"I think a lot of medical people are confused because they do blur it – 'drug resistance is bad' – it's sort of a knee-jerk reaction," added Blower. By treating, she acknowledged, "[w]e've generated a lot of resistant HIV. So what? You always have to balance it against the alternative. If people hadn't been treated, transmission rates would have been higher, and many more people would have died off."

Appendix F

WOMEN AND HIV: THE GENDER PUZZLE

Worrying Reports

For years now, the issue of sex and gender differences has generated a big debate among scientists and the AIDS community, but not enough hard evidence. We know, for example, that women often have lower initial viral load levels than men, but we don't know how important that is for controlling HIV. Different groups of women can have different immune T-cell levels, suggesting that racial or socio-economic factors are at work. We've seen that women with low albumin levels may progress faster to disease. Side-effects are another urgent question mark: women on antiretroviral therapy seem to experience worse or different problems than men – but not always. For example, both sexes typically lose fat in their faces, arms and legs, and buttocks, but gain it in their bellies.

This side-effect of therapy is called lipodystrophy (see Appendix C) and occurs with all the anti-HIV drugs. But some women also see their breast size double or even triple. Is that because women naturally have more fat? Or are hormones the real culprit? It's hard to know, since most early studies were done in men. Whatever the cause, it's a side-effect that's both physically disfiguring and socially uncomfortable, causing some women to experience depression and isolation, and to seek psychological support.

Even when sex or gender differences jump out, it's hard to know what's really causing them, since so many factors could be involved. At the Tenth Conference on Retroviruses and Opportunistic Infections (CROI) in February 2003, Ruth Greenblatt, MD, of the University of California summed up the challenge by remarking that "all cells have a sex."[1] Even at the most fundamental cellular and molecular level, she explained, there are differences between men and women that can impact on how a virus like HIV interacts with our cells, and might explain why women have greater sexual vulnerability to HIV infection than men. The list also includes immunology, genetics, women's lower body weight, pharmacokinetics (how drugs are processed by the body), hormones, pregnancy and interactions with birth control. Then there's life and its daily hurdles – the myriad psychosocial and economic factors that affect women's access to health-care.

The more one looks for a cause, the longer the list grows. But the reason to find out is critical: HIV remains a major cause of death in American women aged twenty-five to forty-four, especially African-American women. It's also a faster-growing global killer of women and girls than men or boys. As Greenblatt put it, the time has come for everyone to emphasize that "HIV is a women's health concern" – period.

Now comes progress – and some sobering news. Enough data has recently come together for frontline researchers to declare an early consensus: the short answer to the complex puzzle of gender differences is *Yes* – Venus and Mars can be different when it comes to HIV and drug therapy. Some of these differences appear significant, others less so. The biggest worry in the area of side-effects is lactic acidosis, which appears far worse in women and girls in some studies. The new data call for urgent follow-up studies to determine why this is happening, and whether treatment guidelines and strategies should be revised for women.

Greenblatt works for the multi-site Women's Interagency HIV Study (WIHS), the largest US observational study of women living with HIV.[2] Two years ago, WIHS researchers began looking at drug side-effects, including lipodystrophy, diabetes and bone problems, and to judge the impact of hepatitis co-infection and drug interactions. Other groups have done specific drug toxicity studies that have yielded further data.

The Emerging Big Picture

In a CROI conference review of the emerging picture, Dr. Kathleen Squires of the University of Southern California Keck School of Medicine presented a 2003 review of all she could conclude about gender and side-effects based on the many large and small studies that had been completed.[3] In the arena of side-effects, the emerging picture shows that women on therapy have a growing degree of lipodystrophy, and the related problems of mitochondrial toxicity and lactic acidosis – especially women with hepatitis C co-infection. They also have increased pancreatitis (pancreas damage). Since many studies lack comparable data for men, it's hard to draw absolute conclusions about the influence of gender, she said.

Interestingly, studies suggest that men have higher triglyceride levels than women, though both sexes have high cholesterol levels and other lipid abnormalities. Both sexes also suffer from bone loss (osteopenia and osteoporosis) and it's too early to say if this is worse in women, especially older or menopausal women. But researchers are worried, since bone loss is often seen in individuals with lipodystrophy, suggesting that a similar mechanism may cause both.[4] Finally, women are at greater risk from nevirapine rash, said Dr. Squires, citing female gender as an independent risk factor for rash.

Lactic Acidosis and Mitochondrial Toxicity

Of all the drug side-effects, lactic acidosis, a rare but potentially fatal problem, has jumped out as disproportionately affecting women and girls (see glossary in Appendix C). Lactic acidosis is caused by elevated lactate levels (hyperlactemia) that cause problems to the muscles and are associated with liver damage, for example. Researchers caution that many people on therapy can have raised lactate levels, and stress the importance of distinguishing this from severe lactic acidosis. Looking at cases to date, Dr. Squires said the majority of cases have occurred in women. She cited an FDA review of 178 cases in 1999, in which two nucleoside drugs were involved. There, 83 percent of lactic acidosis cases were in women. Half the women weighed over 175 pounds, and there was a 55 percent rate of mortality. Since individuals co-infected with hepatitis C have damaged livers, this side-effect is especially risky for them.

Some scientists think the root cause of lactic acidosis and fat distribution problems is mitochondrial toxicity, which is defined as damage to mitochondrial DNA (mtDNA), the energy-producing units of cells. Many studies have noted a decrease in the levels of mtDNA linked to use of nucleoside reverse transcriptase inhibitor drugs (nukes and non-nukes). New reports confirm that d4T appears to be the bigger culprit in mitochondrial toxicity, compared with other nukes like AZT.[5] (The good news is that this mtDNA loss can be *reversed* by discontinuing d4T drug, and substituting d4T with abacavir or AZT.)[6]

Warning: In another update, experts say it's dangerous to use ddI with ribavirin, a hepatitis[7] drug, because this increases the risk of mitochondrial toxicity, especially in people co-infected with hepatitis C.[8]

The Link to Lipodystrophy

More lipodystrophy data has come from an ongoing WIHS sub-study involving 1,057 women, headed by Dr. Phyllis Tien at the University of California at San Francisco. In it, HIV-positive women on treatment had double the amount of fat loss in their face, arms or buttocks (peripheral lipoatrophy) than well-matched HIV-negative women, and double the fat increase in the waist, chest and upper back (central lipohypertrophy). Fat loss happens in both sites, but it's rare to see fat gain and loss at the same time in these women.[9] Reviewing this finding, Dr. Greenblatt said that HIV-positive women on treatment appear to have lower body fat than HIV-negative women, and they show greater fat loss in their arms, legs and buttocks. Another team at the Montefiore Medical Center in the Bronx, NY, compared body fat changes in a group of 120 women, and concluded that use of d4T and being white or Latina were independent risk factors for increased truncal fat and peripheral fat loss. Interestingly, the use of protease inhibitors was not.[10] A number of CROI conference posters also showed that girls were developing a higher degree of lipodystrophy than boys.

Emerging Diabetes Problem?

For now, there's not enough information on insulin resistance and diabetes linked to therapy, but WIHS researchers are worried by preliminary data that are still being analyzed. Their early data are based on self-reporting by women, and suggest a very high risk of diabetes related to HIV therapy, especially for African-American women, though researchers caution that controlled studies are needed to confirm this finding.

For now, the key question of why women may be more prone to drug side-effects is still open to debate. Squires noted that some scientists have asked whether dose and drug concentrations play a role in increased toxicity, since women tend to weigh less than men. It's known that weight affects drug serum levels in the bloodstream. But so do drug interactions, and other factors like hormones. The task of separating out these factors remains difficult.

Concluding her review, Dr. Squires made an emphatic statement that backs what many in the field believe: "There are sex and gender-based differences in toxicity, adverse events and drug and HIV-associated complications." Moving ahead, she called for prospective studies to determine which regimens are best for women, given the toxicity data. That, in turn, could lead to a distinct women's HIV treatment agenda in the coming years.

The news is particularly relevant for women in other countries. New treatment guidelines call for use of all-nucleoside regimens, and for two-nuke, one non-nuke cocktails. Will these spell more trouble for African women or less than the myriad regimens that have been used by US women, including women of color? Given that African women won't be getting protease drugs from the start, they may be able to avoid the severe lipodystrophy that's hit women with long histories of treatment. But we don't know enough about the impact of these drugs on African bodies, including female bodies. There's also the issue of how drugs affect the specific subtype C virus that is prevalent in Africa. Non-nucleoside drugs don't work as well. They include efavirenz, a popular non-protease drug being combined in fixed-dose pills for easy once-a-day regimens.

WIHS researcher Kathy Anastos is a leader in the field of gender-based HIV studies. She's now looking more closely at these side-effects, hoping to tease out gender and race variables that may underline treatment responses in WIHS women. She feels it's critical to study the impact of treatment on the large numbers of now treatment-naive women in developing countries who are beginning to take these drugs. "We need to establish what the baseline of their health is now, even before they begin therapy, to be able to monitor them in a longitudinal study," she said. "We need some parameters for what is considered normal, and then to look from there at how they do on therapy."

She ticked off a few key questions from a long list of things she'd like to know immediately: "What are normal viral load levels in African women? What about their immunity and T-cell levels? Do they get regular Pap smears? What about cancers?" She added:

A lot of people in these countries have been exposed to chronic tuberculosis and malaria and other endemic diseases. That's gonna make these studies more complicated. But we owe it to these women to do this now, especially because we have the benefit of seeing how treatment has affected women here. We're having trouble here with side-effects and we can expect it there since it's linked to long-term therapy. We're gonna need this information to be able to track what's happening in these women and make sure they're getting the kind of care they deserve.

She's eyeing a potential gender-based study in Rwanda that could benefit women who were exposed through mass rape during the civil war. Elsewhere, other researchers are beginning to discuss studies that put women at the center of the global focus on treatment.

Appendix G

WOMEN AND SEXUAL VIOLENCE

On World AIDS Day, December 1, 2003, Human Rights Watch issued a forty-page report cataloging the increase in violence and discrimination against women and girls that is fueling Africa's AIDS crisis.

"Policy Paralysis: A Call for Action on HIV/AIDS-Related Human Rights Abuses Against Women and Girls in Africa"[1] documents human rights abuses that women and girls suffer at each stage of their lives, and that increase their risk for HIV infection. Girls face sexual abuse and violence, in and out of school. Women in long-term relationships risk violence if they insist on condom use or refuse sex. Widows are discriminated against in property and inheritance rights. And women and girls are raped in war and civil conflict, where rape is used strategically as a weapon. "Women and girls in Africa are dying by the millions, partly because their second-class status makes them vulnerable to violence and unsafe sex," said Joanne Csete, director of the HIV/AIDS Program at Human Rights Watch. "In the fight against AIDS, protecting women and girls from sexual abuse and ensuring their equal rights under the law are as crucial as keeping the blood supply clean."

The report sharply criticizes governments for allowing these abuses to continue, and ignoring the critical link between them and HIV/AIDS among women and girls. Legal and judicial remedies for violations of the rights of women and girls are often inadequate or nonexistent. Even where such laws exist, they are poorly enforced. Women and girls who are courageous enough to file complaints are often laughed at or mistreated by officials. "There is near paralysis in African governments' response to HIV/AIDS among women and girls," said Csete. "State failure to protect women and girls from such abuses is fueling the AIDS epidemic in Africa. And studies suggest that this is a global phenomenon. Even Uganda's widely heralded success in fighting AIDS will unravel as long as women face violence when they refuse sex or demand safer sex," said Csete. "These abuses don't go away by themselves; well funded programs are needed. The Global Fund and other donors should promote protection of women's and girls' rights as a central part of AIDS programs."

The report covers abuses in countries throughout sub-Saharan Africa: West Africa (Sierra Leone and Togo), Central Africa (Democratic Republic of Congo), East Africa (Kenya and Uganda) and Southern Africa (South Africa and Zambia).

Recommendations for Action (From "Policy Paralysis")

Three categories of legal, policy and program action are called for to reduce gender inequality as it relates to HIV/AIDS. These are measures to (1) protect women and girls from sexual and domestic violence and ensure prosecution of the perpetrators of those crimes; (2) eliminate gender inequalities related to property, inheritance, divorce, and other areas related to economic dependence; and (3) ensure equal access of girls and women to health and education services. Areas in which legal, policy and program action should concentrate are considered for each of these in turn. Points highlighted below are derived from recommendations previously made by Human Rights Watch as a result of its investigations and in many cases have been the subject of advocacy campaigns in some countries. **All of these measures should be regarded as important elements of national AIDS control efforts.**

1. Sexual and domestic violence

A range of measures should take top priority in an urgent effort to protect women and girls from sexual and domestic violence, including abuse in marriage and other long-term unions. In all cases, measures should be taken to ensure that improvements in statutory law are not undermined by customary or religious law or practice.

General

Programs designed to ensure basic protection against sexual violence and abuse should be high priorities in governments' allocation of financial and human resources. These include:

- nationwide awareness campaigns, including for schoolchildren, of the problem of sexual violence, with locally appropriate illustration of examples of sexual abuse and coercion;
- urgent action to train police, social welfare officers and workers, health workers, legal and judicial officers, teachers and school administrators on the nature and extent of sexual violence and its prevention;
- urgent action to amend laws to include acts of sexual abuse other than rape (which is already included in the law in most countries). Inheritance of widows as marital or sexual partners without their consent and any other forced marriage should be understood as sexual violence.

These measures should include a particular focus on girls and young women who are the most vulnerable in most countries and monitoring mechanisms to ensure their reach.

Domestic violence and marital rape

Sexual violence laws should be amended urgently to prohibit rape in marriage. The marital rape laws in South African law may provide a useful model.[2] These changes should be accompanied by sufficient resources to ensure the enforcement of the laws, training of relevant officials, and prosecution of perpetrators.

All countries should enact legislation and accompanying policy to ensure prohibition of domestic violence, including physical violence that does not include rape. In addition, accompanying policy measures should support the following actions:

- establish a clear and deliberate policy to remedy domestic violence within the justice system (police, local councils, and courts);
- issue guidelines and provide training on appropriate responses to domestic violence issues and enforce guidelines for police intervention in cases of domestic violence, including standardized arrest policies for

perpetrators and the separate categorization of domestic violence in police records;

- ensure police training in appropriate investigative methods for cases of domestic violence, including techniques for interviewing victims, and methods for protecting victims and witnesses from harassment.

- Governments should move to end harmful customary practices such as "wife inheritance" and ritual "cleansing" of widows, including by prosecuting rape and forced marriage cases and by providing education on the harmful effects of these practices.

Police and judicial proceedings

- Create centers where sexual violence can be reported with privacy and sensitivity toward survivors, staffed by trained police, medical personnel and counselors. The experiences of the special sexual offenses courts in South Africa[3] and the child protection units of the police department, while not perfect, have elements that may serve as replicable models.

- Measures should be taken to ensure the rights of witnesses and victims in sexual violence or abuse cases tried in courts. As suggested in the Rome Statute of the International Criminal Court, these may include the possibility of *in camera* proceedings, withholding the victim's identity from the general public, providing protection for the security of witnesses and victims, and providing counseling services within the judiciary. Judicial staff should be trained on the management of sexual violence cases, and efforts should be made to ensure adequate trained women staff members in judicial bodies.

- If national justice systems are not willing or able to prosecute widespread instances of systematic sexual violence, as in situations of armed conflict, they should be prosecuted by the International Criminal Court as its jurisdiction allows.

Other services

- Strengthen support and treatment services for survivors of rape and other sexual violence, including provision of HIV post-exposure prophylaxis (PEP), voluntary and confidential HIV testing, testing and treatment for other sexually transmitted diseases, legal assistance, and other appropriate counseling. Personnel in facilities providing these services should be trained to address the particular needs of children and young women who survive sexual abuse. States should ensure PEP and related medical and legal services are available on an equal basis to all survivors of sexual violence. They should ensure wide dissemination of information about these services (including what they are, why they are important and where to get them) in the general community, as well as among health care providers, police, social workers, teachers, and others likely to be important contact points for sexual violence survivors.

- All governments should ensure nationwide access to affordable male condoms at all times. Governments should improve distribution and access to female condoms and increase awareness of the link between sexual violence and HIV transmission and awareness of HIV reinfection.
- In all countries, ministries of education should work with other relevant ministries and the national AIDS control office to formulate and implement national programs of protection against sexual violence in schools, including strengthening of education on sexual abuse in the formal curriculum, training and binding codes of conduct for school employees, guidelines for schools detailing appropriate responses to allegations of sexual abuse by students, and procedures for disciplining offenders. Mechanisms should be established to monitor schools' records in all these areas, and headmasters or other school directors should be held accountable for failure to respond to allegations or to follow guidelines adopted nationally.
- All governments should strengthen the collection and dissemination of comprehensive national statistics on sexual abuse and domestic violence, detailing the nature and degree of abuse, rates of prosecution and conviction, and the nature of punishment applicable, but using methods that protect the privacy of survivors of these crimes.

Rape of sex workers
- Sex workers who are victims of rape and other sexual violence should have equal standing under the law to bring formal complaints, be received by the police with dignity, and expect prosecution of offenders. The high degree of vulnerability of sex workers to sexual abuse should be included in training programs mentioned above.

Sexual violence in war

- Military personnel in all countries should be trained in prevention of and receive clear orders against any action that might constitute sexual abuse. Military authorities must be held accountable for full investigation of allegations of sexual abuse by their personnel and appropriate prosecution of offenders. The well-being, privacy and dignity of complainants and witnesses must be protected in all proceedings. Civil society should be allowed to operate freely to monitor rape and other sexual abuse and assist the survivors of these crimes. In the case of the Democratic Republic of Congo (and Burundi), pressure is still needed on all parties to the combat to ensure immediate cessation of all sexual violence against women and girls. In Sierra Leone, the government must take urgent steps to ensure the release of girls and women still held as sexual slaves by former combatants, and diligence on the part of all parties is needed to ensure that the Special Court for Sierra Leone will adequately pursue cases of sexual violence and sexual slavery.

2. Gender inequity in property ownership and control, inheritance and divorce

- All countries should amend or repeal all laws that violate women's property rights, including the rights of widows. Countries should hold accountable those authorities who undermine statutory protection of women's equal right to property by applying discriminatory provisions of customary law. Adequate legislation will normally include a presumption of spousal co-ownership of family property and of equal division of property upon the termination of marriage; registration of all marriages in a central registry; equal inheritance rights; a requirement of family consent for transfers of family land and housing; and a clear recognition that payment of dowry is not a legal requirement for any type of marriage. Legal changes should be accompanied by resources that ensure enforcement of the law and establishment of appropriate judicial mechanisms, such as family courts, for prosecution of offenders.
- Governments should undertake nationwide awareness campaigns to inform the public about women's property rights, including ensuring availability of information in local languages about rights to inheritance

and division of family property; writing wills; registering marriages; co-registering property; and the health risks of customary sexual practices tied to property rights, such as the risk of contracting HIV/AIDS. Governments should encourage the sharing of information across sectors, such as by including informational materials on inheritance rights in health facilities and by distributing health-related HIV/AIDS information through women's networks and organizations as well as in police stations and court offices.

- Governments should provide training for judges, magistrates, police, and relevant local and national officials on laws relating to women's equal property rights and their responsibility to enforce those laws and should include women's property rights in the required curriculum of police training academies and law schools.
- Governments should ensure access of indigent women to legal assistance to pursue civil property claims. Governments and donors should support the activities of nongovernmental organizations that provide legal services to women whose property rights have been violated.
- Divorce laws should be amended to reflect the presumption of spousal co-ownership of family property and of equal division of property upon the termination of marriage. They should also reflect equality in the ability to claim wrongful conduct as grounds for divorce. Most importantly, governments must take steps to ensure that provisions of divorce law that recognize women's equality under the law are not undermined by customary law and practice. Authorities failing to respect this principle should be brought to account.

3. Equal access to social services and information

Ensuring equal access to education for girls is the key to protecting them from many of the abuses highlighted in this report and ensuring their access to life-saving information. The Convention on the Rights of the Child guarantees all children free primary education, but this remains an elusive goal in many African countries, especially for girls. Most African governments have made commitments and formulated plans of action around the "education for all" goals established at the education summit in Dakar, Senegal in June 2000, but these have not been backed up by resources and political commitment. In many countries, girls and women face discriminatory barriers in access to health services and information, as noted above. Social service policies and supporting legislation are an essential area of action for redressing gender-based injustices that contribute to risk of HIV/AIDS. In particular:

- Governments should make equal access to education for girls an urgent priority and should understand it as a central element of fighting HIV/AIDS along with measures to ensure freedom from sexual and gender-related abuse in schools. As UNICEF has noted, real progress will not be made in this area until education in general draws more government and donor resources, including to schools in marginalized rural and urban slum areas and generally for better training and compensation of teachers. Until that happens, measures should be taken at least to ensure that girls are not discriminated against in education, including by ensuring equal access to school meal programs that may help children stay in school, stipends for secondary school girls who would otherwise be under pressure to become breadwinners, and legislation that prohibits marriage for girls under age eighteen. Public awareness of the importance of girls' education, including its link to lower risk of HIV/AIDS, should be promoted.
- Governments should amend or repeal all policies and laws that pose discriminatory barriers to women and girls in access to health services and information. Women should not be required to provide evidence of their husbands' permission for reproductive health services.
- Governments should provide training to health care providers to ensure that girls and women receive appropriate, discreet and non-stigmatizing counseling and information on HIV/AIDS and reproductive health concerns. Health sector reform measures should make nondiscriminatory access to services a central part of their activities.

Source: <http://www.hrw.org/reports/2003/africa1203>

Human Rights Watch Reports on Gender-Related Abuses and Aids in Africa

"Just Die Quietly: Domestic Violence and Women's Vulnerability to HIV in Uganda," August, 2003: <http://www.hrw.org/reports/2003/uganda0803>

"Stolen Children: Abduction and Recruitment in Northern Uganda,"
March, 2003: <http://hrw.org/reports/2003/uganda0303>

"Double Standards: Women's Property Rights Violations in Kenya,"
March, 2003: <http://hrw.org/reports/2003/kenya0303>

"Borderline Slavery: Child Trafficking in Togo,"
April, 2003: <http://hrw.org/reports/2003/togo0403>

"Suffering in Silence: Human Rights Abuses and HIV Transmission to
Girls in Zambia,"
January, 2003: <http://hrw.org/reports/2003/zambia>

"We'll Kill You If You Cry: Sexual Violence in the Sierra Leone Conflict,"
January, 2003: <http://hrw.org/reports/2003/sierraleone>

"The War Within the War: Sexual Violence Against Women and Girls in
Eastern Congo,"
June, 2002: <http://hrw.org/reports/2002/drc>

"In the Shadow of Death: HIV/AIDS and Children's Rights in Kenya,"
June, 2001: <http://www.hrw.org/press/2001/06/kenya0625.ht>

"Scared at School: Sexual Violence Against Girls in South African Schools,"
March, 2001: <http://www.hrw.org/reports/2001/safrica>

"South Africa: Violence Against Women and the Medico-Legal System,"
August, 1997: <http://www.hrw.org/reports/1997/safrica>

"South Africa: The State Response to Domestic Violence and Rape,"
November, 1995: <http://www.hrw.org/reports/1995/Safricawm-02.htm>

Reprinted with permission of Human Rights Watch

Appendix H

HOSPICE AND PALLIATIVE CARE

Many individuals with advanced HIV illness in Africa suffer from pain related to end-stage HIV illnesses. The WHO has developed "three-step" palliative care guidelines for pain relief, which were first created for cancer patients and are now used more broadly.

WHO "three-step" Pain Ladder Guideline:
    If pain occurs, there should be prompt oral administration of drugs in the following order: nonopioids (aspirin and paracetamol); then, as necessary, mild opioids (codeine); then strong opioids such as morphine, until the patient is free of pain. To calm fears and anxiety, additional drugs – "adjuvants" – should be used. To maintain freedom from pain, drugs should be given "by the clock," that is, every three to six hours, rather than "on demand." This three-step approach of administering the right drug in the right dose at the right time is inexpensive and 80 to 90 percent effective. Surgical intervention on appropriate nerves may provide further pain relief if drugs are not wholly effective.[1]

Expanding Hospice Care

Expansion of hospice and palliative care programs is an integral part of a multi-sectoral approach to conquering the HIV/AIDS epidemic in Africa.[2] As more than 6,300 people die every day of HIV/AIDS in sub-Saharan Africa, the development of new programs to provide quality end-of-life care is essential. Vast numbers of people die in pain without the relief and support provided by organizations such as hospices. New hospice and palliative care programs must therefore be established to address the needs of this dying population.

The plan of the Foundation for Hospices in Sub-Saharan Africa (FHSSA) for increased hospice access through hospice training was borne out of FHSSA's *International Consultation on Hospice and Palliative Care in Sub-Saharan Africa*, attended by hospice experts from South Africa, Zimbabwe, Kenya, Tanzania, and the United States in 2000. At this consultation, the African and American participants identified the development of hospice programs as integral to caring for the millions dying from HIV/AIDS each year on the continent. Drawing from this Consultation, FHSSA offers a two-pronged approach to hospice expansion through increased training services that is consistent with the WHO's Foundation Measures for Implementing Cancer (HIV/AIDS) Pain Relief Programs: Education/Drug Availability and Government Policy.

The FHSSA identifies the following areas as integral to shoring up training resources for the expansion and provision of hospice and palliative care programs in Africa:

1. Administration and Non-Clinical Models and Training
2. Clinical Service Delivery Models and Training (Palliative Care and Home Care Training)

To this end, the FHSSA is proposing a two-pronged approach building on the hospice structures that already exist in sub-Saharan Africa. The proposed model includes the need for:

1. Multi-National Resource Centers to provide Administrative Training; and Hospice and Palliative Care Clinical Specialty Training (such as Pediatrics and Physician Training).
2. Regional Training Centers to provide Clinical Training in hospice and palliative care to nurses, community caregivers, and volunteers.

Hospice History and Development in Africa

The Hospice movement in Africa started in 1979 with the establishment of Island Hospice in Harare, Zimbabwe. This program and others that followed in South Africa, Kenya, and Uganda were modeled on the principles of hospice care from the United Kingdom, but focused on the provision of *home-based care* for patients and not, as in the UK, on specialized in-patient facilities. The hospice programs started as care for cancer patients and had the capacity to have nurses visiting patients in their homes on a regular basis. But with the advent of the AIDS epidemic, many hospices were forced to modify their programs to meet the needs of the ever-increasing number of AIDS patients in their communities.

Now, to meet the staggering numbers of HIV/AIDS patients, the hospices have well-trained community caregivers (usually volunteers) supervised by nurses to provide most of the home-based care, and day centers to reduce isolation and offer respite for families. In addition, they have modified their approach to address the multi-sectoral needs presented by the pandemic. They have begun taking on community development activities as part of their service models, including expanded services for AIDS orphans, such as bereavement and aftercare planning; food distribution programs; income-generating projects; and collaboration with tuberculosis programs using DOTS. Hospices have significantly refocused their service delivery goals in the face of the HIV/AIDS epidemic. There are currently about 100 hospice programs in sub-Saharan Africa, with at least one formal hospice program located in each of South Africa, Zimbabwe, Uganda, Botswana, Swaziland, Zambia, Malawi, Tanzania, and Kenya.

The FHSSA's Partnership ("Twinning") Initiative now consists of twenty-six partnerships between individual hospices in Africa and their hospice partners in the United States. These partnerships alone have generated almost $100,000 to date for individual hospice programs in sub-Saharan Africa. Direct Grants have been awarded for such projects as hospice and palliative care, training for new hospices in northern Tanzania and southern Kenya, the funding of nursing positions at specific hospices, and general operational funds.

Reprinted with permission of the FHSSA

NOTES

2 Aids and Empire I: A Brief Chronology of Recent Events

1. Mark Schoofs, "AIDS: The Agony of Africa," *Village Voice*, eight-part series reprint, November 9, 1999.
2. Salih Booker and William Minter, "Global Apartheid," *Nation*, July 9, 2001; "Africa's Debt: Fueling the Fire of AIDS," *Africa Action Press Release*. According to research by Africa Action, ten African governments spent more repaying their foreign debt in 2002 than their combined national budgets for health-care and education. Meanwhile, illiteracy plagued the continent and 42 million African school-age children lacked schooling. Without education, people lack skills to secure jobs.
3. "Indian Firm Offers AIDS Cocktail for $1 a Day," *Reuters*, February 9, 2001. At the time Cipla made its revolutionary $360 a year offer, the cost of discounted three-drug brand-name antiretroviral regimens being offered to African countries like Senegal ranged from $1,008 and $1,821 a year. Bob Huff, "What Does R&D Really Cost?" GMHC's *Treatment Issues*, July/August 2001, vol. 15, no. 7/8. Prior to Cipla's entry into the HIV drug field, the multinationals had long persuaded consumers that AIDS drugs cost so much because of the billions they spent on research. When Cipla made antiretrovirals for a fraction of the US price-tag, the true costs – and massive profits – of the multinationals were revealed.

   It's true that drug development is risky and expensive; there are many drug failures for each successful wonder drug. But the companies also get tax credits and benefit from accelerated FDA approval of ARV products, which spells savings, Huff found. With patent laws that provide a twenty-year monopoly on products, they get a lot of time to more than recoup their initial investments.

Huff reported that it cost about $65 million to bring a new drug to market in the US in 2001, according to Public Citizen, a Ralph Nader consumer watchdog group – a figure far lower than an oft-quoted industry claim of $179 million. That's because big companies factor in lost profits – what they might have made while their investments were tied up according to a review of drug costs by Huff. That year, Bristol-Myers spent $1.9 billion – only 10 percent of its total drug revenue – on R&D, but spent three times that – $5.6 billion – on marketing and administration (M&A). Overall that year, the big drug companies enjoyed profits twice those of Microsoft, to name a comparable company that spends around 40 percent of its revenues on R&D and M&A.

Today, profits remain solid, despite inroads by generic competitors. Ten multinational companies own 40 percent of the global drug market, estimated at $400 billion in 2002. Almost 90 percent of that market is in the US, Western Europe and Japan. While Asia's technological capacity to make drugs has sharply increased, Africa's has steadily declined.

4. Tina Rosenberg, "How to Stop the World's AIDS Crisis: Look at Brazil," *New York Times Magazine*, January 28, 2001.

5. Donald McNeil, Jr, "U.N. Disease Fund Opens Way to Generics," *New York Times*, October 16, 2002.

6. Naomi Koppel, "WTO Talks End Without Subsidy Agreement," *Associated Press*, June 22, 2003.

7. "Access Denied," a special Human Rights Watch report on the impact of the global gag rule, co-sponsored by Population Action International and Human Rights Watch, among several groups, released October 2003. The Mexico City Policy was first announced at the 1984 Mexico City Conference on Population. "Access Denied" found that the policy had severely harmed reproductive health clinics, including five that closed in Kenya. Groups like Lesotho Planned Parenthood Association no longer received any donated condoms from

USAID. Nor did leading providers of reproductive health services in another thirteen countries, including Ethiopia and Zambia. "In short, thanks to the closure of medical clinics and reductions in supplies wrought by the policy, more Africans will contract HIV, more mothers will transmit it to their babies and more of the population will die," concluded PAI in its report.

8. Jim VandenHei, "Drug Firms Boost Bush's AIDS Plan," *Washington Post*, May 1, 2003. According to VandenHei, "Top White House officials have encouraged corporations, especially those with direct business interests in Africa, to support Republican lobbying efforts aimed at passing Bush's AIDS initiative in Congress."

9. Ibid. According to VandenHei, drug companies such as Bristol-Myers Squibb and Abbott are among the biggest supporters of the Bush global AIDS bill. Not surprisingly, both companies have major AIDS drug programs in Africa. The pharma companies and other multinational firms were initially asked to cough up as much as $250,000 each to join two pro-Bush lobbying groups to help win passage of the bill. Most eventually contributed around $25,000. GOP strategist John Vandenheuvel admitted, "All the major multinational pharmaceuticals have some type of [AIDS] program they are already using and would like to have it utlilized as part of the [Bush] plan."

10. *New York Times*, July 12, 2003.

11. Interview with Bill Haddad, August 2003.

12. The clause promoting genetically modified food was slipped in as an eleventh-hour action that stunned many activists. By the time they heard about it, it was too late to remove it, according to critics. Senate Majority Leader Dr. William Frist, who introduced the GM clause, is well known in Washington as a lobbyist for the agribusiness giant Monsanto, one of the big six GM producers. Lori Wallach and Michelle Sforza, *Whose Trade Organization? Corporate Globalization and the Erosion of Democracy*, Public Citizen Foundation, 1999. Genetically modified (GM, or GE – genetically engineered) foods include grains and seeds in which genes are selectively introduced. In the US, products containing genetically modified organisms are completely unregulated, according to Wallach and Sforza of Public Citizen, a consumer watchdog group. Their 1999 research shows that Monsanto, for example, requires

farmers who buy their GM seeds to agree not to save the seeds. The biofood giant recently developed sterile or "terminator" GM seeds that can only be activated by use of a chemical. The seeds that such crops produce do not germinate. India is among several developing countries that have banned entry of terminator genes into India, the Public Citizen duo reported.

In recent years, several African countries (Zambia, Zimbabwe, Mozambique, Malawi) have balked at accepting GM foods produced by US biotech agricultural firms, convinced these may not be environmentally safe and could overtake native agricultural strains, and thus hurt domestic farming. As with AIDS drugs, the war over food patents is being fought within the WTO. After 2005, when the deadline on patents is expected to be applied, India and others opposed to GM foods may have new battles to fight over GM food and food aid. The Bush administration strongly backs GM food exports to developing countries and has denounced Europe's rejection of bioengineered food. "Congress and the Administration have repeatedly acknowledged that a major reason they support filing a WTO case against Europe's GM food policy is because they fear that Europe's policies are influencing Africa and other regions to reject American GM food," conclude Wallach and Sforza.

13. On July 30, 2003, AIDS activists targeted top White House advisor Karl Rove, a key player allied with big pharma in the WTO generics fight.

3   Brazil's AIDS Model: A Global Blueprint?

1. The prediction of the collapse of South Africa was made on the basis of a mid-2003 World Bank estimate. Since that time, South Africa has remained mired in debate over President Mbeki's opposition to antiretroviral treatment. But in September 2003 Mbeki capitulated, following a meeting and an offer of financial aid from former US president Bill Clinton. The William Jefferson Clinton Foundation is now helping South Africa to draw up a national scale-up plan that includes treatment, which the government is backing, although Mbeki and his health minister, Manto Tshabalala-Msimang, remain privately – some say publicly – opposed to the plan. In the flurry of events that have fol-

lowed, South Africa's Congress, civil society, NGOs and activists have moved quickly to implement access to treatment. If all goes according to plan, its success could prevent the apocalyptic World Bank prediction. Much will depend on political jockeying by Mbeki and his allies and, on the other side, on the continued vigilance and protest activities of the Treatment Action Campaign and its allies, who fervently embrace the treatment plan. Helen Epstein, "AIDS: The Lessons of Uganda," *New York Review of Books*, July 17, 2003.

2. Tina Rosenberg, "How to Stop the World's AIDS Crisis: Look at Brazil," *New York Times Magazine*, January 28, 2001; "The Brazilian STD and AIDS Programme," a document published by the Brazilian STD and AIDS Programme, 2000; "The Brazilian Response to HIV/AIDS," a document published Brazilian Ministry of Health, Secretariat for Health Policies and the National Coordination for STD and AIDS, Brazil, 2000.

3. "Brazilian National AIDS Program Receives 2003 Gates Award for Global Health," Press Release, *Global Health Council Newsletter*, May 28, 2003.

4. "US–Brazil Joint Venture on HIV/AIDS in Lusophone Africa," US Department of State Fact Sheet, June 20, 2003.

5. "Worldwide Protest Against AIDS Medicines Patents on the Increase," *WOZA Internet*, Johannesburg, February 27, 2001.

6. Lori Wallach and Michelle Sforza, *Whose Trade Organization? Corporate Globalization and the Erosion of Democracy*, Public Citizen Foundation, 1999.

7. "Brazil: US Protects Drug Companies," *Associated Press*, May 2, 2001.

8. The production of several nucleoside drugs allowed Brazil to provide three-drug combination therapy at a fraction of the cost of importing such drugs. Once Brazil produced non-nucleoside drugs, it had generic non-protease combinations available for patients who were less ill, based on WHO guidelines that advocate the use of alternative first-line non-protease drugs for treatment-naive individuals who are not seriously ill with AIDS.

9. "US Drops Brazil AIDS Drugs Case: Demand for Cheaper AIDS Drugs Has Sparked Protests," *BBC News*, June 25, 2001. As the BBC report noted, the Bush administration dropped its lawsuit against Brazil during the three-day United Nations General Assembly Special

Session on AIDS, UNGASS, in New York. Defending its actions, the Brazilian government, led by President Fernando Henrique Cardoso, accused the Bush administration of launching an attack on its successful AIDS program and of being overly influenced by the multinational brand-name AIDS drugs producers. In April, the UN Human Rights Commission added its weight to those protesting the US lawsuit when it overwhelmingly voted to support a Brazilian resolution calling for universal medical treatment for people with HIV and AIDS. "White House Drops WTO Claim Against Brazilian Patent Law," *Wall Street Journal*, June 26, 2001.

10. Interview with the author, late June 2003.

11. Elizabeth Becker, "US Suspends AID to 35 Countries Over New International Court," *New York Times*, July 2, 2003. Becker noted that the Bush administration is concerned about current war crimes indictments filed in Belgium against several serving US officials related to their roles in the 1991 Gulf War, including Vice President Dick Cheney and Secretary of State Colin Powell. In response to the US aid cutoff, Richard Dicker, a director of Human Rights Watch in New York, said that the suspension of military aid amounted to a defeat for the international court – and a departure of sorts. "I've never seen a sanctions regime aimed at countries that believe in the rule of law rather than ones that commit human rights abuses," he told Becker.

12. Warren A. Kaplan, Richard Laing, Brenda Waning, Libby Levison and Susan Foster, "Is Local Production a Way to Improve Pharmaceutical Access in Developing and Transitional Countries? Setting a Research Agenda," a draft document circulated for review and publicly available on the internet, by researchers from the Boston University School of Public Health, April 23, 2003. According to the authors, "Smaller countries with fewer resources and a weak industrial base are unlikely to be viable in the global pharmaceutical market." Their preliminary conclusion was that it is economically unfeasible for many developing countries to produce medicines domestically, since local production is often unreliable and does not necessarily result in cheaper medicines for local consumers. It would be economically wiser for such countries to build up other aspects of the industrial sector or stimulate the existing market for drugs, than embark on local production, including state production of generic AIDS drugs. Further, if local production of such

drugs is adopted by many countries, the result may be less, not more access, to lifesaving medicines, since there are no economies of scale in having a production facility in each country. State-controlled local production is "ill-advised," they find, an analysis echoed by some WHO experts (Bennett, Quick & Velasquez 1997).

13. Interview with the author, late June 2003, in Brasilia. Rech's comments have been backed by those of other Brazilian officials, who say the country does not have the current capacity for global export.

14. *Associated Press* and *Kansas City Star* reports, September 26, 2003. In late September, Eric Noehregberg, director of international trade and market issues for the International Federation of Pharmaceutical Manufacturers' Association, concurred with a view of Brazil's limited capacity to manufacture drugs for export to other countries.

15. The new fixed-dose pills, according to Brazilian officials, are: AZT-3TC-NVP; 3TC-ddI-Sustiva; d4T-3TC; Ritonavir-Saquinavir; Indinavir-Ritonavir.

16. Interview with Norberto Rech, late June 2003.

17. M.A. Loewy, J.C. Brava, "Free HIV Drugs in Brazil Have Boosted AIDS Survival, *Reuters*, July 25, 2003.

18. Interview with Paolo Teixeira, June 2003.

19. *AIDS* 2003, vol. 17, no. 11: 1675–82.

20. "Free HIV Drugs in Brazil Have Boosted AIDS Survival," *Reuters*, July 25, 2003.

21. "Quality of the Brazilian AIDS Program Will Be Defended at the World Bank," report by Brazilian Ministry of Health, Health Surveillance Secretariat, National STD/AIDS Programme, June 6, 2003. This report, made available to the media, summarized Teixeira's presentation of the results of the Brazil program to World Bank managers and others who met on June 17 and 18 to assess the results of a number of treatment programs funded by the World Bank in African and Caribbean countries. According to several Brazilian health officials I spoke to during my July visit to Brasilia, the government decided to make the study results available to counter criticism by several high-level US experts, including Robert Gallo and Luc Montagnier, the co-discoverers of HIV. The duo had expressed reservations about Brazil's AIDS program, and concerns about levels of resistance globally. They allegedly urged World Bank officials not to back global treatment pro-

grams, according to my sources. "It is outrageous, but we have the evidence to prove they are wrong," Teixeira told me in July, as the fallout of the war-of-words over resistance continued behind closed doors.

"Brazilian AIDS Program Activities on HIV Drug Resistance, Monitoring and Prevention," a report by the Brazilian Ministry of Health, Executive Secretariat, National STD/AIDS Program, April 10, 2003. The report describes the results of several studies done by HIV-BresNet, a National Network for Drug Resistance Surveillance. These include prevalence studies of drug resistance mutations in HIV-positive patients failing antiretroviral therapy (study results from 1998 and 2000), and localized studies in Rio de Janeiro and Brasilia in drug-naive groups, including blood donors and AIDS patients.

22. Brazil has moved to remedy this gap. In November, the government launched a program of free HIV testing in public hospitals, with the goal of reaching 3.6 million people by the end of 2004. Their research showed that 40,000 Brazilians didn't know their HIV status. Meanwhile, the epidemic was spreading fastest among women aged thirteen to twenty-nine. Source: "Brazil Launches Free HIV Testing Campaign," *Reuters*, October 30, 2003.

23. Unpublished interview with *POZ* reporter Cindra Feuer, June 2003.

24. Ibid.

25. Interview with the author, late June, 2003.

26. Ibid.

4   Tipping the Scales: India and Generic Drugs

1. Jon Cohen, "HIV/AIDS in Asia: A Special Report," *Science*, September 19, 2003. Science staff reporter Cohen is also author of a much-heralded exposé of AIDS vaccine research, *Shots in the Dark: The Wayward Search for an AIDS Vaccine*, W.W. Norton & Company, 2001. In this series, he reports from Laos, Vietnam, Thailand and Cambodia.

2. The Lawyers' Collective was started by Anand Grover, a lawyer and human rights advocate who has become a leading defender of HIV-positive individuals. His legal team has offices in Mumbai and New Dehli, and is concentrating on fighting HIV discrimination cases. It is also working on patent issues and lobbying the government to ensure that Indians with HIV get access to low-cost generics and care.

3. In the week of February 27, Muslims in Gujarat state had rioted and set fire to a train full of Hindu pilgrims, killing fifty-nine and setting off a chain of events that led to the deaths of thousands of Muslims and the loss of homes for many more. These acts of revenge had followed violent clashes between Hindu pilgrims who had demolished a sixteenth-century mosque in Ayodhya, and planned to build a temple there. Many critics accused far-right nationalist Hindu leaders of the ruling Bharatiya Janata Party government of helping to foment the attacks and of doing little to stop police attacks on Muslims in the aftermath of the train attack.

See Project Ploughshares' December 2002 Armed Conflict Report on India. In a summary of the fundamentalist politico-religious wars of 2002, it stated:

> In February [2002], 59 Hindus were burned alive in a train stationed in Godha and traveling to a religious site sacred to both Hindus and Muslims, an incident that incited a series of reprisal killings from both communities, including a three day anti-Muslim riot in which up to 2,500 people, mostly Muslims, were killed, and another 100,000 people were forced to relocate to relief camps within Gujarat state. State police and officials of the ruling BJP [Bharatiya Janata Party] were accused of participating in, and even orchestrating, the riots. In September, Muslim extremists attacked a Hindu temple in retaliation, killing 30 Hindus, an act that Indian officials blamed on Pakistan. After a brief respite, violence increased during September state elections.

Others say 35,000 people were displaced in the weeks after the February 27 Godha train massacre, in which mostly Hindu women and children died. ("Riots in India Leave Hundreds Dead, Thousands Homeless," *News & Letters*, a Chicago-based newsletter, April 2002.)

4. Amy Waldman, "Anxiety Rises in a Muslim Enclave Near Bombay," *New York Times*, September 1, 2003. As Waldman reported, tensions were rising again in India following two bombings in late August that took place in downtown Bombay. At the time, no arrests had been made, but Muslim militants were being blamed. For their part, Islamic groups blame India's ruling BJP party for the attacks on Muslim Indians, who make up 14 percent of the country's population of 1 billion. In 1992 and 1993, over 1,000 Muslims died in what are

called the Bombay riots, or clashes with Hindus (and as Amnesty International noted in a special report on the ongoing religious-political tensions in India, 2,500 died in the 2002 clashes). Waldman notes that Muslims in India are often viewed as being different from Muslims in Islamic countries. Many Muslims have migrated to Mumbra, a suburb of Bombay. "They did not join Al Qaeda; they did not surface in training camps in Afghanistan. They lived in secular India, as opposed to its Islamic neighbor Pakistan, and most see India's democracy and Constitution as providing them with sufficient rights and redress." But Islamic extremism is growing, and includes members of the now-banned Students Islamic Movement of India, which police blame for five smaller bomb killings in buses, trains and markets between December 2002 and July 2003.

5. Habib Beary, "India's Eunuchs Demand Rights," *BBC News*, September 4, 2003. Hijras are born male but identify themselves as female and live in close communities. Bangalore alone is home to about 2,000 hijras. A majority work as prostitutes and experience a lot of discrimination, including numerous illegal detentions and harassment by police in Karnataka state. An estimated 500,000 to 1 million hijras live in India. "The Constitution gives rights on the basis of citizenship and not on the grounds of gender," says Babu Matthew, a human rights activist and professor at the National Law School of India. Hijras have begun to organize for their social and political rights. In 2000 the first hijra MP was elected to Parliament (March 6, 2001, BBC report).

In 2001 a sensitive documentary about India's hijras was also released to critical acclaim. *Bombay Eunuch* was made by co-directors Alexandra Shiva, Sean MacDonald and Michelle Gucovsky, and explores, among other subjects, the heavy impact of HIV on hijras and the widespread discrimination they face in India.

6. The name of India's famous port city was changed in the mid 1990s as part of a continuing effort to cast off vestiges of its colonization by European powers. But even residents interchangeably refer to Mumbai and Bombay. Mumbai's name derives from Mumbadevi, a stone goddess of Buddhist monks and deep-sea fisherman; Bombay comes from Bom Bahia, or Good Bay, a Portugese name given to the Indian coastal settlement by Francis Almeida in 1508.

7. Hetero, for example, obtained FDA approval in 2002 to market five

generic products: omeprezole, tizanidine, fosinopril, cotrimoxazole (Bactrim), and itraconazole, according to company officials (source: author interviews with company officials in Hyderabad). The latter two are used to treat, respectively, HIV-related pneumocystis pneumonia and HIV-related fungal infections. Ranbaxy had more than twenty-five products approved by the US FDA by March 2002, according to Ranbaxy company literature and interviews with company officials in Hyderabad.

8. Stephane Lucchini et al., "Decrease in Prices of Antiretroviral Drugs for Developing Countries: From Political 'Philanthropy' to Regulated Markets?" *Economics of AIDS and Access to HIV/AIDS Care in Developing Countries: Issues and Challenges*, edited by Jean-Paul Moatti et al., a book in the series Collection Sciences Sociales et Sida, published by the Agence Nationale de Recherches sur le SIDA, Paris, 2003.

9. Interview with the author at Cipla headquarters in Mumbai, March 2002.

10. Ibid.

11. Interview with the author, March 2002. Raizada added,

> Even if you came down to making finished dosage form, there might be only three or four countries with industry capability: Brazil, Argentina, South Africa with limited ability, and maybe Egypt. And that's where it stops. When it comes to Asia, Thailand can do API [active pharmaceutical ingredients] and FP [finished product], India yes – and lastly there is China. China doesn't have the technology for API, but it has the technology and capability to produce formulations.

12. A fall 2002 Harvard analysis of patents on fifteen antiretroviral drugs in fifty-three countries by Amir Attaran concluded that in most of Africa, only two HIV drugs are patented, except for South Africa, where over a dozen drugs are patented. In East African countries, only four or five drugs are patented.

13. As of August 2003, the list of generic antiretroviral drug suppliers had greatly increased, though the WHO had only approved products by four. My own research turned up these companies, though private companies in other countries, including in Eastern Europe, Asia and Latin America, are contemplating entry. Multiple sources and individuals contributed to this list, including the WHO, MSF, Ralph Nader's

Consumer Project on Technology, Health GAP, the ANRS, individual company reports, and interviews with representatives I contacted at these companies. For updates, check the websites of MSF, Health GAP, CP Tech, UNAIDS, and the WHO's list of prequalified manufacturers.

Asia

India: Cipla, Ranbaxy, Hetero, Aurobindo, Matrix, Zydus Cadila Healthcare, Sun Pharma, EAS-SURG, Strides, MacLeods, IPCA, Torrent, RPF Life, Micro Labs, Sol Pharma, Pure Health Products, East India, Kerran, Dr. Reddy's.

South Korea: Sahchully, Korea United Pharm, LG Chemicals.

Thailand: Government Pharmaceutical Organization (GPO), T.O. Chemecal.

China: Desano Shanghai, Northeast General (with another ten poised to jump in by the end of the year).

Vietnam: Stada Viet Nam.

Latin America

Brazil: Far-Manguinhos, FURP, Lafepe, Iquego, IVP; also private producers: Microbiologics, Labogen.

Argentina: Richmond Laboratories, Panalab, Filaxis.

Mexico: Apotex, Pisa, Protein.

Costa Rica: Stein.

Columbia: Protein.

Cuba: Genetic Engineering Biotechnology Center.

Western Europe

Spain: CombinoPharma, Andromaco.

Middle East

Egypt: Nile.

Africa

Morocco: Gellenica.

South Africa: Aspen PharmaCare.

Benin: Pharmaquick.

Kenya: Cosmos, Laboratory, Allied.

14. In August 2003 South Africa's government agreed to develop a national treatment program and has enlisted the help of the William Jefferson Clinton Foundation to help develop a comprehensive plan. Details are discussed in the concluding chapter of this book.

15. As of April 2002, Cipla had finished BE studies on eight HIV drugs and

two fixed-dose combination tablets. It is now doing post-marketing studies of the drugs. Hetero initially had trouble recruiting volunteers for BE studies because of the stigma of AIDS. "They were ignorant and afraid of getting HIV," Reddy related. "We had to work a lot to educate them and this caused delays." Hetero had completed BE studies on five antiretrovirals and a two-nuke AZT-3TC combo then. So had Ranbaxy, which was marketing two double-nuke combinations at different doses in mid 2002. Ranbaxy had completed BE for seven products by then, and hoped to have BE data on four more by June 2002, including a three-drug combination, 3TC/d4T/nevirapine. Summary documents on these completed BE studies were shown to me in April 2002 to prove the tests had been done, and the products were approved by domestic regulatory agencies. The other companies are also completing BE studies. More information can be obtained on the progress of their development by going to the websites of the individual companies.

16. Cipla had early results of a clinical observational study of its combination tablets containing nevirapine with two nucleoside analogs (either AZT/3TC or d4T/3TC) in March 2002. The study was carried out by two Indian doctors in 347 treatment-naive patients (296 males, 51 females) attending HIV care centers in two cities, Pune and Ahmedabad. The progress of the trial cohort was evaluated using clinical monitoring and CD4 and CD8 cell counts, but not viral load tests. On average, patients began treatment with a mean baseline CD4 count of 144. After a year, 64.6 percent of patients had CD4 count increases of 20 percent, and little difference was noted between the different nucleoside analog arms. Overall, twenty-three people in the study developed opportunistic infections and six died. As for toxicities, 10.5 percent of the cohort developed rashes, including four who had Stevens-Johnson syndrome, which the study authors associated with female gender. Based on these results, the researchers concluded that nevirapine, being the third cheapest drug in India, "can be positioned as a first-line HAART option for antiretroviral-naive patients."

17. Interviews and private e-mail correspondence with the author, October 2001 to September 2002. "They didn't have the manufacturing process for finished dosages or the information about how to turn APIs into tablets," Hetero's Reddy noted in 2002 about Brazil's Far-Manguinhos. "We have scientists there to simultaneously train and

help to do finished product, and we transferred finished dosage formulations and technology to these manufacturing units. We gave them the analytical method, for example, how to compare to innovator products, how to keep on par with innovator products, et cetera."

18. Interview with the author in Mumbai, March 2002. According to several other physicians I interviewed, corruption among doctors and the influence of drug money in medicine is an enduring problem in India – as it is in many countries, including the US. "These doctors get paid money to use the drugs," admitted Shoshank Joshi, a leading Indian doctor in Bombay. "It's true for the generics as well. It is a way for the doctors to line their own pockets because, as you know, Indian doctors don't make a lot of money compared to what doctors make in America." The same was true for pharmacists, he added. He cited cases he knew of where drug companies had openly paid doctors, or bribed them with paid trips to conferences and other perks, in exchange for prescriptions of their generic products. "Cipla works with some doctors, Ranbaxy with others – everyone does it," he explained. Cipla officials told me in interviews that it was not uncommon for private doctors who managed pharmacies to come to Mumbai to directly negotiate drug purchases, and avoid the cost of shipping the drugs or paying customs taxes. Such small-scale purchases are limited to use by the patients of the physician, but it seemed like there was little oversight as to the eventual use or resale of these drugs by other patients.

19. Interview with the author, Mumbai, March 2002. Follow up e-mail correspondence, summer 2002 and spring 2003.

20. Interview with the author, spring 2002. Since this time, Stern has regularly berated the generic companies for failing to provide their low-cost drugs to Latin American nations, and has publicly shared his e-mail correspondence with activist allies.

21. The drugs for Honduras were purchased by the late Dr. Roberto Trejo, a pioneering physician who treated HIV patients in a poor area. Trejo contacted me shortly after my return from India, asking if I could help his organization buy generic drugs directly from Cipla. At the time, the main physician's organization getting the drugs this way was MSF. He had tried once to e-mail Cipla but gotten no response. He was desperate as several patients were dying, and none could afford the cost of even discounted brand-name drugs. I passed on the contacts I had and

wrote to Cipla's doctors directly, assuring their representatives that Dr. Trejo was a legitimate physician who would only distribute the drugs freely to his patients, not sell them or ask patients to pay for treatment. As we waited, he wrote two or three times, asking me to pressure the company to assure speedy delivery of the shipment. I know he lost more than one patient in the interim, but the drugs immediately worked to save others when they did arrive. I kept his triumphant e-mail, announcing the arrival of the drugs and including his words of thanks, pinned to my wall for a year. It was one of those small actions that made me feel how easily we can sometimes make a critical difference in another person's life.

Early in 2003 I was shocked when Richard Stern wrote to tell me Dr. Trejo was murdered in Honduras by unknown assailants, leaving behind a wife and children and a community of people living with HIV. In Honduras he was known as a champion of the poor, a Honduran patriot, and a doctor, who had crossed over to become an activist, as he put it, out of moral necessity.

22. "South African Generic Drug Maker to Produce Country's First Generic Antiretroviral Drug," *Associated Press*, August 6, 2003.

23. Transparency in this case means that drug bids (called tenders) are open and there are no secrets or closed-door deals being made. This level of openness allows for real competition among manufacturers and allows consumers to evaluate their products and manufacturing processes.

24. Author interviews with Brazilian health officials and generic manufacturers, June 2003.

25. Warren A. Kaplan, Richard Laing, Brenda Waning, Libby Levison and Susan Foster. "Is Local Production a Way to Improve Pharmaceutical Access in Developing and Transitional Countries? Setting a Research Agenda." A draft document produced for RPM+ and circulated for peer review by health policy analysts at the Boston University School of Public Health, April 23, 2003. According to the authors, "Smaller countries with fewer resources and a weak industrial base are unlikely to be viable in the global pharmaceutical market." Their preliminary conclusion was that it is economically unfeasible for many developing countries to produce medicines domestically, since local production is often unreliable and does not necessarily result in cheaper medicines for local consumers. It would be economically wiser for such countries

to build up other aspects of the industrial sector or stimulate the existing market for drugs, than embark on local production, including state production of generic AIDS drugs. Further, if local production of such drugs is adopted by many countries, the result may be less, not more access to lifesaving medicines, since there are no economies of scale in having a production facility in each country. State-controlled local production is "ill advised," they find, an analysis shared by some WHO experts (Bennett, Quick & Velasquez, 1997).

26. Several examples of US aid sanctions were mentioned to me by Brazilian health officials, MSF, Health GAP, and James Love, director of the Ralph Nader watchdog group on trade, the Consumer Project on Technology (CP Tech). The Brazilians provided this information as background only, not wanting to go public in a denunciation of the Bush administration during their delicate negotiations during the August 2003 WTO talks. Among the countries that reportedly backed down from making generics was the Dominican Republic.

27. Interview with the author, September 2003.

28. Remarks to the press by Jim Yong Kim on 3×5 roll-out, November 2003.

5   Cuba Fights AIDS Its Own Way

1. "Cuba: Epidemiological Fact Sheet," Global HIV/AIDS and STD Surveillance, UNAIDS, 2000.

2. Bush Administration Threatens Freedom to Travel," *Global Exchange Newsletter*, Fall 2003, Issue 56; Claudia Marquez Linares, "Free Trade Won't Free Cuba," Op-Ed, *New York Times*, November 6, 2003.

3. Richard Stern, "AIDS and Human Rights in Cuba: A Personal Memoir," *Gully*, online current affairs magazine, May 2, 2003.

4. Victor F. Zonana, "Cuba's AIDS Quarantine Center Called 'Frightening,'" *Los Angeles Times*, November 4, 1988.

5. "Cuba's AIDS Prevalence Rate Low, Although Prevention Methods 'Aggressive, Controversial,'" *Denver Post*, March 23, 2003.

6. Karen Wald, "Cuba's AIDS Patient #1 Dies," *NY Transfer News Collective*, October 4, 1995. Wald is an American activist and journalist who has spent years traveling and reporting in Cuba. Although she

is an open supporter of Cuba and strongly defends its AIDS program, she is also well aware of criticism of its policies. In this report, she discussed why long-time sufferers like Maria Julia and her husband had chosen to remain inside the Santiago de las Vegas sanatorium, and provided details of the evolution of life for those inside: "Patient Number One, Reynaldo Morales and his wife did not choose to leave. Having gone through the shock of adjusting to sanatorium life, they were settled and enjoyed the pampering they got from doctors inside. They also had a great deal of flexibility to leave the facility – admittedly more than some."

7. In a study titled, "Between the Devil and the Deep Blue Sea: Development and HIV in Cuba," analysts Jafari Sinclaire Allen (a Columbia University anthropologist in Cuba and the US), Llane Alexis Dominguez Estrada (a Cuban artist and HIV advocate), and Joseph Simon Mutti (a British journalist specializing in HIV/AIDS issues who lives and works in Cuba), wrote about conditions during the "Special Period":

> In the early 1990s, as the island's economic crisis broadened into an appalling 30 percent drop in GDP after the fall of the Soviet Union and the Eastern European bloc, Cuba sought a way to prevent its economy from collapsing. By 1993, as the Special Period reached its height, Cubans began to show signs of malnourishment. It was obvious that Cuba had to attract hard currency to survive. Moreover, in order to flourish in a global special period of the capitalist model of development throughout the Caribbean and elsewhere . . . while maintaining the gains of the Revolution, it would have to nurture industry, re-educate workers through technological transfer, and repair worn infrastructure – especially in the capital, Havana. This would have to be achieved in the face of an intensification of the US blockade that not only embargoed trade with Cuba, but also isolated Cuba from the international community and global economy. Cuba would also have to tackle its inefficient and unsophisticated administrative practices and top-down leadership style.
>
> Cuba's challenge is unique in its political peculiarities, but not in terms of the worldwide drive for poorer nations to meet the demands of the emerging global financial system. Just as its Caribbean neighbors had been forced to choose tourism to cope with financial hardship

caused by shifting global markets, Cuba made the decision to open itself up to holiday-makers from abroad. President Castro lamented that he wished Cuba could export its beaches, and that to invite tourism was like making a pact with the devil. Nonetheless, the pact was made, the Ministry of Tourism began to court foreign investors, and modernization plans were put in place.

It has been argued that during the Special Period – when food and necessities such as soap and cooking oil have been scarce – sex workers have had to sell sex or starve. Observers now say that government food programs . . . have improved things slightly, though most sex workers still inhabit a purgatory called "survival." Yet if the financial desperation of the Special Period were the sole reason for sex work, we should have observed a steady decrease in the practice since the advent of food programs in 1998. This has not been the case. A more pragmatic view looks at the position of sex workers in the global economy – and compares their motivations with those of Cubans in similar situations who do not choose sex work. Development organizations will have to look beyond food programs as a way of protecting sex workers and the rest of the Cuban population from HIV/AIDS.

8. You can't blame Cuban health officials for being worried about misrepresentations by the Western, and especially US press. The mainstream US media coverage of the sanatoriums has been almost completely critical, and often lurid. Ironically, Perez was frankly quite disappointed by my own story about the sanatorium and Cuba's AIDS picture, first published in the *amfAR Treatment Insider*, especially since he'd offered me so much of his time and been so open in his conversation with me in 2002. He felt it was too critical and that the comments made by Cheo and other critics were inaccurate. As promised, I'd sent my initial story draft to him and other Cubans I interviewed prior to publication for fact checking, and to make sure I had accurately represented their views and comments. It's so easy to slant stories, so, as I do with all my interview subjects, I reassured them in advance that if we taped our interviews, I would give them a chance to review any material referring to our conversations.

On principle, many journalists and editors (and in fact my own editor at *amfAR*) disagree with the decision to show any material to interview subjects beforehand; they are concerned that it leads to self-censorship or threats of lawsuits by interview subjects. I take a different view (though I have been threatened over the years). I think it makes me a more accurate reporter. I will consider changing my remarks if I am given solid evidence that I have made a factual error, but not because they may reflect critically on that person. As I told Perez, I'm not afraid of people disagreeing with my reporting or conclusions.

Still, I understood his disappointment. After all, he has worked very hard and very successfully to change negative aspects of the HIV program, often with a lot of opposition by his colleagues in the government. What I didn't tell him was that I had actually been told more horror stories by critics, which painted a far more damning picture of the early AIDS program. Some of the accusations related to more recent events. But since I hadn't had time to verify such charges independently, or get any concrete evidence to back up or refute them, I hadn't published them. I had only published statements by individuals that were corroborated by other individuals, or when they could offer some documentation of the alleged wrongdoing.

9. In later conversations, former residents said they knew people who had lost their jobs, despite official policy forbidding workplace discrimination against those with HIV.

10. "China SARS Plan Slammed," *BBC News 24 Special Report*, May 16, 2003. "This is completely out of line with international practice and is sending the wrong message to the population," said Nicolas Becquelin, research director of Human Rights in China (HRIC) at the time, referring to the law calling for the execution of quarantine violators.

11. "Cuba's AIDS Prevalence Rate Low, Although Prevention Methods 'Aggressive, Controversial,'" *Denver Post*, March 23, 2003.

12. Interview with Cuban epidemiologists, Havana, 2002.

13. "I don't feel safe talking to you with other people around," Cheo explained when I met him at the Monserrate support group and requested an interview. "You never know who is listening and who will tell the authorities." Even now, he explained, Cubans were not supposed to speak to foreigners, unless they worked for the tourist ministry. Doing so could risk harassment by the authorities. "I especially shouldn't be speaking with you because you're a journalist from America," he added, smiling. "No one is going to come and arrest me, but I don't want to give them any reason to be suspicious, either."

Several other activists I met in Cuba shared his concerns. Although life in Cuba has greatly relaxed, they carry memories of the not-so-distant past, when contact with foreigners was policed.

14. Manuel is a pseudonym for a man I met at the Monserrate support group in Havana. He requested anonymity because he had not disclosed his status to co-workers, and out of a fear of reprisals if his identity was disclosed.

15. Wald, "Cuba's AIDS Patient #1 Dies."

16. In 1980 Fidel Castro released thousands of Cubans from jails, including many gay men who had been locked up for the crime of homosexuality – or suspected homosexuality. Gays were deemed social undesirables by Castro, along with prostitutes and criminals. A large number of Cuban gays and lesbians left Cuba during the Mariel boatlift from April to October, when 125,000 Cubans fled the Port of Mariel for Miami, where they were given safe haven. This chapter of Cuban history is dramatised in a now-famous 1993 novel *Before Night Falls*, by Reinaldo Arenas, a gay, HIV-positive Cuban writer who was a fierce anti-Castro dissident and was imprisoned in the El Morro prison. In 1990 Arenas was broke, dying of AIDS and living in obscurity as a writer when he committed suicide in his Hell's Kitchen apartment in Manhattan, New York.

17. A pseudonym (see note 14).

18. For more information on the Montserrate HIV support group, contact Monserrate church officials or Fernando de la Vega by email at <dei@cocc.co.cu>. Within Cuba, information can be obtained from local AIDS prevention organization and hotline GP-SIDA or CCIETS-SIDA on Calle 27 between avenues B and C, headed by Dr. Rosaida Ochoa. To get involved in supporting treatment access, contact AIDS Treatment Access Cuba, a recycling project based in New Mexico <www.cubasida.net> or AID for AIDS <www.aid4aids.org>.

19. As Cubans pointed out to me several times, it's cheaper – and safer – to build new, sound buildings than refurbish old ones and get them up to code. The contrast between Old Havana's crumbling but charming streets and sections of the city boasting new, modern buildings is one of the most striking aspects of the capital city. But it also attests to the severe shortage of housing that isn't in some way falling apart.

20. Anita Snow and Paul Elias, "Cuba Seeks New Drug Markets," *Associated Press*, 2002.
21. "HIV/AIDS in Cuba: An Overview," pamphlet by the AIDS Treatment Access Cuba project, Santa Fe, New Mexico <www.cubasida.net>, itself a program of Disarm Education Fund.
22. Interviews with Drs. Perez and Millan, IPK.
23. Snow and Elias, "Cuba Seeks New Drug Markets."
24. "Cuban Co-operation with South Africa Could Include Patent-Busting AIDS Drugs," *SAPA-AFP*, March 28, 2001.
25. "Further Moves on Cuba's Entry into the Generic Market," *IRIN*, March 28, 2001.
26. For a different and more positive report on the 2003 Foro, see Carol Amoruso's June 23, 2003 summary on the Hispanic Village website: <www.IMdiversity.com>.
27. Stern is a US journalist and HIV treatment activist who lives in Costa Rica, where he edits a regional Spanish-language HIV treatment newsletter. He was the community representative on Costa Rica official delegation to a UN General Assembly Special Summit on AIDS (UNGASS). In a May 2, 2003 article entitled "AIDS and Human Rights in Cuba: A Personal Memoir," Stern wrote of his reaction to the jailing of journalists and the execution of dissidents:

> It's easy to see news of an event such as this on TV, and to "condemn it," as the international human rights community did in this case. But being right there, at that moment, surrounded by decent and hard-working Cubans, some with AIDS, some not, it was chilling to think that this event had occurred three miles from where I was, just a few hours earlier, and that Cuba's President, who condoned these executions supposedly ordered by a judge, was to appear and give the closing address at the conference the following day.
> (Article posted on *Gully* online magazine, May 2, 2003)

28. Claudia Marquez Linares, "Free Trade Won't Free Cuba," Op-Ed, *New York Times*, November 6, 2003. Linares is married to Osvaldo Alfonso Valdes, head of the Democratic Liberal Party of Cuba. In her op-ed she argued that the ongoing attempt by US senators to pass an amendment easing the new Bush restrictions on US travel to Cuba would not benefit ordinary Cubans, nor the jailed dissidents, only the Castro

regime and top officials of the Communist Party. As of November, her husband faced eighteen years in a cell two-yards-square at the high-security prison of Guanajay. Valdes was among the first dissidents to be arrested, shortly after he met with US Congressional representatives to discuss reforms in Cuba, and the possibility of ending the embargo and increasing trade between the US and Cuba.

29. "Bush Administration Threatens Freedom to Travel," *Global Exchange Newsletter*, Fall 2003, Issue 56.

30. "WTO Members Propose Greater Flexibility for Compulsory Licensing of Essential Drugs," June 27, 2002, News Archives, The Bureau of National Affairs, Inc.

6 HIV Medicines Come to Rural Haiti

1. Paul Farmer, *The Uses of Haiti*, Common Courage Press, 1984, updated 2003, pp. 360–75.

2. For a comprehensive, highly readable portrait of Haiti in the post-Duvalier period leading to Aristide's election, see journalist Amy Wilentz's excellent account, *The Rainy Season: Haiti Since Duvalier*, Simon and Schuster, 1989. Aristide's own speeches and political views can be found in a small book entitled *In the Parish of the Poor: Writings from Haiti*, Orbis, 1992.

3. Peter Dailey, "Haiti: The Fall of the House of Aristide," *New York Review of Books*, March 13, 2003; Roger Fatton Jr., *Haiti's Predatory Republic: The Unending Transition to Democracy*, Lynne Rienner, 2003.

4. D. Robert and R. Machado "Haiti: Economic Situation and Prospects," Inter-American Development Bank, Country Economic Assessment, 2001. For details see: <http://www.iadb.org/regions/re2/sep/ha-sepg.htm>. The embargo began in 2000 and suspended $500 million of promised foreign-aid development money by the Bush administration and European allies, and froze $146 million in IDB loans, including $22.5 million for medical supplies, $54 million for clean water programs, and money for education programs. It quickly left Haiti economically paralyzed. Worse, Haiti has had to pay millions of dollars in interest and "commission" fees to the IDB for loans it can't access. Many NGOs and traditional donors followed Bush's lead and curtailed

their activities there, causing a further decline in services to Haiti's rural poor, including health-care.

5. Paul Farmer, *Pathologies of Power*, University of California Press, 2003, pp. 124–6; 180–93. In this book, Farmer also warns of the consequences of establishing DOTS programs for tuberculosis without focusing on resistant TB, a strategy that can result in TB patients with resistant strains being treated with the wrong drugs. This leads to a treatment failure that also creates more drug resistance. This insight should be kept in mind now as DOT HIV programs are rolled out.

6. Anne-christine d'Adesky, "Silence + Death = AIDS in Haiti," *Advocate*, 577: 30–6.

7. Dailey, "Haiti: The Fall of the House of Aristide"; Fatton, *Haiti's Predatory Republic*.

8. "Haiti: Inter-American Development Bank Continues to Block Health Loans – Approves Grants to NGO for HIV/AIDS," *PRNewswire*, November 30, 2001.

9. Ibid.

10. Peter Greste, BBC News, 2000; "Haiti: the Role of the International Community," Human Rights Watch World Report, 2000; Jeffrey Kahn, "Haiti's AID Crisis Timeline," unpublished internal review of impact of international embargo on Haiti prepared for Partners In Health, January 19, 2001; George Gedda, "Haiti Faces Demand to Deal with Flawed Election," *Associated Press*, May 28, 2001.

11. Paul Farmer, Mary C. Smith Fawzi, Patrice Nevil, "Unjust Embargo of AID for Haiti," *Lancet*, February 1, 2003, vol. 361; Carl Hiaasen, "U.S. Denies Crucial Funds to Help Haiti," op-ed, *Miami Herald*, June 16, 2002. As Hiasen remarked, the embargo marks a shift in US policy. In the four years prior to the aid blockade, the US spent $300 million on humanitarian aid to Haiti – about $10 a person. He noted that the fourteen Caricom Caribbean nations and the US Congressional Black Caucus had urged Bush to free up funds for Haitian medical clinics, drinking water and education. But in May 2002, US Ambassador Lino Gutierrez declared that access to aid loans "will remain limited because the government of Haiti refuses to adhere to the most basic principles of good governance."

12. "Harvard Professor of Medicine Laments Human Impact of Financial

Embargo on Haiti," Interview with Paul Farmer, *Haiti Bulletin*, December 2001.

13. "Haiti's AID Crisis Timeline," internal document prepared for Partners In Health. According to a PIH analyst, Japanese chargé d'affaires Tsuyoshi Ebihara told reporters that "Japan was offering the aid because 'the precarious situation of the Haitian people' should not be influenced by Haiti's political problems" (*Agence France-Presse*, April 19, 2001).

14. Tracy Kidder, "Why do We Punish the Haitian People?" op-ed, *Washington Post*, August 7, 2002; Farmer, *The Uses of Haiti*. In this critical study of US foreign policy toward Haiti, Farmer provides a detailed overview of recent events that have contributed to Haiti's vicious cycle of poverty and dependence on foreign aid.

15. Kim Ives, "The Unmaking of a President," *Dangerous Crossroads*, an anthology published by the North American Congress on Latin America (NACLA), South End Press, 1995.

16. In July 2003, Aristide further annoyed US officials by demanding reparations against France, its former colonizer, from whom it asked for $22 billion in restitution, reported Canute James in the *Financial Times*, July 14, 2003. The bid for reparations came a month after Haitian banks agreed to loan Aristide's government $30 million to pay arrears to the IDB.

17. William Finnegan, "The Economics of Empire: Notes on the Washington Consensus (How the White House, the World Bank and the I.M.F. Impoverish the World on America's Behalf)," *Harper's*, May 2003. "The idea that open markets and increased trade lead invariably to economic growth may be sound in theory, but it has repeatedly failed the reality test," wrote Finnegan in his blistering, well-sourced review of Washington's neoliberal economic policies of the recent past. As he noted, IMF programs have had an overall deleterious effect on economic growth in participating countries: "And the World Bank's declared mission of reducing poverty has been a bust so far. More than a billion people are now living on less than one dollar a day – the figure in 1972 was 800 million – while nearly half the world's population is living on less than two dollars a day." It's become standard practice for the World Bank, IMF and other bilateral lenders, he stated, "to make new loans to deeply indebted countries in order to avoid the embar-

rassment of non-performing loans. Because it helps condemn the world's poor to a fate of permanent debt, the Bank's self-description as a 'pro-poor' development agency is at best self-deluding."

18. "SAP: The Outcome of a Policy of Capitulation," *Haiti Info*, February 11, 1995, vol. 3, no. 11.

19. Michael Dobbs, "Free Market Left Haiti's Rice Growers Behind," *Washington Post*, April 13, 2000.

20. Ibid. Dobbs found that structural adjustment policies in the agricultural sector had destroyed the livelihood and productivity of rice growers in the fertile Artibonite valley, where some residents said they were starving. "You can't expect a country like Haiti to compete on world markets immediately," Mark Weisbrot, co-director of the Center for Economic and Policy Research in Washington, told Dobbs. "If you look at the countries that have succeeded in dramatically lowering their per capita incomes – countries like Japan, South Korea and Taiwan – you'll find they all did it under some kind of protection." Critics have concluded that structural adjustment has further impoverished Haiti, and have come up with recent data to prove it. In "The Economics of Empire," journalist William Finnegan writes, "A recent study found that IMF programs have had, overall, a negative effect on economic growth in participating countries. And the World Bank's declared mission of reducing poverty has been a bust so far."

21. Greg Chamberlain, "Haiti's Second Independence," *Dangerous Crossroads*, a NACLA anthology, South End Press, 1995. Aristide was later denounced by former allies on the Haitian left for selling out to the US when he agreed to have US troops occupy Haiti as a condition of his return to power from exile in 1994. Everyone knew Aristide had little choice: if he refused the US offer of help – and troops to maintain security and keep his Duvalierist foes from regaining power – he remained in exile. To some on the political left, that would have been preferable to a US occupation, however temporary. See also "SAP: The Outcome of a Policy of Capitulation." In a full and complete capitulation before the US and other powerful countries who run the all-powerful Washington multilateral banks, President Jean-Bertrand Aristide and his government have signed the country up as the most recent passenger on the sinking ship of "structural adjustment," wrote

members of the Haitian Information Bureau who published the biweekly *Haiti Info*, an alternative news agency based in Fort Lauderdale, Florida. *Haiti Info* noted that the January 31 loan agreement merely formalized an earlier agreement, made in August 1994, whereby members of the Aristide team, led by Prime Minister Smarck Michel, agreed to "neoliberal" reforms, including the privatization of publicly owned industries, the reduction of all tariffs to zero the reduction of the public payroll by half (cutting 22,000 jobs), "micromanagement" of social services (a shifting away from state to private and/or "non governmental"-provided services. Additional source: *Haiti Info*, August 1994, vol. 2, no. 2.

22. "Harvard Professor of Medicine Laments Human Impact of Financial Embargo on Haiti," *Haiti Bulletin*.

23. "Haiti: Inter-American Development Bank Continues to Block Health Loans," *PRNewswire*.

24. Ibid.

25. "Haiti: IMF Deal May Free Up Funds," *Miami Herald*, May 14, 2003.

26. AIDS groups include SOFA – the Society of Women with AIDS; ASON – Association de Solidarite National; GIPA – Greater Involvement of People Living with AIDS; and a nascent gay rights group, GRASADIS ("Thanks to Ten," a reference to the estimated 10 percent of gay people in most societies).

27. Paul Farmer et al., "Community-based Approaches to HIV Treatment in Resource-Poor Settings," *Lancet*, 2001, vol. 358, no. 9,279; WHO Tuberculosis Control, "The DOTS Strategy: an annotated bibliography" compiled by the Global Tuberculosis Programme and the Regional Office for South East Asia, Geneva, Switzerland, WHO, 1997.

28. Interview with the author, August 2001.

29. Ibid.

30. Angela Garcia, "Epidemics, Politics and Discourse: The Hegemony of Directly Observed Therapy in the Treatment of AIDS," unpublished manuscript, Harvard University, 2002.

31. Haitian HIV patients have a name for accompagnateurs: "zanj yo" – angels. Their dedication is remarkable and fosters close relationships between patients and PIH staff – the extended family model. "We are all members of the same community, so these are our brothers and

sisters," said one accompagnateur. "We are all in the same boat living here." Source: author interviews with Cange HIV clinic patients and staff, August 2001.

32. Interview with the author, August 2001.

33. Almost 4,000 locals from the Cange clinic catchment area had HIV in 2001, and Farmer estimated that 10 percent would not live more than a few months without antiretrovirals. But even that figure was a best guess. Even with all the encouragement at Zanmi Lasante, the stigma surrounding AIDS had kept all but a handful from publicly revealing their HIV-positive status at that time.

34. Interview with the author, August 2001.

35. Ti Ofa hadn't warned his wife that he was going to come out publicly as HIV-positive at the Cange forum. He was a bit worried about the repercussions. But he had to testify, he said, because he felt a responsibility to his community and to the project. He wants to spread the message of hope. "I am not afraid, I am not hiding. I want to live and take care of protecting others. I tell them, if you don't want to disclose, you can find another means, but you can protect yourself and others."

36. Interview with Dr. Leandre, August 2001.

37. Abstract B10598, Fourteenth International AIDS Conference, Barcelona, Spain, July 7–12, 2002.

38. Interviews with Paul Farmer, May 2000, August 2001, May and June, 2003. For a full biography of Paul Farmer and the Haiti project see Tracy Kidder's new biography, *Mountains Beyond Mountains*, Random House, 2003.

39. Ian James, "New AIDS Fund Brings Hope to Haiti," *Associated Press*, April 7, 2003.

40. Correspondence with Paul Farmer, May and June, 2003.

41. Correspondence from Dr. Bill Pape and Dr. Rose Irene Verdier, Ghekio, May 2003.

42. Correspondence with Paul Farmer, May and June, 2003.

43. "Gheskio HIV/AIDS Treatment Scale Up at the National Level," an unpublished document prepared by Gheskio, May 2003.

44. "Government of Haiti Comprehensive HIV/AIDS Care and Treatment Plan (The Plan)," draft document circulated for review and prepared by the William J. Clinton Foundation HIV/AIDS Initiative, May 2003. One of the Foundation's first successes was in the Bahamas,

where Ira Magaziner, a top aide to Clinton during the White House years, succeeded in cutting a deal to slash the price of generic HIV drugs from $3,600 a year per person to $500. In a major coup, Magaziner talked four Indian generic manufacturers into slashing their antiretroviral prices to $0.50 a day in October 2003; Michael Norton, "American Officials Launch Bush's AIDS Initiative in Haiti," *Associated Press*, July 22, 2003.

45. The Clinton Initiative aims to assist hard-hit developing countries in the implementation of integrated care, treatment and prevention programs that can reverse the course of the epidemic. The Foundation forms partnerships with interested countries, providing assistance in developing national care and treatment plans, building the indigenous human capacity and physical infrastructure necessary to implement these plans, procuring needed drugs and mobilizing international resources to implement the country plans. The Foundation is working with the International AIDS Trust, headed by Sandra Thurman, another former Clinton aide, to mobilize political leaders to support global AIDS care, treatment and prevention efforts.

46. Ibid.

47. Ibid.

48. Interview with the author, August 2001.

49. In 2002 Gheskio saw 16,000 patients; 4,500 were given HIV care and 300 were given antiretroviral drugs. It is the largest TB facility in Haiti; some 2,500 patients required TB screening in 2002, and 1,500 were treated with TB drugs, according to Dr. Pape.

50. Jean Pape and Warren Johnson, "Epidemiology of AIDS in the Caribbean," *Bailliere's Clinical Tropical Diseases*, vol. 3, no. 1, pp. 31–42.

51. David Gonzales, "A Haitian Doctor's Success in the Fight Against Disease," *New York Times*, December 22, 2002.

52. Anne-christine d'Adesky, "Haiti: Scaling the Mountains: AIDS Vaccine Trial Begins in the Western Hemisphere's Hardest-hit Country," *IAVI Report*, April/June 2001.

53. While Haiti moves ahead to fight AIDS, internal and external political opposition to Aristide continues to contribute to civil strife. The once fanatical popularity of "Titid" among progressives has steadily fallen. A coterie of one-time allies broke from the Fanmi Lavalas party to form Democratic Convergence, an opposition political group. They

hope to electorally unseat the Aristide camp. But to ordinary Haitians, Aristide continues to be viewed as a near-God. That's why, despite widespread disappointment at Haiti's stalled economy and at Aristide's inability to break the logjam, Haitians in the street retain respect for the man who helped *dechouke*, or uproot, Duvalierism. Meanwhile, Aristide's critics reserve no great love for Uncle Sam. Progressives continue to view the carrot-and-stick of foreign aid for health programs – AIDS included – with suspicion.

Aristide's enemies include Democratic Convergence, as well as other political aspirants who accuse him of being a demagogue, and of betraying Haiti's commitment to democracy by refusing to share his power once in office. They blame his followers in La Fanmi Lavalas for acts of violence, including assassination, against political opponents. Some critics have even publicly accused some of the president's closest aides of being drug traffickers. Meanwhile, a coterie of former military men and members of Haiti's elite who fervently hate Aristide are doing what they can to foster political dissent against him.

Aristide's supporters charge that the US is seeking to further destabilize Haiti by tacitly backing his opponents. Rumors of a possible coup have been circulating in Haiti for months – but then, they periodically do in this strife-torn nation. Of course, coups do happen, and Aristide has been the victim of one already. So he's got reason to worry. All of this makes Haitians jittery, and does little to foster economic stability.

54. Open letter from Paul Farmer on the May 7 attacks, circulated via e-mail to PIH supporters, May 7, 2003.

7   Two Mexicos: One Urban, One Rural

1. B.D. Estrada et al., "Health Status Characteristics of HIV/AIDS Patients in the US–Mexico Border Region," Abstract ThPe8222, XIV International AIDS Conference, Barcelona, Spain, July 7–12, 2002.
2. Interview with the author, Mexico City, June 2002.
3. This contributes to a high rate of maternal death pre- and post-partum in pregnant women, due to hemorrhage and a lack of assistance at delivery. According to official figures, out of 370,000 births in Mexico in 2002, around 2,000 took place without help from trained professionals.

But out of sight of everyone, women in Oaxaca often give birth in the bush, or at home, relying on birth attendants or family members to help them. Last year there were 1,200 maternal deaths annually in Mexico, and rising. Secretary of Health Julio Frenk Mora recently admitted that the increase, which is higher among indigenous women, "reflects poverty and inequality." His remarks were published in a July 22, 2003 article in *La Jornada* by reporter Carolina Gomez Mena, entitled "Cada Ano Mueron 2 Mil Mexicanas Por Complicacion de Parto o Embarazo."

4. Interview with the author, Oaxaca, June 2002.

5. Interview with the author at offices of La Red Mexicana, Mexico City, June 2002. La Red operates a small office in a quiet residential neighborhood of the capital and relies on a small staff and volunteers. It receives grants from European AIDS organizations but has limited funding. It focuses on providing treatment information and education to city residents and does advocacy work with other NGOs.

6. Jenaro Villamil, "Contra el SIDA, Ni 1 percent Del Gasto Oficial Para El Rescate Bancario," *La Jornada*, June 5, 2002.

7. Interview with the author, June 2002. His statistics are based on data from the hospital.

8. Personal correspondence with the author, June 2003. Dr. Volkow-Fernandez is one of the leading physicians working with women who have HIV, and has conducted epidemiological studies on the evolution of the epidemic among different groups in Mexico.

9. Ibid. In response to my inquiry regarding any progress in Mexico's AIDS fight compared with 2002, Dr. Volkow-Fernandez cited poverty as a continuing barrier to care for HIV-positive individuals at Mexico City's top medical institutes. Although AIDS drugs and HIV services may be free or subsidised, depending on what program is involved, patients often can't afford the fees charged, and may not return to access HIV drugs or follow-up care.

10. J.C. Rosas et al., "Education and Prevention Program on AIDS in Rural Communities of Mexico and Central America," Abstract No. Mo.D.1901, International AIDS Conference, July 7–12, 1996.

11. Interview with the author, Puerto Escondido, June 2002.

12. Interview with the author, Paris, July 2003.

13. Interview with HIV-positive activsts in Oaxaca City from Frenpavih, June 2002.

14. Interview with the author at Coesida's offices, Oaxaca City, June 2002.
15. "Servicios de Salud de Oaxaca: Casos de SIDA Por Municipio 1986–2001," published by Servicios de Salud de Oaxaca: Direccion de Prevencion Y Control de Enfermedades, December 31, 2001.
16. Rapid tests for HIV provide a same-day result, compared with standard HIV antibody Elisa tests, which can take up to two weeks. The introduction of rapid testing in some clinics allows doctors at the Coesida clinic to provide better services to patients who come from outside the city. Those who test positive can then be provided with same-day health-care and referrals to specialists, if needed. Around the world, rapid tests are increasingly being used in pregnant women, and in settings where hospitals or clinic services may be limited. The downside of rapid testing is that, ideally, it should follow pre-test counseling for HIV. The quick results of a rapid test may not allow individuals to be emotionally prepared for their test results. On the other hand, rapid tests results can reduce the number of people who now fail to return for the results of standard HIV tests.
17. Interview with the author, June 2002.

8   Uganda: Sparing the Next Generation

1. Helen Epstein, "AIDS: The Lessons of Uganda," *New York Review of Books*, July 17, 2003.
2. UNAIDS, Report on the Global HIV/AIDS Epidemic, July 2002.
3. Elizabeth Bumiller, "Uganda's Key to White House: AIDS," *New York Times*, June 11, 2003.
4. "Uganda: Government Decentralizes Access to anti-AIDS Drugs," *IRIN HIV/AIDS Weekly*, Issue 35, July 13, 2001. This report refers to a recent Unicef study of AIDS mortality in Uganda, where the agency notes that AIDS was responsible for 12 percent of deaths in Uganda in 2001, surpassing malaria and other diseases among individuals aged between fourteen and forty-five. An estimated 1.7 million children under fifteen had also lost one or both parents to AIDS. At the time Unicef predicted that, despite a growing population, Uganda will have 2 million fewer people of working age by 2010. Already life expectancy has dropped from 54 percent to 43 percent due to AIDS.

5. Epstein, "AIDS: The Lessons of Uganda." Epstein notes that Uganda's successful prevention program remains an exception in Africa, where "many HIV prevention programs have proven suprisingly unsuccessful." In her view, Uganda succeeded due to a variety of factors, including "enlightened policies" by the government, an "unusually active" response to HIV/AIDS by ordinary people, and programs that emphasized straight talk about sex and the effects of AIDS in local communities. While Ugandans are "not usually compassionate people," and HIV stigma persists, the country's strong social networks have allowed this more open discussion of sexual and HIV issues than elsewhere in Africa, Epstein suggests. According to a July 2001 Unicef report on Uganda, major nationwide prevention campaigns have influenced young people, contributing to the falling rate of HIV infections among pregnant teenagers, which dropped from 20 percent in early 1992 to less than 5 percent in 1998.

6. Ibid. According to Peter Okwero, a World Bank health specialist, Uganda reduced adult HIV infection rates from 18 percent in 1995 to 8.3 percent in 1999, but the decline has slowed.

7. The Third Conference on Global Strategies for the Prevention of Mother to Child Transmission, Kampala, Uganda, September 10–14, 2001.

8. Miriam Rabkin and Wafaa El-Sadr, "Saving Mothers, Saving Families: The MTCT-Plus Initiative," a draft document about the MTCT-Plus Initiative, Mailman School of Public Health, Columbia University, 2003.

9. "A Focus on Women," an official satellite conference of the Conference on Global Strategies for the Prevention of Mother-to-Child Transmission, Kampala, Uganda, September 10–14.

10. Epstein, "AIDS: The Lessons of Uganda."

11. Amolo Okera, Joseph Serutoke, Elizabeth Madraa and Elizabeth Namagala, "Scaling Up Antiretroviral Therapy – Ugandan Experience," A Draft Case Study, one of a WHO series on Perspectives and Practice in Antiretroviral Treatment, published by the World Health Organization, May 2003. According to the authors, while there is evidence of a decline in new infections, the number of people already infected with HIV and progressing to AIDS is increasing.

12. Peter N. Mugyenyi, "Antiretroviral Access in Uganda – When and

Where to Get It," Presentation made at the First African Great Lakes Conference, Entebbe, Uganda, September 6–9, 2001.

13. A.K. Ammann et al., "Prevention of Perinatal HIV Transmission," an updated report prepared for an *amfAR* Continuing Medical Education Symposium titled "Focus on Women: Challenges in the Prevention and Treatment of HIV/AIDS," 2002.

14. Joep Lange et al., "The PETRA Study: Early and Late Efficacy of Three Short ZDV/3TC Combination Regimens to Prevent Mother-to-Child Transmission of HIV-1," Oral Abstract no. 17, Third Conference on Global Strategies for the Prevention of HIV Transmission from Mothers to Infants, Kampala, Uganda, September 9–13, 2001; Jay Ross et al., "HIV and Infant Feeding: Modeling the Balance of Risks," Poster 305, Third Conference on Global Strategies for the Prevention of HIV Transmission from Mothers to Infants.

15. Saul Onyango and Michele Magoni, "Implementing PMTCT Programs: Challenges and Lessons Learned," Poster Abstract no. 306, Third Conference on Global Strategies for the Prevention of HIV Transmission from Mothers to Infants.

16. Francois Dabis et al., "Assessment of the Peri-Partum and Post-Partum Interventions to Prevent Mother-to-Child Transmission (PMTCT) of HIV-1 and Improve Survival in Africa: The DITRAME PLUS ANRS 1201/1202 Project in Abidjan, Cote D'Ivoire," Poster presentation no. 212, Third Conference on Global Strategies for the Prevention of HIV Transmission from Mothers to Infants.

17. Michele Magoni et al., "Feasibility and Effectiveness of the Prevention of Mother-to-Child Transmission Program in an Urban Hospital in Kampala, Uganda," Oral Abstract no. 16, Third Conference on Global Strategies for the Prevention of HIV Transmission from Mothers to Infants.

18. Interview with the author, September 2001.

19. Pius Okong et al., "Male Involvement in Perinatal Transmission in Uganda: the 11th Hour," Poster presentation no. 406; Naomi Rutenberg, et al., Horizon Populations Council, "Involving Men in the Prevention of Mother to Child Transmission of HIV," Poster presentation no. 303, both from the Third Conference on Global Strategies for the Prevention of HIV Transmission from Mothers to Infants.

20. Interviews with the author, September 2001.

21. "Just Die Quietly: Domestic Violence and Women's Vulnerability to HIV in Uganda," Human Rights Watch report, August 2003.

22. Ibid.

23. "What Women Want from this Conference," *AIDS Today*, July 9, 2002, a daily newsletter of the Fourteenth International Conference on HIV/AIDS in Barcelona, July 2002.

24. Interviews with the author, September 2001; follow-up correspondence 2003.

25. Interview with the author, September 2001. Florence, an HIV-positive woman and mother, asked that her family name be withheld as she had disclosed her HIV status only her immediate family.

26. Interviews with the author, September 2003. According to counselors at Hope After Rape, a Kampala-based organization that co-sponsored the Focus on Women satellite conference, rape can make it much harder for women to seek immediate care and testing services for HIV, due to their trauma. It is also linked to the delay in seeking testing in women who become pregnant due to rape. This observation has been made by women HIV advocates in other studies.

27. "Shattered Lives: Sexual Violence During the Rwandan Genocide and its Aftermath," Human Rights Watch report, September 1996.

28. Samantha Powers, "Rwanda: The Two Faces of Justice," *New York Review of Books*, January 16, 2003; Anne-christine d'Adesky, "Rwanda, HIV and Rape," *POZ magazine*, January 2003; Liisa K. Hyvarinen, "Sisters in Pain: A Killer Still Stalks in Rwanda," *Atlanta Journal-Constitution*, November 17, 2002.

29. Hutus – including, in a savage irony, the female former head of Rwanda's Ministry of Women's Affairs – are being tried before the UN's International Tribunal in Arusha, Tanzania, and in popular courts in Rwanda. But justice is slow: only a handful of tribunal cases have been reviewed; the 100,000 backlog could take generations to try. Even more outrageously, the tribunal provides antiretroviral drugs and care for accused rapists who are PWAs, but denies this to the raped women. How can this be? Tribunal officials say they are responsible for caring for detained defendants but not their victims.

30. Interview with the author, July 2003.

31. Rabkin and El-Sadr, "Saving Mothers, Saving Families: The MTCT-Plus Initiative." The foundations supporting the MTCT-Plus

Initiative (2003) were: Bill and Melinda Gates Foundation; William and Flora Hewlett Foundation; Robert Wood Johnson Foundation; Henry J. Kaiser Family Foundation; John D. and Catherine T. MacArthur Foundation; David and Lucille Packard Foundation; Rockefeller Foundation; Starr Foundation; United Nations Foundation.

32. Uganda Global AIDS Program Country Report, Center for Disease Control and Prevention website, August 2003.
33. "AIDS and Malaria Cost Uganda a Billion Dollars, Says President," *Associated Press*, November 19, 2002.
34. Uganda has a tiered system of district health clinics. The designation "IV" means a clinic run by doctors or specialists that offers a higher level of medical services than smaller facilities run only by nurses or community lay health workers.
35. Okera et al., "Scaling up Antiretroviral Therapy."
36. Ibid.
37. Ibid.
38. Interview with the author, July 2003.

9   Morocco's Bold Experiment

1. K. Ghalib, "Islam, AIDS and Human Rights: A Framework for Understanding and Change," Abstract no. 44151, International AIDS Conference, 1998; Arye Barkai, "Africans and HIV," Letter to the Editor, *New York Times*, August 13, 1998.
2. "E. E. Elharti et al., "Result of HIV Sentinel Surveillance Studies in Morocco During 2001," Abstract no. MoPpC2014, Fourteenth International AIDS Conference, July 7–12, 2002, Barcelona, Spain; "SIDA – Solidarite," *Bulletin d'Information*, Avril–Mai, 2002, a newsletter of the Association de Lutte Contre le Sida, ALCS, Casablanca, Morocco; Kim Murphy, "Regional Outlook: Arabs Waking Up to AIDS. Spread of Virus Alarms Regional Health Officials, but it Remains a Disease of Fear and Shame," *Los Angeles Times*, March 24, 1992.
3. R. Bensghir et al., Infectious Diseases Unit of Casablanca, Morocco, "Antiretroviral Therapy in Limited Resource Countries   Example of Morocco," Abstract no. MoPeB 3231, Fourteenth International AIDS

Conference; K. Alami et al., "National Strategic Plan of HIV/AIDS Control in Rabat, Morocco," Abstract no. WePeF6729; L. Marih et al, "Monitoring for Efficacy of HAART in Limited Resource Settings," Abstract no. B10534; A. Choquairi, "Combining Different Approaches for HIV Prevention in a Low-prevalence Setting: The Case of Morocco," Abstract no. F11795.

4. Studies suggest that during the brief flu-like period of acute infection with HIV, a person may have a high amount of circulating virus in their blood and body fluids, which increases their risk of passing on the virus to a partner during unprotected sex. Once the body's immune system kicks in, viral levels fall. Existing rapid tests for HIV can help detect cases of acute infection.

5. Elharti et al., "Result of HIV Sentinel Surveillance Studies in Morocco During 2001." Also from the same conference, see: Hakima Himmich et al., "Incidence of AIDS-related Opportunistic Infections in Patients With and Without HAART in Morocco," Abstract no. B10331; Rose Marie Marque, "HIV/AIDS IEC for Young People in Secondary and Technical Schools, Essaouira, Morocco," Abstract no. ThPEF7956; R. Lamzaini, "Integrating HIV into Development Interventions: The Case of the National Literacy Programme in Morocco," Abstract no. MoPeG4267. For earlier reports on the course of HIV in Morocco, see: M. Mehadji Zahraoui et al., "Epidemiological and Clinical Aspects of HIV Infection in Morocco," Abstract no. PO-B01-0908, International AIDS Conference, July 6–9, 1993; S. Benjelloun et al., "Sexual Transmission of HCV in Morocco," Abstract no. PO-BO8-1292, International AIDS Conference, July 6–9, 1993; L.E. Manhart et al., "Sexually Transmitted Diseases (STD) in Three Types of Health Clinics in Morocco: Prevalence, Risk Factors and Syndromic Management," Abstract no. MO.C.1627, International AIDS Conference, July 7–12, 1996; J. Mahjour et al., "HIV Seroprevalence in Tuberculosis Patients in Morocco," Absract no. MO.C.1645, International AIDS Conference, July 7–12, 1996.

6. A. Choqairi, "Breaking the Silence Around Sex Work in Morocco," Abstract No. ThPeD7664, Fourteenth International AIDS Conference.

7. Interview with Drs. Hakima Himmich and Rajaa Bensghir, July and August, 2002.

8. Although I've been to other countries where Islamic law dictates that

the sexes are segregated, it was a renewed shock to encounter this to such a degree in Morocco, since it is regarded as the most modern of Islamic states. I found my day-to-day experiences there sobering and depressing from the point of view of being a woman, albeit a Western visitor. Men continue to rule public spaces in Morocco: there are rarely women sitting in the public cafés where men sit, for example. It was almost impossible for me to walk with a female friend in cities like Fez without being repeatedly accosted by men who insisted women should not do so without a chaperone. In Fez, these warnings were issued with hostility, even violence.

Of course, daily life is different for Moroccan women than for a Western tourist. Many women are highly educated and accomplished and hold important positions in government and society. Drs. Himmich and Bensghir are good examples of leaders in the health-care field. But a number of women I talked to acknowledged that the ingrained sexism I was encountering in the streets was not reserved for Westerners. The feminist Islamic movement in Morocco has been vocal and quite active for decades, but the rise of fundamentalism has worked against it. During my visit to the old section of Fez, I encoun-tered a number of women, some heavily veiled, some quite young, silently kneeling in the streets, begging. I was told by my male escorts that these were women who had been divorced by their hus-bands and cast out by their families. Several had small children with them. There were women like that all over Fez, one young man told me. Once they were divorced, no man wanted them. Like the Berber women in Sefrou, these women were socially outcast by devout Moroccans.

In conversations with a number of young men and women there, I heard how painful the social segregation is for both sexes. One man in his twenties talked about how impossible it was for him or his broth-ers to have women friends when they were growing up. It had distorted their views of women, he felt. Like many of his friends, he had sought out prostitutes at a relatively young age for his sexual initiation. In spite of some general awareness of AIDS, this cultural habit had not changed in Morocco, he felt. It made me think that, to be effective, new HIV programs aimed at sex workers should make sure they reach out to younger boys, as well as men who are their clients.

9. Hakima Himmich, "Femmes et Sida: la Vulnerabilité des Maghrebines," unpublished paper, March 8, 2002.

10. Jerome Hule, "Global Fund Gives 14 Nations $480 Million," *Panafrican News Agency*, April 25, 2002.

11. Note de Presentation, Association de Lutte Contre Le Sida (ALCS), 2002.

12. Rachel Zimmerman, "Glaxo Unveils Another Price Cut for AIDS Drugs to Poor Countries," *Wall Street Journal*, June 11, 2001; personal correspondence, Hakima Himmich, ALCS and Marie de Cenival and Gaelle Krikorian, ACT UP–Paris, June 2002. Even with the discount deal, Morocco had failed to access these drug purchases quickly. In a frustrated e-mail, Himmich informed ACT UP and other treatment activists:

> GSK [GlaxoSmithKline] and Boehringer have granted the same prices to Morocco as sub-Saharan countries, but to benefit from them we must order antiretrovirals not in Morocco, but from their export services abroad, a procedure which is totally incompatible with the established purchasing methods of the Moroccan administration. For this reason, the Ministry has not yet received the antiretrovirals for which it had sought tender in 2001 and 2002 . . . Like all other countries who have subscribed to the [UNAIDS] ACCESS [initiative], we are seriously shortchanged by the limited number of low-cost antiretrovirals.

13. Hakima Himmich, "Journées de Reflexion Sur L'Acces Aux Medicaments Génériques Contre le VIH/SIDA [Meeting on Access to Antiretroviral Medicines Against HIV/AIDS]," a discussion paper presented at a meeting on generic production, March 16–17, 2002.

14. Y. el Mansouri et al., "Ocular Damage During HIV Infection at the University Hospital Center in Morocco (Apropos of 400 cases)," *Bulletin of the Society of Exotic Pathology*, 2000.

15. "Girls, 14, Convicted on Terror Charges," *Agence France-Presse*, September 30, 2003. As AFP reported, a juvenile court in Rabat sentenced twin fourteen-year-old sisters to five years in prison for plotting terrorist attacks. They were arrested in August 2003 and accused of planning suicide attacks, along with eighteen adults accomplices, in

an upscale neighborhood. The attacks were said to be aimed against the royal family.

16. Most, if not all, of the May 16 suicide bombers came from Sidi Moumen, a dangerous, sprawling urban slum on the outskirts of Casablanca, which is rife with poverty, crime, drug dealing and prostitution. There, the government's slow reforms appear to have done little for residents. This has created a vacuum for religious leaders who denounce what they call the King's pro-Western reforms – economic policies they say favor a handful but not the great majority of Morocco's poor citizens. Many Arab pundits feel the actions of the Bush administration and its allies have given powerful ammunition to Islamic hardliners everywhere. New round-ups of suspected terrorists took place in Morocco in the days after May 16, and it's not likely the threat will go away. Instead, newspapers there chart the Arab world's mounting anger.

10   Aids, Apartheid and South Africa: The Challenges of Survival

1. Samantha Power, "The AIDS Rebel," *New Yorker*, May 19, 2003. In her profile of Zackie Achmat, Power provides a political and social context for recent developments in the movement to provide AIDS medicines there, and an analysis of President Mbeki's actions and inactions.

2. AZT's high cost was one reason TAC joined the ANC in 1997 and supported the government's plan to begin using generic HIV drugs, with help from Fidel Castro. As Power explains in her article, that move was fought by thirty-nine big pharma companies, who collectively joined a lawsuit to prevent access to lower-cost generics. By March 2000, TAC had scored a major victory when Glaxo halved the price of AZT. A year later, South Africa won its lawsuit against the multinationals. But by then, Mbeki had been handed a book, "Debating AZT," that said AZT was toxic and suggested HIV was not the cause of AIDS. Prior to the July 2000 global AIDS conference in Durban, Mbeki convened a panel of thirty-three scientists, many of them in the dissident AZT-is-poison camp. A year later, when Boeringher Ingleheim offered South Africa free donations of nevirapine to stop maternal transmission of HIV, Mbeki refused the offer. Eventually, South Africa's highest court ruled that Mbeki's government was violating its own constitution, and forced

the state to give the drug to pregnant mothers, writes Power. Nevertheless, the stage was set: access to drugs was openly fought by the Mbeki administration. The battle forced TAC to increase street protests, and eventually drew the support of civil society, isolating Mbeki and his closest aides. The blocking of treatment lasted until August 2003, when TAC's civil disobedience protests and other actions, including intervention by former US president Bill Clinton, persuaded a still-defiant Mbeki to concede. Today the government is rolling out a national treatment program using free generic antiretrovirals. But millions perished due to Mbeki's actions, which TAC dubbed "culpable homicide."

3. Power, "The AIDS Rebel."

4. William Finnegan, "The Poison Keeper," *New Yorker*, January 15, 2001; Heather Hogan, "Apartheid Atrocities Unravel in Basson," *Mail and Guardian*, May 26, 2000; "Secrets of Apartheid's Death Machine Surface During Trial," *Reuters*, May 19, 2000. For a comprehensive review of this chapter of South African history, see Tom Mangold and Jeff Goldberg, *Plague Wars*, MacMillan, 1999. For an early report, see De Wet Potgieter, "Apartheid's Poison Legacy," *Covert Action Quarterly*, Winter 1998, no. 63. Complete transcripts of the hearings of the Truth and Reconciliation Commission are available on the internet at <http:www.woza.co.za.trc>.

5. Inteview with Glenda Gray, September 2001, in Kampala, Uganda.

6. "100,000 South African Mothers Have Had Nevirapine: AIDS Expert," *South African Press Association*, August 3, 2003.

7. The PHRU unit have also worked closely with their own hospital's Reproductive Health Research Unit (RHRU), directed in 2000 by Helen Rees. It brings its own extensive experience in international trials and partnerships – for instance, as a reproductive health research site for the WHO and a participant in the UNAIDS-sponsored multicenter study of nonoxyl-9 as a microbicide. Another collaborator is the AIDS Unit at the National Institute for Virology in Johannesburg, headed by Lynn Morris, whose newly-established Southern African Regional Laboratory is doing much of the immunology work for vaccine studies.

8. "South Africa Approves its First HIV Vaccine Trials," *HIV/AIDS VAX*, a newsletter bulletin of the International AIDS Vaccine Initiative, edited by Emily Bass.

9. "Microbicide Initiative Launched," *MRC News*, March 2003, vol. 34, no. 1, Press Release, Medical Research Council of South Africa.

10. More information on the status of current and future microbicide trials is available from The Alliance for Microbicide Development <www.microbicide.org> and the Global Microbicide Project.

11. Interview with Glenda Gray in Boston, February, 2003.

11   Carletonville: Research in the Eye of the Storm

1. B. Williams and C. Campbell, "Carletonville: Working Together for Health," Focus 10 lecture, Helen Suzman Foundation, 2000.

2. Claire Keeton, "Anglo Leads in Treating HIV-positive Miners," *Sunday Times* (South Africa), January 19, 2003.

3. Janette Bennett, "Anglo's Far Reaching Plan Shows the Way," *Sunday Times* (South Africa), December 1, 2002.

4. Ibid.

5. Wambui Chege, "AngloGold Rolls Out AIDS Drugs to South Africa Staff," *Reuters NewsMedia*, April 8, 2003.

6. Ibid.

7. Interviews with Mercy Makhalemele and local women from Durban townships who knew Gugu Dlamini, July 2000, in Durban.

8. Interview with Eric Goosby in March, 2003.

9. The project is run under the auspices of the Council for Scientific and Industrial Research. The project is co-funded with Gold Fields, another mining company, and Harmony. In all, five mining companies have established AIDS workplace programs in the country, including Gold Fields, DeBeers, and AngloPlat. They are supported by insurance companies such as Metropolitan and Old Mutual.

10. Interview with van Dam, Fall, 2000.

11. Michale Grunwald, "A Small Nation's Big Effort Against AIDS," *Washington Post Foreign Service*, December 2, 2002.

12. Ibid; also oral presentation by Ernest Darkoh on Masa Program and early results, IAS Conference, Paris, France, July 2003.

13. They include Coca-Cola and Heineken, Exxon Mobil and British Petroleum (BP), DaimlerChrysler and Ford, Standard Chartered Bank, and South Africa's national electricity utility, Eskom. Appropriately, the mining and extraction companies are heavily represented, includ-

ing AngloGold, Gold Fields, DeBeers, and Botswana's Debswana. In India, Tata Iron and Steel, Bajaj Auto and RRR Industries are active members; in Thailand, Rohm Apollo Electronics has joined. Along with major multinational drug companies are rivals like Indian generic producer Cipla. Communication giants as Viacom, MTV and AOL Time Warner are also involved.

14. Today, over thirty-six medical insurance providers are part of the AFA program, and other companies like Debswana and Rand Water have signed on with Medscheme. As of early 2003, over two-thirds of AFA's 12,000 patients were taking HIV medications. The average patient's age was thirty-four years, and 62 percent were women; over a third began the program with CD4 T-cell counts below 200. The results are quite promising, showing clinical benefits to patients, good adherence to therapy and a significant, sustained reduction in hospitalization costs. This is especially impressive since a majority of hospitalized patients had full-blown AIDS. Medscheme has determined that costs can be further reduced if people access the AFA services earlier.

15. Since the Rwandan Heineken subsidiary also bottles Coca-Cola, a plan is brewing to establish a joint treatment project with the soft drink company, starting with two clinics in Kigali. Coca-Cola began rolling out treatment for its employees last year. For many years it has partnered with Population Services International (PSI) to implement its AIDS prevention programs in southern Africa. "We're in a discussion about how the partnership could work," said Eric Goosby, CEO of Pangaea. "It's about using and not recreating or duplicating any systems of care, but maximizing the systems that are there already and expanding their purview to include Coca-Cola employees and distributors." The other critical partner is the government. In Rwanda, the government is backing a national scale-up of treatment and recently teamed up with another new player, the William J. Clinton Foundation, to get it moving.

16. *South African Press Association*, August 18, 2003. At that time, there was no identified funder for the program, but the trucking industry was pressing forward with the plan.

17. PharmAccess was contracted to roll out the Coca-Cola treatment program, and a US non-profit organization, Family Health Inter-

national, agreed to provide prevention services. GlaxoSmithKline is also contributing to the effort.

18. Although PharmAccess chair Joep Lange said that he is pleased with Coca-Cola's progress, Lynch promised that Health GAP will increase the pressure "to make sure Coke delivers on its promise to workers."

19. Michale Grunwald, "A Small Nation's Big Effort Against AIDS," *Washington Post Foreign Service*, December 2, 2002.

20. Botswana, Cameroon, Ivory Coast, Ghana, Kenya, Mali, Nigeria, Rwanda, South Africa and Tanzania. Working with ITAC, the GBC will identify service providers in government, business and international agencies who could be tapped to help with the scale-up effort.

21. The companies are: Anglo American, Bristol-Myers Squibb, Chevron Texaco, DaimlerChrysler, Eskom, Heineken, Lafarge, Pfizer and Tata Steel. They will expand activities in several countries: Cameroon, Botswana, Ghana, India, Kenya, Nigeria and Russia.

22. Tamar Kahn, "HIV-Positive Workers Wary of Programme," *Business Day* (South Africa), December 1, 2003.

12   Russia's Post-Perestroika Pandemic

1. Thomas Maugh II, "Former Soviet Bloc Hit by Skyrocketing HIV Rates," *Los Angeles Times*, November 29, 2001. At this time, Maugh reported, the former Soviet Union had the fastest-growing HIV infection, with a fifteen-fold increase in the past three years, according to United Nations estimates. The highest rates were in the Ukraine and Russia, but experts thought the epidemic was "grossly underreported." "We never thought it could come to these levels in Europe," said Peter Piot of the UN Program on AIDS at a Moscow press conference, adding, "This is the first time that any European country has seen this level of infection," a reference to Ukraine's statistics. "The window of opportunity to avert a major epidemic in this region is narrowing, if it is not already closed." There were 40,000 new infections in the first half of 2001 in Russia alone, compared with only 11,000 total cases reported three years previously. Many were among drug users. But among newly detected cases in 2001, the ratio of men to women had shifted from 4:1 to 2:1, a trend that reflected the shifting pattern of the epidemic from drug users to their sexual partners and to commer-

cial prostitutes. Consider the statistics: in 1987, before the fall of Communism, syphilis rates were 4.2 per 100,000; at the close of 2001, there were 157 cases per 100,000. That compared with 2.2 cases per 100,000 in the US – a record low; Gary Shteyngart, "Letter from Russia: Teen Spirit," *New Yorker*, March 10, 2003.

2. Author interview with Ilya Kolmonovsky, May 2003.

3. As Communism fell, billionaire financier George Soros began heavily investing in the former Soviet bloc (Laurie Garret, *Betrayal of Trust*, Hyperion, 2000, pp. 164–71). Soros established the Open Society and its offshoot, the Soros Foundation, which promoted a human rights agenda and helped promote cultural exchanges and dialogue between citizens and policymakers from East and West. The Open Society also supported nascent pro-democratic organizations. The Soros Foundation quickly focused on the escalating problem of drug addiction, and has been instrumental in advocating progressive drug treatment programs, including harm-reduction and needle-exchange programs.

When I was in Moscow, a UNAIDS official described with irony how the Soros Foundation managed to launch needle exchange programs in Russia, a country that takes a punitive attitude toward illegal drug users. Russia bans the use of methadone and does not allow citizens to buy syringes from pharmacists. According to one official who requested anonymity, Russian health officials were quick to accept offers of aid from the Soros Foundation, and few people in the rest of the government paid attention to the fact that the grants supported harm reduction programs that included controversial needle exchange programs. When other government officials found out, they opposed the programs. But it was too late: the government did not want to risk public scandal by discussing the issue and they did not want to alienate George Soros. Almost overnight, Russia saw dozens of needle exchange programs spring up aimed at helping those at risk from HIV – making it a pioneer in the field of drug addiction and AIDS.

4. "HIV Prevention and Treatment Efforts in Eastern Europe and the Former Soviet Union," *IATEC Update*, July 2003, p. 28.

5. "Health Promotion in Russian Prisons: New Approaches," an educational video documentary by Virgjil Kule, co-produced by the AIDS Foundation East–West and Médecins Sans Frontières, 2001. This film

was reviewed by the Main Directorate of Corrections (GUIN) and recommended for distribution.

6. Tsekhanovitch, a former historian, joined Médecins du Monde a few years ago. MDM was started by the physicians who founded Médecins Sans Frontières. MDM has operations in many parts of the world. In Russia, it has focused on the plight of orphans, particularly street children, and now sex workers and drug users. MDM began its AIDS outreach projects in St. Petersburg on a shoestring budget. After debates over the political position of the agency, Tsekhanovitch and his colleagues decided to opt for institutional independence from MDM and launched Humanitarian Action. The move allows the group to take more open positions on policy issues and speak out with more freedom, explained Tsekhanovitch in 2002. He said his denunciation of certain government officials and policies related to drug users and prisoners had alienated some peers. But Tsekhanovitch was adamant about the need to speak out: "Why should we call it a democracy if people are afraid to give their opinions? I consider it my duty as a citizen to speak the truth."

7. Prison surveys in Russia have found that sex and injection drug use are commonplace activities in prisons, although they are forbidden. Since these activities are banned, neither condoms nor syringes are available in prisons. There is little medical treatment available outside several projects run in four regions by AFEW and its allies. Those who have HIV are often isolated and face stigma from prison authorities. The escalating rates of TB, and especially resistant TB, in prisons have led TB experts to declare the HIV–TB problem in Russian prisons to be a health emergency. Studies by a number of groups have shown that the risk of contracting TB inside Russia's prisons is dangerously high. For more information, see AFEW's website <www.afew.org>.

8. Michael Wines, "Rise of HIV in Russia is Quickening, Official Says," *New York Times*, May 22, 2003.

9. "In Kalingrad, which was the first city where the epidemic exploded, they began to test all drug users," explained Tsekhanovitch, "but to test users who don't want to do it is absurd – they all escaped and they tested the general population that was not touched yet. This was maybe 1995 or 1996. Millions of dollars were spent on testing and they detected nothing."

10. "The surveillance system is not useful if you don't have controlled sites or control groups among the highest-risk groups," said Pedro Chequer at the UNAIDS Moscow office. He worried that low estimates are missing more serious cases. "They say they have 240,000 people but that AIDS cases are less than 1,000 – that's not possible," he added. He helped set up the much-lauded national AIDS treatment program in his country. "Look at Brazil: it has reached 700,000 HIV cases, and confirmed 130,000. So," he shrugged, "something is not right there." But Dr. Pokrovsky, Russia's top numbers man, argued that the low AIDS caseload reflects HIV's late appearance in the region. Chequer knows what he is talking about when it comes to global AIDS, though: he was a key figure who helped Brazil's government to develop its model national treatment program, and has been advising many governments on their own programs.

11. Kasia Malinowska Sempruch, "HIV Prevention and Treatment Efforts in Eastern Europe and the Former Soviet Union," *IATEC Update*, July 2003, vol. 3, no 1. pp. 6–7, see also statistics, pp. 18–20.

12. Nicholas Eberstadt, "The Future of AIDS," *Foreign Affairs*, November/December 2002.

13. Ibid. It's important to point out that Eberstadt is a politically conservative foreign policy analyst who holds the Henry Wendt Chair in Political Economy at the American Enterprise Institute, a far-right think tank; he is also Senior Adviser to the National Bureau of Asian Research. This piece was culled from a longer study prepared with Lisa Howie. For more results, see <www.AEI.org/scholars/eberstadt.htm>. For additional views on US foreign policy toward Russia, particularly its economic future, see Michael Mandelbaum's article, "Westernizing Russia and China," *Foreign Affairs*, May/June 1997.

14. Garrett, *Betrayal of Trust*. Garrett notes the flight of capital was matched by the largest peacetime brain-drain in history, including doctors, scientists, technicians and teachers who fled to the West to get higher-paying jobs.

15. Paul Farmer, *Pathologies of Power: Health, Human Rights and the New War on the Poor*, University of California Press, 2003. As discussed in the Haiti chapter, Farmer's organization, Partners In Health, helped pioneer treatment for resistant TB using second-line drugs. Farmer and his colleagues, including physician Jim Kim, worked closely with

Russian prison health officials and other groups like Médecins Sans Frontières to develop pilot TB programs in some of the most heavily affected prisons. "Just as they said you can't treat AIDS in Haiti, they said you can't treat prisoners with resistant TB in Russia, but we've shown them it can be done," Farmer told me in 2002. "The situation is really scary and it's only going to get worse because it's not really being dealt with, although you've got some great people over there trying to do something."

16. Janine Wedel, "The Harvard Boys Do Russia," *Nation*, June 1, 1998. Wedel is also the author of *Collision and Collusion: The Strange Case of Western Aid to Eastern Europe 1989–1998*, St. Martins Press, 1998.

17. Ibid. Other Harvard members included the university's current president Lawrence Summers, David Lipton, another PhD, and academics at the Harvard Institute for International Development (HIID). Various members of this Harvard group began working in Ukraine and elsewhere in the region in the early 1990s. According to Wedel, the HIID actually got its first grants from the elder Bush's administration, and in all secured US AID grants and other monies totaling $57.7 million to work in Russia – all but $17.4 million without competitive bidding. Much of it, claimed Wedel, was funneled to Chubais and the Moscow-based Russian Privatization Center (RPC) that he founded and led in 1992. Wedel's research shows the RPC received some $45 million in USAID loans, along with millions from the European Union, Japan and other countries, including $59 million in World Bank loans and $43 million in European Bank for Reconstruction and Development loans that Russian taxpayers must now repay.

18. "Consensus Statement on Antiretroviral Treatment for AIDS in Poor Countries by Individual Members of the Faculty of Harvard University," *Topics in HIV Medicine*, 2001, 9: 14–26.

19. My information about the William Jefferson Clinton Foundation is based on a mid-2003 interview with Ira Magaziner, Clinton's right-hand man at the White House, who has been recruited to lead the Foundation's HIV/AIDS initiative. He told me Clinton decided to begin the initiative after several meetings with African leaders and potential donors, where they discussed Clinton's interest in issues related to poverty and development. Unless major action was taken around AIDS, all efforts at poverty-reduction were fruitless, leaders

told Clinton. The Foundation is promoting a public–private business-oriented approach to helping hard-hit countries and their governments develop comprehensive national AIDS plans that include treatment. In 2003, a cadre of business volunteers were working closely with government officials in the Bahamas, Haiti, Rwanda, Mozambique and South Africa, among other countries; several had signed agreements to launch the programs. Clinton is using his extensive personal contacts to secure new funding sources for these programs from European governments and untapped donors. Magaziner has helped broker better deals on generics and other drugs for countries like the Bahamas.

In October 2003, Magaziner and his team scored a major coup for the Foundation by getting four generic producers – Cipla, Ranbaxy and Matrix of India, and AspenCare of South Africa – to produce generic drugs for those in poor countries for as little as 38 to 50 cents a day per person. The initial agreement covers two commonly used combinations: d4T, 3TC and nevirapine; and AZT, 3TC and nevirapine, both first-line non-protease regimens used in treatment-naive AIDS patients in resource-poor settings. This reduces by half the cost of the first combination to $132 a patient a year, down from $255 a year. African countries involved include Mozambique, Rwanda, South Africa, Tanzania; and Caribbean countries involved include Bahamas, Dominican Republic, Haiti, Antigua, Barbuda, Dominica, Grenada, St. Kitts, Nevis, St. Lucia, St. Vincent, the Grenadines, Montserrat, Anguilla, British Virgin Islands. See Lawrence Altman's article, "Clinton Group Gets Discount for AIDS Drugs," *New York Times*, October 24, 2003.

20. Helen Epstein, "Can AIDS Be Stopped?" *New York Review of Books*, March 14, 2002. In this review of recent events in the arena of global AIDS and access to cheaper drugs, Epstein, a talented science journalist who has written several important articles on AIDS in Africa, notes Soros' turnaround on globalization and how he's now focused on global health:

> In his new book *George Soros on Globalization* (Published by Public Affairs, 2002), Soros concludes that international finance and trade have outstripped the capacity of sovereign states to manage the politics of globalization. Especially neglected has been the provision of global public goods, things needed by everyone but not produced by the mar-

ketplace, such as clean air and disease control. Instead of proposing to dismantle the WTO, the World Bank, and the IMF, Soros would like to see them strengthened, and complemented by stronger global institutions in social fields like health, such as the World Health Organization, and labor standards, such as the International Labor Organization. Successful globalization, he argues, requires effective global institutions devoted not only to finance and trade, but also to public health, human rights, environmental protection, and other public goods.

21. Interview with the author, St. Petersburg, May 2003. Musatov is one of a limited number of physicians with experience treating HIV patients with antiretroviral drugs, and he is moving to share that knowledge with other doctors. In our conversations, Musatov discussed the need for Russian AIDS organizations to learn more about the activities of other frontline groups working with HIV-positive addicts, particularly innovative models of outreach, care and treatment.

22. I visited Children's Hospital No. 3, a city institution, after a brief interview with Galina Tyuleneva, MD, a pediatrician and head of the hospital. She oversees the care of HIV-positive infants who are housed in two of the orphan wards there. Tyuleneva was candid about the fiscal budget crisis that is limiting the care that the hospital can provide to the orphans, and asked me to inform agencies and donors abroad about the critical needs of the hospital and issues related to care of HIV-positive orphans in Russia.

23. These observations were made after a visit to the clinic run for street children by Humanitarian Action in St. Petersburg, and staff interviews with physicians and counselors there.

24. According to Roman Dudnik of AFEW, and MDM's Tsekhanovitch, among others, the government's ban on methadone is a major obstacle to helping drug users get off drugs and into care. The government's AIDS programs do not provide treatment for active drug users, creating a catch-22. Many advocates have called on the Putin government to reconsider the policy on methadone maintenance, which has proved to be effective as a means of helping drug users kick heroin. But the issue is not merely one of government obstruction. According to Tsekhanovitch, the Russian drug mafia also opposes the use of methadone, which would lower the demand for heroin. "The drug mafia is

incredibly powerful here," said Tsekhanovitch. "They call the shots more than people think." According to Sergei, an ex-soldier who had just kicked heroin when we met at MDM's offices in St. Petersberg, it's much harder to get methadone on the streets than heroin or other illegal drugs; it's more expensive than heroin.

25. Interview with the author, Moscow, May 2003. Dr. Pokrovsky has become even more outspoken on Russia's need to act quickly on the AIDS front, but remains the spokesperson for the government's AIDS effort. He is very well educated with respect to updates in the science and research of HIV, and is conducting clinical trials to determine how Russians are responding to antiretroviral treatment. Many AIDS activists remain very critical of Dr. Pokrovsky, who they view as the architect of national and state AIDS policies that they oppose.

26. Interview with the author at AFEW's offices in Moscow, May 2003. Dudnik, a gay man, is one of the better-known HIV-positive activists in Russia. He works closely with Western European and US AIDS activists and has taken a leading role in organizing a regional network of treatment activists.

27. Interview with the author, May 2003, Moscow. Gessen is a well-known Russian-American journalist and author who reported on gay and lesbian issues as a staff journalist of the *Advocate* in the late 1980s, before returning to Russia after Communism fell. She continues to cover AIDS issues and has been outspoken about the Putin government's failure to respond with urgency to the epidemic, as well as its war in Chechyna. She joined the staff of *Itogi* magazine, an affiliate of *Newsweek*, as its senior investigative reporter, and covered the war in Kosovo and the ongoing conflict in Chechnya.

28. Interview with the author in Moscow, May 2003.

29. Russia submitted a Round 3 GFATM proposal to get $88,742,355 for a five-year plan to provide AIDS and TB services in ten regions. The proposal was submitted by a consortium of twenty-five government and NGO representatives, which Pedro Chequer of UNAIDS helped to pull together into an Advisory Council. This group could become the Country Coordinating Mechanism, or CCM, to the Global Fund if the grant is approved. The grant would seek to prevent 3.5 million infections in youths, and would target vulnerable groups such as drug users, sex workers and prisoners. It would also be used for public edu-

cation campaigns and to help treat more of the estimated 1.7 million HIV-positive individuals in these regions. The TB portion of the grant requested $10,800,827 for a program in the Tomsk Oblast region, where 13.5 percent of new TB cases are resistant. The goal is to treat registered TB cases and reduce new cases by scaling up the 1995 DOTS program there, and the 2000 DOTS Plus program that is aimed at drug resistant TB. Some 16,000 prisoners in the Tomsk Oblast region were set to receive TB treatment if the money was awarded: thousands with drug-sensitive TB would get first-line drugs, through a DOT program; 950 prisoners with MDR-TB would be offered treatment using second-line drugs in a DOTS-Plus program. The latter model was developed by, among others, Paul Farmer and Jim Kim's Partners in Health group in Haiti, Peru and Russia's prisons. For more information, see the Global Fund website: <www.gfatm.org>.

30. In a private interview, a top Russian official in the Ministry of Health who is an epidemiologist told me that there are tensions within the government between officials, who favor generics, and Russia's leading medical association, which has strong ties to the pharmaceutical industry. As elsewhere, Russia's doctors benefit from their ties to the drug industry, which offers them money to travel to conferences and upon whom they depend for money and drugs to conduct clinical research. But he conceded that the global momentum favoring generics might sway those at the top, as long as such a move was not too politically risky.

31. Interview with the author, Humanitarian Action offices in Moscow, May 2003.

32. Ibid. Sergei requested that I print only his first name in any news articles. When we met at Humanitarian Action's offices in Moscow, he had only been off drugs for a short while, but was already active as a support group leader. His experience of being discriminated against in the military has left him angry and determined to try to reform military policies around HIV, and to increase education for young men doing their military service. "There was no information available to us about AIDS," said Sergei of his time in the army. "The government has a responsibility to provide that education."

33. *Associated Press*, September 10, 2003.

13   AIDS: A New Model for Global Public Health

1. Abstract MoPe3225, Fourteenth AIDS Conference, Barcelona, Spain, July 7–12, 2002.
2. T. von Schoen Angerer, D. Wilson, N. Ford and T. Kasper, "Access and Activism: The Provision of Antiretroviral Therapy in Developing Countries." *AIDS*, 2001, 15 (supp 4).
3. Abstract WEOrB, Fourteenth AIDS Conference, Barcelona, Spain, July 7–12, 2002.
4. "ARV Simplification Off the Beaten Track for High-Prevalence Countries," recommendations from an MSF Workshop, MSF Campaign for Essential Medicines, September 20, 2003. Report submitted in November 2003 to the World Health Organization for consideration regarding WHO's revised guidelines for use of HIV drugs in resource-poor settings and their 3×5 scale-up global treatment plan.
5. "WHO International Consultative Meeting on HIV/AIDS Anti-retroviral Therapy," Report of the Meeting, Geneva, May 22–3, 2001. Although many experts have weighed in on these guidelines, Basil Vareldzis from the WHO's HIV-AIDS department outlined the agency's new initiative to simplify antiretrovral therapy in order to facilitate a rapid scale-up at this May 2001 meeting. It laid the groundwork and marked the first steps of what has become the WHO's 3×5 global AIDS treatment plan.
6. "Scaling Up Antiretroviral Therapy in Resource-Limited Settings: Guidelines for a Public Health Approach," WHO Department of HIV/AIDS 2002; Revised US Federal Health and Human Services Guidelines for Anti-HIV Treatment, 2002 and 2003.
7. "ARV Simplification Off the Beaten Track for High-Prevalence Countries."
8. "Care, Treatment and Support for People Living with HIV/AIDS," Report on the Global HIV/AIDS Epidemic, WHO, 2002.
9. The WHO's "Pain Ladder" guidelines state:

> If pain occurs, there should be prompt oral administration of drugs in the following order: nonopioids (aspirin and paracetamol); then, as necessary, mild opioids (codeine); then strong opioids such as morphine, until the patient is free of pain. To calm fears and anxiety, additional

drugs – "adjuvants" – should be used. To maintain freedom from pain, drugs should be given "by the clock," that is every 3–6 hours, rather than "on demand." This three-step approach of administering the right drug in the right dose at the right time is inexpensive and 80–90 percent effective. Surgical intervention on appropriate nerves may provide further pain relief if drugs are not wholly effective. (Source: World Health Organization, 2003).

10. The FHSSA backs a "twinning" model that links hospices and groups in developed countries with those in less developed countries. It is also focusing on funding community-based hospices and providing support for regional training centers. South Africa and Zimbabwe have strong hospice associations, and they are helping other nascent groups in Uganda, Kenya, Zambia and Botswana, who have formed the African Hospice and Palliative Care Association (AHPCA).

11. Peter Sarver, "Palliative Care Comes Front & Center for Sub-Saharan Africa," FHSSA newsletter, August 2002.

12. "ARV Simplification Off the Beaten Track for High-Prevalence Countries."

13. For more details on managing drug-related side-effects, see Emily Bass's 1999 overview, "The Good, The Bad and The Ugly," *HIV Plus* magazine, June 1999. Several agencies and universities provide excellent updated information on HIV-related treatment issues, including the WHO, the CDC, and UNAIDS; Johns Hopkins University School of Medicine; the University of California's website <www.HIVInsite.org>, <www.hopkins-aids.edu>; and the University of Alabama at Birmingham (UAB).

14. Bone problems – namely avascular necrosis – appear to be on the rise among a subset of US and Western European patients, most with long treatment histories. Bone problems have also been seen in heavily treated children, some of whom develop bone fractures after years on therapy.

15. Anne-christine d'Adesky, "Studies Warn of Global Drug Resistance," *amfAR Treatment Insider*, April/May 2002. According to Richman, "There is a significant increase by genotype, by phenotype, any way you look at it. One-drug and multi-drug . . . resistance has gone up substantially." Now comes early clinical evidence of the outcome of

failing therapy. "We are seeing such patients develop traditional AIDS-related complications," said Stephen Deeks of the University of California at San Francisco, sounding the alarm. Deeks has been following 200 to 300 people with MDR-HIV who began failing therapy back in 1997, and are running out of salvage therapy options. "It's beginning to look like those patients that the clinic was full of in the mid 90s. Such patients are clearly happening as a result of prolonged virologic failure. There is a huge delay in the onset of that failure and [in when symptoms occur], but it definitely does happen."

Clinical signs of failure include progressive loss of CD4 cells and appearance of HIV-related lymphoma and opportunistic infections – though not mycobacterium avium complex (MAC) or cytomegalovirus (CMV). Deeks is quick to point out that the number of people with MDR viruses who fail therapy is low compared with how many do well on regimens. "Among those with drug resistance, a significant proportion – perhaps half – achieve durable benefit as long as they remain on therapy," he stressed. But he worries that the other half mark a trend.

16. Drug resistance is a natural by-product of Darwinian evolution. By its nature, HIV mutates every time it reproduces, producing changes or "point mutations" in the amino acid structure of key viral enzymes (or proteins like protease and reverse transcriptase). If these mutations occur at a site where HIV drugs act, the drugs' effect can be significantly reduced, and the virus becomes at least partially drug-resistant.

Drug-resistant HIV has an advantage over drug-sensitive HIV. As long as therapy allows some replication, the mutated HIV will rapidly predominate over the initial HIV, though it may remain a minor population or peter out entirely when no drugs are present. If HIV with early drug resistance can survive, it will continue to evolve and accumulate more mutations, leading to further drug resistance. David Gilden, "NCI Conference Considers Specter of Widespread Drug Resistance," *amfAR Treatment Insider*, February/March 2002.

17. This report on resistance was presented at the International AIDS Society Conference in Paris, July 2003. These findings came from a Dutch study of 1,633 HIV patients in seventeen European countries

between 1996 and 2000, led by scientists at the University of Utrecht in the Netherlands.

18. The majority of patients were carrying the subtype B virus, which is prevalent in the US and Western Europe (subtype C is common in Africa). According to one researcher, patients carrying subtype B viruses were four times more likely to get a resistant infection than those with other subtypes.

19. Du Venage, *San Francisco Chronicle*, August 29, 2003.

20. Personal correspondence with the author, 2002. In a national survey of genotypic resistance in 225 Brazilian patients failing HAART, researcher Mauro Schecter, MD, of the AIDS Research Laboratory at Hospital Universitario Clementino Fraga Filho, found that "85.3 percent of these individuals had genetic mutations in reverse transcriptase, protease or both." In a pilot study in Schecter's lab, 12 percent of thirty-nine treatment-naive individuals had mutations associated with resistance, while 90 percent of them presented polymorphisms (variations) in these regions. Such polymorphisms are "not yet described as resistance mutations," related Marisa Tavares of the Brazil team.

21. In a July 2000 survey, 78 percent of patients in Uganda taking 3TC had resistance to that drug; 20 percent of those treated with AZT had resistance to AZT; one of two patients taking a protease inhibitor regimen had protease inhibitor resistance; and a dual AZT/3TC resistance was also found in some patients. In the Ivory Coast, 57 percent of patients surveyed had resistance to one or more drugs. AZT resistance was detected in 43 percent of patients and 3TC resistance in 15 percent. But resistance to non-nucleoside drugs was reportedly rare, reflecting the low use of those drugs at that time.

22. "There was a study in Thailand where they were treating with ddI and d4T and 10 percent of patients [with genotyped HIV] had a 151M mutation [which lowers susceptibility to most nucleoside analogs]," said Daniel Kuritzkes, MD, an HIV expert at the University of Colorado Health Sciences Center, in 2002. "That was after one to two years of follow-up. Resistance occurs promptly and predictably." That's certainly true when only a single drug or two drugs are used; Du Venage, "Incidence of Drug-resistant HIV Strains May Increase in Africa with Increased Availability of Antiretroviral Drugs," *San Francisco Chronicle*, July 29, 2003.

23. Anne-christine d'Adesky, "Poor Countries Need Faster, Cheaper, Better HIV Monitoring," *amfAR Treatment Insider*, February 2002.

24. "Fuzeon: Important Advance, No Magic Bullet," *amfAR news*, summer 2003.

25. At the recent Paris International AIDS Society meeting, researchers reported that Trizivir was less effective than other first-line non-protease regimens (AZT/LMV/3TC/ABC vs AZT/3TC/EFV vs AZT/3TC/ABC/EFV). The clinical trial (ACTG 5095) by Roy M. Gulick, MD, from Weill Medical College of Cornell University in New York City, involved 1,100 patients and found that Trizivir was "demonstrably inferior to each of the two efavirenz-containing regimens."

Another study by Dr. Charles Farthing of the AIDS Healthcare Foundation found Trizivir didn't work as well in treatment-naive patients. He openly called on the Food and Drug Administration to withdraw approval of Trizivir. Other activists charged that Farthing and his organization had a political reason for attacking Trizivir, as they had been denied access to GlaxoSmithKline's drugs for AVH's international programs. The AIDS Treatment Activist Coalition, a US-based alliance of treatment activists, denounced Farthing's actions and instead demanded that the FDA re-label Trizivir to reflect the latest studies, and do additional research to clarify its role in combination therapy.

There's also a problem of anemia in very ill patients, due to chronic malaria or malnutrition, who should not take AZT – and thus Trizivir. Yet, as Indian doctors confided to me, some of their colleagues were ignorant of this and put patients on Trizivir because it was what was available. Patients with anemia are often switched to d4T, but this drug poses problems too.

From a scientific point of view, the news about Trizivir also means it isn't as good a choice for the bulk of people now going on treatment in the developing world, since people with AIDS and very ill patients tend to have high viral loads and poor immune health, which requires more potent regimens, often including protease inhibitors.

26. *Journal of Acquired Immune Deficiency*, November 1, 2003.

27. Abstracts WePeB5868, B10598, TuPe5208, ThPe7376, Fourteenth AIDS Conference, Barcelona, Spain, July 7–12, 2002.

28. Donald McNeil, *New York Times*, September 4, 2003. He noted that an

entire African family may help to pay for a relative's drugs, creating greater social and familial incentives and support for patients to adhere and benefit from treatment.

29. Philip P. Pan, "CHINA: Some Chinese with AIDS Abandon Free 'Cocktail,'" *Washington Post*, November 11, 2002.

30. The most common regimen used was a non-protease combination of nevirapine, ddI and either AZT or d4T. For those who failed these regimens, efavirenz and Combivir were available as salvage regimens, but not protease inhibitors.

31. David Bansberg et al., *AIDS*, September 5, 2003. This one-year study involved monitoring of 148 HIV-positive participants, the majority urban, homeless residents of shelters and low-income, single-row occupancy hotels, or participants in free meal programs. In other words, America's urban poor with HIV. Many of them are African-Americans with histories of drug and alcohol abuse, and mental illness. They are not the face of AIDS patients who typically grace advertisements for HIV drugs across San Francisco and major US cities: healthy-looking gay men climbing up mountains thanks to antiretroviral drugs.

32. "Many patients with excellent, even perfect, pill-taking are living longer with resistant virus than those who do not take enough medication to select for resistant virus," concluded Bansberg. Activists have been struggling with the news too. "I think they're just saying that high adherence doesn't preclude the development of resistance and that people with less adherence may gain some clinical benefits from drugs," said Gregg Gonsalves, a treatment advocate and policy director at Gay Men's Health Crisis, a US NGO in New York, in an e-mail discussion with other frontline treatment activists.

> They also say there is a threshold where too-low adherence will result in little clinical benefit. I think the message to patients still is: be as adherent as possible, higher adherence is better and associated with better outcomes. For doctors the message may be: don't preclude patients from receiving ART because you think they may not have the ability to be perfectly adherent. They will get some benefits from the drugs, and even your most adherent patients will develop resistance down the line, if they are not completely virologically suppressed.

33. Abstract MoOrC1103, Fourteenth AIDS Conference, Barcelona, Spain, July 7–12, 2002.

34. Laure Montouch, Jacques Corbeil, Douglas Richman, "Recombination Leads to the Rapid Emergence of HIV-1 Dually Resistant Mutants Under Selective Drug Pressure," Proc. Natl. Acad. Sci. USA, June 1996, vol. 93, pp. 6,106–11; Anne-christine d'Adesky, "Double Jeopardy," OUT magazine, October 1997; Mark Schoofs, "Who's Afraid of Reinfection," POZ magazine, May 1997; Edwin J. Bernard, "Further Evidence of Superinfection Found in African Sex Workers and Swiss Drug Injectors," AIDSMAP, July 15, 2003; Emma Ross, "Scientists Document Increasing Reports of Superinfection," Associated Press, July 16, 2003; "HIV Coinfection, Reinfection and Superinfection," I-Base, 2003; Tim Murphy, "Losing Control," POZ magazine, October 2002.

35. Alarmed, researchers feel that dual infection could spell trouble from the start. Why? Because having more than one virus at the start may generate a more diverse viral pool in the body. Studies suggest that viral diversity makes it harder for the immune system – aka, antibodies – to bring acute HIV infection under control. The marker of control is a viral "set point." In the South African study the women who progressed faster had much higher set points and more viral diversity when compared with twenty-eight other women in the study.

36. Grobler presented his data on dual infection and superinfection at the South African AIDS Conference in Durban in August 2003.

37. So far, there's no evidence of a genetic defect that would predispose the South African sex workers to more rapid disease, however.

38. Farmer worries about people taking "drug holidays" who then get exposed to a second infection through unsafe sex or sharing needles. "Structured treatment interruptions were, last I checked, an experimental therapy," he stated in September 2003. "We don't recommend them outside of research protocols for patients with advanced disease."

39. Abstract 948, International AIDS Society Conference, Paris, France, July 13–17, 2003.

40. "Scaling Up Antiretroviral Therapy in Resource-Limited Settings." According to the WHO, immune restoration syndrome occurs in 30 percent of TB patients and is characterized by fevers, lymphadenopa-

thy, worsening pulmonary lesions, and expanding lesions of the central nervous system.

41. Oral Presentation, International AIDS Society Conference, Paris, France, July 14, 2003.

42. "Tests May Fail to Detect TB in AIDS Victims," *Reuters*, January 14, 1992. The dime-shaped standard five-millileter bump on the skin that indicates a positive exposure in an otherwise healthy person may be smaller. That finding prompted doctors at Johns Hopkins School of Public Health in 1992 to call for changing the definition of a positive test to two milliliters or larger for advanced HIV patients. Not all care providers are aware of this information.

43. One study in Senegal showed that HHV-8 virus is present is children in Senegal, despite low rates of KS. But in Brazil, rates of KS are creeping up in patients on HIV therapy. In countries where intravenous drug use is a major route of HIV's spread, leishmaniasis remains an early OI in HIV patients. Other developing country studies suggest that anti-HIV drugs do work against central nervous system non-Hodgkin's lymphoma, but not T-cell lymphomas. One report from Canada has global implications for both treatment and prevention: it found that anal humanpapilloma virus was "nearly universal" in the men with HIV they studied. It's long been known that HPV in women with HIV often persists despite HIV therapy. Other OIs reported at the Paris meeting included fungal infections of fluconazole-resistant candida *albicans* in Pune, India; upper respiratory candidiasis in Russia, histoplasmosis in Argentina, leprosy, and a new HIV-related OI not seen in the West: penicillosis, which turned up in southwest Indian HIV patients going on therapy. Bacterial infections included another newcomer: lingual bacteriosis, linked to thrush. There were also viral infections linked to cancers, such as HHV-8, a herpes virus associated with Kaposi's Sarcoma.

44. "Care, Treatment and Support for People Living with HIV."

45. Working Draft, "TB – Not Reading This Article Could Cost Your Life," document circulated by ACT UP New York TB Working Group, 1990s.

46. This rules out the use of the TB drug rifampicine with preferred first-line drugs like nevirapine. Another TB drug, rifabutin, is used as a substitute for rifampicine, and efavirenz can be a substitute for nevir-

apine. But like HIV drugs, TB drugs are often lacking. Compared with HIV, adherence to TB drugs is viewed as harder by physicians. Current HIV guidelines advocate starting with TB drugs first in individuals with active TB, but that depends on how badly they need to start antiretroviral therapy.

47. AZT can cause anemia, also a common feature of TB, while d4T is linked to higher incidences of lactic acidosis. Meanwhile, efavirenz isn't recommended for pregnant women. Rifampicin also lowers the dose of nevirapine by 31 percent.

48. "Tuberculosis: A New Antibiotic Appears Effective Against Multidrug-Resistant Strains," *Tuberculosis Weekly*, June 11, 2003. The study showed linezolid worked against strains that were resistant to eight to twelve TB therapies. "They were in a lot of trouble and we had run out of treatment," reported William Rom, MD, professor of medicine and environmental medicine at NYU School of Medicine. "Trying the linezolid was a real act of desperation." He added that there is a continuing need for new antibiotics for TB, and called on the WHO to begin large-scale clinical trials of the drug.

49. "Global Alliance at Full Steam for New TB Drugs," *Bulletin of the World Health Organization*, 2002, 80:6. The Global Alliance is promoting a private–public partnership model for drug development to ensure cheap drugs will reach consumers, along the lines of the model used by the International AIDS Vaccine Initiative to develop HIV vaccines. It estimates that the global market for TB drugs will be worth around $450 to $700 million by 2010. That's three times higher than the average $200 million threshold that companies estimate make it financially worth investing in drug development for a disease.

50. Gavin Yamey, "Malaria Researchers Say Global Fund is Buying 'Useless Drug,'" *British Medical Journal*, November 2003. An analysis in November showed that in four countries that accounted for 82 percent of Global Fund spending on malaria – Uganda, Nigeria, Ethiopia and Sudan – chloroquine was used alone, not combined with a second malarial drug such as sulfadoxine-pyrimethamine, which is more effective.

51. Ibid. Activists quickly blamed the Global Fund for backing such ineffective regimens, but officials there argued that, as with antiretrovirals, they do not dictate the drugs governments buy. The WHO is respon-

sible for laying out guidelines for treatment of malaria, as it is with HIV and TB, they told activists from Health GAP. That's true, but the Global Fund does choose which grants to support. Why are they financing ineffective programs that increase the prospect of malaria resistance? In response to the furor caused by this report, the WHO appears to be taking some action to ensure that more effective malaria regimens are adopted.

52. Kathy Anastos, the lead WIHS researcher in the Bronx, has been developing a simplified protocol for a longitudinal study of treatment effects in treatment-naive women for possible use in a Rwandan project. I have also been involved in developing this draft protocol.

53. "Policy Paralysis: A Call for Action on HIV/AIDS Related Human Rights Abuses Against Women and Girls in Africa," Human Rights Watch summary report, December 2003.

54. A.K. Ammann et al., "Prevention of Perinatal HIV Transmission," an updated report prepared for an *amfAR* Continuing Medical Education Symposium titled, "Focus on Women: Challenges in the Prevention and Treatment of HIV/AIDS," 2002. Joep Lange et al., "The PETRA Study: Early and Late Efficacy of Three Short ZDV/3TC Combination Regimens to Prevent Mother-to-Child Transmission of HIV-1," Oral Abstract no. 17, Third Conference on Global Strategies for the Prevention of HIV Transmission from Mothers to Infants, Kampala, Uganda, September 9–13, 2001; Jay Ross et al., "HIV and Infant Feeding: Modeling the Balance of Risks," Poster 305, Third Conference on Global Strategies for the Prevention of HIV Transmission from Mothers to Infants, Kampala, Uganda, September 9–13, 2001.

55. "ARV Simplification Off the Beaten Track for High-Prevalence Countries."

56. Ibid. According to the MSF report, "First-line protocols for pediatric patients should mirror those of adults at all levels of care (levels I, II, III] (of the WHO Staging System for HIV infection). This is particularly difficult because of the lack of appropriate pediatric formulations, particularly for children under 10 to 15 kilos." What are needed are fixed, low-dosage or breakable tablets that would provide alternatives to current liquid formulations, which are difficult to use due to "complexity of three different drugs, lack of adequate dose measurement,

volume, storage, bad taste, etc." In addition, "[p]owders are considered impractical (texture, lack of pure water). Such breakable tablets should be capsules that can be mixed with food, or fixed-dose concentrated liquid formulations in small volumes and with weight-based dispensers," they suggested.

57. "Care, Treatment and Support for People Living with HIV."

58. *Associated Press*; *New York Times*, October 8, 2003. Lekota estimated that 20 to 22 percent of the military is HIV-positive, and said that the government was working to reduce the number of HIV infections. He blamed supporters of the former apartheid regime for trying to destabilize the government by saying that the military is "ravaged" by HIV/AIDS. In response, TAC spokesperson Pholokgolo Ramothwala said, "It is disappointing for a person who is chairman of the ANC and minister of a department most affected by AIDS to say something as irresponsible as this. As a minister, he should be leading the fight against HIV, yet he is misleading the country."

59. What's important here is that these men have families and they are also mobile. In areas of conflict such as Rwanda and Congo, rape and mass rape are increasingly linked to the spread of HIV from soldiers and paramilitary groups. Based on what we already know from the Great Lakes region of East Africa, urgent attention is needed to halt this chain of transmission. In Rwanda, it only took a 100-day genocide in 1994 to expose over 250,000 to HIV. A similar pattern may be repeating itself in the Congo. In November 2003, human rights workers revealed that thousands of Congolese women are turning up in health clinics who were raped and sexually mutilated by warring groups in recent months. Similar reports about the link of war and rape to HIV have been released every few months by Human Rights Watch and other groups in a number of regions and countries. They provide plenty of evidence for what we find when testing becomes available: fresh explosions of HIV among women linked to ongoing civil conflicts.

60. Stan Houston, "Justice and HIV Care in Africa – Antiretrovirals in Perspective," *IAPAC* quarterly journal, Spring 2003. In a critical and at times skeptical overview of the global scale-up plan, Houston, an associate professor of medicine from the University of Alberta, Canada, notes that advocates of HIV prevention worry that funding treatment programs will take away from prevention efforts.

There are reports from Western countries and anecdotal reports from Africa, suggesting that the perceived availability of effective treatment can reduce uptakes of prevention messages so vital to any effective response to the HIV epidemic. There is widespread concern that a focus on treatment may distract governments from the necessary commitment to HIV prevention – the natural tendency for clinical care to trump public health when spending decisions are made is all the more likely to manifest in the context of an issue as emotive as HIV.

Houston raises the issue that drove a wedge between prevention and treatment activists during the UNGASS meeting, and continues to stir debate. At UNGASS, world leaders agreed that prevention and testing go hand in hand, and should be regarded as complementary strategies.

61. It took them a long time to get the first two of their twelve sites in sub-Saharan Africa and Thailand up and running in Uganda. It's taken time to engage local communities in the effort; without doing that, the programs won't be taken up and become self-sustaining. This is the reality of implementing new programs. It's taken time to train counselors and outreach workers, to establish a procurement system for low-cost drugs, and so on. Like treatment, the first steps are the hardest; after that the payoff shows as the numbers accessing services exponentially increase.

62. Patricia Kahn, "IAVI Outlines R&D Plans for Next Two Years," *IAVI Report*, July–September 2002; Patricia Kahn and Emily Bass, editors, *HIV/AIDS VAX*, an IAVI Report Bulletin, September 2003, vol. 1, no. 2. As with treatment, vaccine researchers believe they may have to create a vaccine cocktail that both induces immune responses and provides specific immunity to a range of HIV subtypes. Haiti has moved into phase III vaccine trials. In the South African vaccine trials, one study will test an experimental vaccine known as AVX101, developed by AlphaVax; the second will test a vaccine combination called HIVA.MVA and will take place in South Africa and Europe. Many scientists are very excited about the second vaccine, based on early animal and human studies.

63. VaxGen was supported by the CDC, the vaccine manufacturer and Thai authorities. It tested a vaccine made from a genetically engineered

version of the core protein on HIV's surface, glycoprotein 120, or gp120. The vaccine cannot cause an infection in humans, but was thought to induce an immune system response that might control viral replication.

64. When I was in Mexico City, Dr. Patricia Volkow-Fernandez, a leading doctor who treats HIV-positive women, showed me reams of documents that she has collected regarding her – still unproven – theory that early HIV cases in Mexican women stem from their having been paid blood donors to largely unregulated commercial plasma centers. These centers were in operation until not long ago, she claimed. She showed me pictures of women with bruises on their arms from regular weekly or monthly donations of blood. In some cases, the whole family was surviving on the sale of their blood to these local businesses, which then exported the blood abroad. The blood was "pooled" to make plasma products and contaminated with HIV, she found.

  Her as-yet-unpublished research suggests a pattern linking early AIDS cases in Mexico to Zaire and other parts of Africa where there were commercial plasma centers. Volkow-Fernandez continues to argue that contaminated blood products are still being exported into the US and other countries because the FDA does not screen and test all blood-derived products as they do drugs. As an example, she cited the blood products used to make serum hepatitis B vaccines used in the US. At last count, she was hoping to publish her research in a peer-reviewed, reputed medical journal, but was sharing her concerns and data with colleagues, hoping to provide others with an opportunity to refute or confirm her initial findings.

65. "China Health Minister Official Puts HIV/AIDS Patients at 840,000," *Agence France-Presse,* November 5, 2003.

66. Jim Yardley, "China Offering AIDS Drugs to the Poor," *San Francisco Chronicle*, November 8, 2003.

67. Lawrence K. Altman, "Spread of AIDS Outpacing Response," *New York Times*, November 26, 2003.

68. We need to know, for example, what constitutes "normal" health, normal T-cell levels and "normal" liver function levels in South Africans with chronic exposure to malaria, TB or hepatitis.

69. Sonia Shah, "Globalizing Clinical Research," *Nation*, July 1, 2002. The FDA doesn't require drug companies to notify the agency before they

move their research overseas; nor does the agency track research in other countries after it has approved new drugs. In the realm of HIV, drug companies go to countries like Mexico where they can do trials quickly with minimal investment, and get positive results that will allow them to market the drug in some new fashion. It's all about markets and profit shares, not patient health. A key reason for this is that Mexican AIDS patients, like South Africans or Thais, are clean guinea pigs – in other words, they are treatment-naive. In the US, people have been on therapy for over a decade. They have complicated treatment histories and side-effects that make them less useful to scientists trying to track efficacy. According to Shah, China, India and Taiwan are among the governments "bending over backward" to lure drug companies to conduct research and make products in their countries. They offer them tax breaks and other incentives like buildings in which to do their clinical research.

70. V. Josse et al., "The Ethical Problems that Therapeutic Research Arouses in Africa: Particularly the Trials Promoted by the ANRS (French AIDS Research Agency)," ACT UP–Paris.

14   AIDS and Empire II: The Cost of Delay

1. The WHO objects to any suggestion that they are embracing a lower standard of care for poor countries. In a written defense of the agency's low-tech treatment guidelines for limited-resource settings, Craig McClure, director of the International AIDS Treatment Access Coalition (ITAC) and a member of the WHO's working group on the 3×5 global treatment plan, said:

> I disagree that there is a higher standard of care being advocated for the richer nations. WHO is prepared to respond to this accusation as follows: a public health approach to HIV/AIDS puts the emphasis on clinical monitoring of patients, and on investing in the community support required to help people adhere to their medication. High-tech monitoring tools are no substitute for information, education and support. If the industrialized world had adopted a public health approach to treating HIV/AIDS, we would not see the high levels of drug resistance, nor the low levels of patient adherence, that we see today.

2. "WHO International Consultative Meeting on HIV/AIDS Anti-retroviral Therapy," Report of the Meeting, Geneva, May 22–3, 2001. See p. 19 for "Major Outcomes" of this key meeting, which helped launch the 3×5 plan.

3. See Jon Cohen's series, "AIDS in Asia," *Science*, September 19, 2003.

4. Oral presentations of WHO 3×5 goals and progress by Joep Lange, IAS, Paolo Teixeira, the WHO, and Craig McClure, ITAC, at the International AIDS Treatment Coalition Partners' Meeting, July 2003.

5. Richard Ingham, "Donors Scrutinize Global Fund's Work – At Least Half a Billion Dollars Needed," *Agence France-Presse*, July 16, 2003.

6. Kevin McElderry, "EU Pledges Dollars on AIDS as Africa Joins G8 Summit," *Agence France-Presse*, June 2, 2003.

7. Steve Sternberg, "Thompson Urges Nations to Match US Commitment to Fight AIDS," *USA Today*, June 4, 2003; Tommy Thompson, Opinion Piece, *St. Louis Post-Dispatch*, October 20, 2003. In a response to an October 19 *Post-Dispatch* editorial, HHS Secretary Thompson, the chair of the Global Fund board, argued that the US was the "unmatched leader" in contributions to the Global Fund. The October 19 editorial criticized the fact that, at the time of this writing, the global fund was not planning to issue new grants over the following eight months, due to a lack of funds for round 3 grants. It accused the Bush administration of being partly responsible for the Fund's liquidity problems. Thompson argued that the US has invested $622 million to the Global Fund – 37 percent of the total paid into the Fund. (See capsule news summary, *Kaiser Daily HIV/AIDS Report*, October 21, 2003.)

8. Elizabeth Becker, "US Unilateralism Worries Trade Officials," *New York Times*, March 17, 2003.

9. Maureen Grope, "Tobias Says Ties to Industry Won't Affect AIDS Job," *Indianapolis Star*, October 1, 2003. Tobias and his wife are major contributors to the Republican Party, who donated at least $97,000 to federal candidates and parties, almost all Republicans.

10. Jeffrey Sachs, Op-Ed, *Washington Post*, April 2001: "Americans would not shrink from the $5 per American that prevention and treatment would cost this year. . . . The biggest risk is not cold-heartedness but simple inattention. There is also a nagging doubt . . . that AIDS is just

too big and costly to address. It's time for these doubts to be put to rest by the evidence."

11. Stephanie Nolen, "Global Fund and Games," *POZ* magazine, January 2003. "These attempts at rationing beforehand," Nolen quoted Sachs, "are to make donors look good while the poor die silently."

12. Ibid. In October 2002, Feacham drew heavy criticism from activists and Global Fund delegates when, at the closing of a Global Fund board meeting, after many delegates had left, he abruptly announced that the Fund would reduce its 2003 pledge goal from $3.6 billion to $2 billion. Activists charged that the US and Britain had forced his hand, but were angry he had diplomatically capitulated, rather than letting the Global Fund fail, which would expose the lack of donor commitment. Feacham also publicly butted heads with Sachs over the decision to lower country expectations of funding to match the actual purse size of the Fund. Others praise Feacham for his stewardship in these shark-infested waters, arguing that some in the US would be happy to see the Global Fund fail. Feacham continues to defend his pragmatic actions. "How far beyond our means can we make promises? If we start scaling up HAART therapy, and then suddenly cut off treatment – that is life and death. You can't make promises you can't keep." Of course that's exactly what the world did at UNGASS, and continues to do by reluctantly nickel-and-diming the Global Fund.

13. Critics are demanding that other critieria besides GNP be used to determine eligibility for the grants. One suggestion is the rate of HIV infection or other disease indicators. After all, a country like Mexico or Thailand may have pockets of wealth, but many people live in desperate poverty there, and many people have HIV. As the picture stood in November, most of the Latin American and Caribbean countries were being left out of future funding by the Global Fund.

14. The CCMs are supposed to include an array of groups including government and non-government representatives, NGOs, and – importantly – people with HIV and AIDS. In some countries, they do. In Uganda, for example, activists like Milly Katana have assumed an important role in campaigning on the needs of her colleagues, including poor women in rural areas.

15. Personal interviews with Paolo Teixeira, Bernard Schwartlander and Jos Perriens of the WHO; Craig McClure of ITAC; May and June, 2003.

16. When I was in India, officials at several generic companies were fuming about the long delay in getting the agency's nod, and were anxiously awaiting a chance to prove their new products were up to snuff. Representatives from the International Dispensary Association, MSF and Partners In Health also privately confided their criticism of what they viewed as the WHO's foot-dragging around the issue of access to generic HIV drugs.

17. Unpublished preparatory discussion paper, Health GAP strategy meeting, October 26, 2002.

18. Dr. Schwartlander recently left the WHO to work for the Global Fund, but played an important role at the WHO, where he helped shape HIV treatment guidelines and focused on technical challenges related to the management of the disease in resource-poor settings. See "WHO International Consultative Meeting on HIV/AIDS Antiretroviral Therapy."

19. The result is that consumers in countries will not be able to feel as confident about the quality of domestically produced generic AIDS drugs as about those approved by the WHO.

20. Personal interviews with Paolo Teixeira, Bernard Schwartlander and Jos Perriens of the WHO; Craig McClure of ITAC; May and June, 2003.

21. Personal conversations with generic manufacturers in India and the US, June 2002.

22. That amount actually represents a drop of $1 billion because, Thompson and other US officials maintain, they were told by African leaders that the money won't be well spent, since African countries aren't prepared to deliver treatment yet.

23. The coronavirus linked to SARS is a particle-borne virus, one that is carried in droplets of saliva, but is not air-borne.

24. Nicole Itano, "South Africa Gears Up for AIDS Fight," *New York Times*, November 20, 2003.

25. NGOs aren't the only ones affected by this common problem. It's true of the activist camp too. Although many grassroots players advocate unity, they practice exclusivity, and do little to share what they are learning with others. Instead, they hoard their funds, newfound expertise and resources, limiting their value to countries and communities. The reality I encountered in many countries is that groups and individuals, large and small, tend to work together out of necessity and

personal interest rather than common cause, even when the agenda is as important as global AIDS.

26. Some argue that the charitable branches of pharmaceutical companies like Bristol-Myers Squibb and Merck, through their foundations, provided seed money to jumpstart treatment programs, and have offered not only discounts on drugs but free drugs on a small scale to various groups. That may be, but their price-gouging on the big drug issue also completely overshadows these smaller acts of charity. These groups belong to the GBC, and helped get that organization off the ground. Now a much larger array of companies is part of the GBC. With new private–public alliances being rolled out as part of national treatment scale-up programs, there are clear avenues for businesses to step in and make a difference.

27. In Malawi the government had planned to buy drugs for 25,000 people using Global Fund money, based on the price of patented drugs. When they recalculated that amount using the costs of generic products, 50,000 people were suddenly eligible for treatment. Clearly, the switch to generics can greatly multiply the number of people accessing treatment. A number of countries, like Uganda and Senegal, have opted for a "hybrid" supply of both brand-name and generic drugs procured from multiple suppliers in order to negotiate the cheapest prices. Most are using non-protease regimens, including the most popular drug on the global market, the fixed-dose combination generic pill, Cipla's Triomune. In Cameroon, the cost to patients in July was around $15 a month. In Senegal, it was free.

The slashing of the price of Combivir was also hailed as a major step toward multiplying access. Another example comes from Latin America, where a strategy of pooled procurement and open bidding between generic and patented drugs resulted in the Andean agreement, which will increase access to 150,000 people. And of course the Clinton deal on generics will allow access for many more by dropping the price of generics to a historic low of 38 cents a day per person – something even the generic companies didn't imagine a few months ago.

28. It calls for using simple, standardized drug regimens and fixed-dose pills such as those promoted by the WHO in its new HIV guidelines.

29. Daniel Raymond, "Pooled Procurement: Learning from Tuberculosis," *amfAR Treatment Insider*, September 2003. Another TB group called the

Green Light Committee is seen as a model for supervising use of second-line AIDS therapies. It remains to be seen whether these new mechanisms will provide a streamlined process or a new layer of bureaucracy. Some critics are worried about giving insider groups like the Green Light Committee too much control over the purchase and distribution of alternative drugs. But the recent Andean Agreement showed that pooled procurement is effective in promoting low drug prices, access to generics and, most importantly, open, competitive bidding and a degree of transparency regarding drug prices, which benefits consumers and governments. Given the WTO's new decision granting some nations access to generics, the status of the Andean Agreement is a bit unclear as it relates to better-off developing countries like Mexico, which don't qualify for the deal benefiting the poorest African nations.

30. Unpublished draft of the WHO 3×5 plan, October 27, 2003. Today there are some models that suggest a different system might be established for drug pricing and development – private–public non-profit initiatives, like the one developed by the International AIDS Vaccine Initiative. This model uses grants to support basic and academic research, with the caveat that any promising vaccines that emerge, and may then be marketed by large companies, will be placed within pricing and delivery structures that guarantee their affordability and accessibility. A similar model is being developed for the WHO's new diagnostic initiative. The recognition that academic research creates many drugs, which are then sold by companies, has changed the public attitude toward the high prices being charged by drug companies. Recently a US group, the AIDS Healthcare Alliance, sued drug companies for profiteering through AIDS drugs, since they had not developed several of them.

31. *New York Times*, September 27, 2003.

32. Warren A. Kaplan, Richard Laing, Brenda Waning, Libby Levison, Susan Foster, "Is Local Production a Way to Improve Pharmaceutical Access in Developing and Transitional Countries? Setting a Research Agenda," a draft document produced for RPM+ and circulated for peer review by health policy analysts at the Boston University School of Public Health, April 23, 2003. According to the authors, "Smaller countries with fewer resources and a weak industrial base are unlikely to be viable in the global pharmaceutical market."

33. Recent evidence shows NAFTA critics are right: a November Carnegie report issued in time for the FTAA found that economic conditions have worsened in Mexico due to NAFTA.

34. Asia Russell, Health GAP Letter to Gloria Blue of USTR on "Public Health and Access to Medicines and the Second Draft of the Free Trade Area of the Americas Agreement," February 28, 2003. Russell cites a Joint Study by the WHO and the WHO Secretariat on WTO Agreements and Public Health (2002), p. 90, paragraph 170.

35. Doug Palmer and Kristen Roberts, "US Pushes Ahead with Bilateral Trade Pacts at FTAA," *Reuters*, November 18, 2003.

36. In 2002, the Bush administration forced the UNFPA to lose $34 million in financing, even after the State Department concluded the UN agency had not knowingly supported such a pro-abortion or involuntary sterilization policy in China.

37. For their part, State Department officials said the move "wasn't an ideological decision, it was a legal decision," and criticized the relief groups for refusing funds that were tied to an anti-abortion agenda: "We had hoped they would show more humanitarian statesmanship that that," one State Department official told the *Times*. Across the world, activists and many NGOs spoke out against the Bush policy – a harbinger of things to come, many predicted.

38. The plan follows Bush's 2002 $500 million Mother-and-Child HIV Prevention Initiative to prevent maternal HIV transmission – the plan that's been put in place in Haiti.

39. According to a May 1, 2003 *Washington Post* report, a number of multinational drug companies that make antiretroviral drugs were invited to join two pro-Bush lobbying groups backed by the President and his aides to help secure support for Bush's global AIDS bilateral initiative. The Coalition for AIDS Relief went to bat for the Bush plan outside Congress. It is chaired by several GOP heavyweights and funded by Coca-Cola, ChevronTexaco and General Motors, among others. Each company coughed up $25,000 to back the program – just a tenth of a hoped-for $250,000 contribution that coalition officials had asked them to donate.

40. "America's national ambition is the spread of free markets, free trade and free societies," notes a White House press release announcing the launch of the volunteer corps. Regarding the volunteer mission: "These goals – advancing against disease, hunger and poverty – will

bring greater security to our country. They are also *the moral purpose of American influence* [my italics]. They set an agenda for our government, and they give idealistic citizens a great cause to serve."

41. These groups accused the Bush administration of "manipulating the southern Africa food crisis to benefit their GM food interests and of using the UN to distribute domestic food surpluses which could not otherwise find a market," according to an October 7, 2002 report in the *Guardian* newspaper.

42. GM products are patented, and local farmers must pay annual fees to use these seed types, according to research by Public Citizen, a US consumer watchdog group. Monsanto's products include "terminator" or sterile seeds that can be activated to grow only by use of a specific chemical, and produce crops that never germinate. That means farmers have to buy seeds every year. The US recently offered $266 million of GM maize to southern Africa. Swaziland, Lesotho and Mozambique have accepted GM food aid, but Zambia, Malawi and Zimbabwe have refused it, fearing damage to their domestic agriculture. Andrew Natsios, head of USAID, claimed "We offered non-GM food but they all declined to accept it . . . We would have preferred to send non-GM wheat, or rice, but they only wanted maize. We tried to source non-GM maize but the industry said they could not guarantee that it was GM-free." But Zambian and Malawi officials countered that they could easily source non-GM food locally if they had the resources. Andrew Natsios is famous in AIDS circles for a major slip of the tongue, on June 9, 2001, when he publicly declared that poor Africans cannot manage HIV therapy because they don't even use watches to tell time. His implicitly racist comments provoked global outrage. He now heads the lead agency for Bush's global AIDS initiative.

43. "China Health Minister Official Puts HIV/AIDS Patients at 840,000," *Associated Press*, November 6, 2003; Brad Adams, "Waiting for Death in China," *Asian Wall Street Journal*, September 3, 2003.

44. Draft document, "WHO Estimated Number of People Under ARV by 2005 with Existing Programs," WHO, November 14, 2003.

45. "The Global Fund to Fight AIDS, Tuberculosis and Malaria," Annual Report, 2002/2003.

46. "A Commitment to Action for Expanded Access to HIV/AIDS Treatment," International AIDS Treatment Access Coalition document,

2002; statistics culled from "Coverage of Selected Health Services for HIV/AIDS Prevention and Care in Less Developed Countries in 2001," WHO, 2002.

47. Data reported from several case studies of antiretroviral treatment scale-up programs during oral presentation, July 14, 2003, International AIDS Society Conference, Paris, France.

48. *United Nations Integrated Regional Information Networks*, December 9, 2003. The most affected regions of Congo were the provinces of North and South Kivu, Maniema and Orientale, in the east and northeast of the country. PNLS director Jack Kokolomani told IRIN that prevalence of the epidemic among people aged between fifteen and forty was 15 to 19 percent higher than in many other countries. "The vast majority of people who die today from AIDS in our country are aged between 15 and 40. Infection begins very early, around 10, 11, 13 or 14 years," he said. In a report publicized during UN World Aids Day on December 1, 2003, PNLS reported that precocious sexuality was the reason for the high rate of infection. "Experts say 83 percent of patients are infected throught sexual intercourse. Some [individuals] confessed in the survey to having started having sexual intercourse at around the age of eight, nine and ten years," Kokolomani said. "Most began between 12 and 14. Fifty percent of young people will have had their first sexual relationship by the age of 16."

Due to this threat, PNLS has started to sensitize the public, pointing to the example of churches and different religious communities in Congo which have set up an inter-denominational committee to fight HIV/AIDS. Within this framework, Methodist pastor Daniel Ngoy Mulunda questioned the message coming from the churches that abstinence was the way to fight the pandemic. "Our message that you shouldn't use condoms has failed, you cannot continue to preach morality and abstinence to people who are ill," he said on World Aids Day, referring to a declaration made by a conference of African churches – Conference des Eglises de toute l'Afrique (CETA) – during a meeting in Cameroon held between 22 and 29 November.

49. The drugs will be provided through service points in every health district within a year, starting in the metropolitan provinces, and in every local municipality within five years, extending to remote outposts.

50. *San Francisco Chronicle*, November 20, 2003.

51. Activists in Central and South America have been pushing for access to treatment. As of November 2003, the government of Panama was treating for free all of the 1,200 HIV-positive citizens who had registered with the public health system and qualified for therapy, according to a health official. Surprisingly, the government has opted to use only a brand-name three-drug cocktail that cost up to $1,200 a year. An estimated 120,000 people are HIV-positive, and the government assumes up to 2,000 may need therapy now, but haven't been identified.

In Guyana, another emerging success story, the government has put 2,000 people on therapy, and now makes several antiretrovirals; the government hopes that all HIV-positive people will be on treatment. In Honduras, access has steadily increased, but has far to go. In the summer of 2002, activists finally persuaded the government there to begin offering treatment at three centers. Prices fell from $1,400 a year for a three-drug cocktail to $900, the price when Honduras secured round 2 Global Fund money. The government also kicked in $2 million to begin developing national resources to implement treatment. Two more treatment centers opened. The price of diagnostic tests fell, from $50 for a T-cell test to just $4, in November 2003.

By then, access had increased from a single patient on antiretroviral therapy in July 2002 within the public health system, to 1,345 individuals. Doctors there are seeing fifty patients a week now, up from thirty a few months ago. They hope to put another 1,000 on treatment as quickly as they can be screened. An estimated 200,000 Hondurans are HIV-positive. Things are less active in Paraguay and Uruguay, where activists say there is a need not only for drugs but for all sorts of assistance. In Columbia and Argentina, access through the public health system is increasing, but activists complain that the drugs being used to treat those in the social security system are of dubious quality. As I described in Mexico, activists in these countries complain that governments are purchasing locally produced "similares" or copy-cat antiretrovirals that have not been tested for quality, rather than high-quality WHO "prequalified" generic drugs like those produced by Cipla and Ranbaxy. Local generics are priced lower than foreign generics, and in some cases the Indian and other generic manufacturers haven't submitted paperwork to register their drugs in a given country. Until they do, the drugs can't be purchased.

"We are demanding that our government provide us with an assurance of quality, but so far they refuse to show us the data," said Julio Cesar, a Columbia AIDS activist attending the Panama Global Fund meeting. "We know some of these similares are of very bad quality and are very toxic. We are demanding access to treatment as a right, but it must be a medicine that works and is not going to harm us." Some activists feel the failure of governments to adopt strict measures to ensure that only quality drugs are used will undermine the global effort and give ammunition to big pharma supporters who claim generics aren't as good as brand-name drugs. "We know the Indian drugs that the WHO has approved are of excellent quality," countered Cesar. "The issue here unfortunately, once again, is one of profit and corruption. The government is trying to save money but it is jeopardizing the health of people with HIV by refusing to care about quality."

There are other complaints. Latin American activists from a dozen countries report that although AIDS awareness is increasing, it is still very limited within the general public. Outside cities, people lack access to HIV tests and medicines for OIs. Although first-line drugs are becoming more available, there's a lack of second-line drugs. And everywhere the stigma of HIV remains a major impediment facing HIV-positive individuals and groups – as does homophobia, often cited by activists as the shadow issue that has yet to be seriously addressed by governments and civil society; one that represents a fundamental barrier to AIDS prevention work.

Afterword

1. Aryeh Neier, *War Crimes – Brutality, Genocide, Terror and the Struggle for Justice*, Times Books/Random House, Inc., 1998, p. 55.
2. Ibid., p. 121.
3. Ibid., p. 213.
4. Paul Farmer, *Pathologies of Power*, University of California Press, 2003, pp. 42–50, 137–59.

Appendix B   Low-Cost Monitoring Tools

1. Second IAS Conference on HIV Pathogenesis and Treatment, Paris, July 2003, Abstract no. 1,234.
2. Ibid., Abstract no. 1,229.
3. Ibid., Abstract no. 1,237.

Appendix D   Factors Affecting Adherence

1. S. Weiser et al., "Barriers to Antiretroviral Adherence for Patients Living with HIV infection and AIDS in Botswana," *J Acquir Immune Defic Syndr*, 2003, 34, pp. 281, 288.
2. J. I. Nwokike, "Baseline Data and Predictors of Adherence to Anti-retroviral Therapy in Maun General Hospital (MGH), Maun, Botswana," Second International AIDS Society Conference on HIV Pathogenesis and Treatment.
3. I. Laniece et al., "Determinants of Adherence Among Adults Receiv-ing Antiretroviral Drugs in Senegal," ANRS 1215 Cohort Study. Second International AIDS Society Conference on HIV Pathogenesis and Treatment, Paris, 2003, abstract 1,118.

Appendix F   Women and HIV: The Gender Puzzle

1. Tenth Conference on Retroviruses and Opportunistic Infections, February 10–14, 2003, Boston, Massachusetts.
2. WIHS was set up in 1993 to track HIV in women and tackle the gender puzzle, then expanded in 2000. The study is racially diverse, involving a large group of African-American women in their mid-thir-ties who are very poor, with no health insurance. Some have a history of drug use and co-infections such as hepatitis C and STDs like herpes. Overall, domestic violence has emerged as a pervasive risk factor for HIV infection, and depression is common in this group.
3. K. Squires, Oral Presentation, Tenth Conference on Retroviruses and Opportunistic Infections, February 10–14, 2003, Boston, Massachusetts.
4. Ibid., CROI Abstract no. 764.
5. Ibid., CROI Abstract no. 739.

6. Ibid., CROI Abstract no. 728.
7. Ibid., CROI Abstract no. 763.
8. Ibid., CROI Abstract no. 765.
9. Ibid., CROI Abstract no. 736.
10. Ibid., CROI Abstract no. 735.

Appendix G   Women and Sexual Violence

1. Reprint Courtesy of Human Rights Watch. For a full copy of this report, go to HRW's website – <http://www.hrw.org/reports/2003/africa1203>.
2. See South Africa, Domestic Violence Act, Act No. 116 of 1998, Section 1 (defining complainant to include "any person who is or has been in a domestic relationship with a respondent and who is or has been subjected or allegedly subjected to an act of domestic violence," and "domestic relationship" to include marriage recognized by any law, custom or religion, and relationships "in the nature of marriage," including same-sex relationships).
3. An early experience is the Wynberg Court in Cape Town, where prosecutors are specially trained in sexual violence cases. By 1995, the Wynberg court was achieving a 20 percent higher conviction rate in rape cases than in other courts. See description in Human Rights Watch, "Violence Against Women in South Africa: State Response to Domestic Violence and Rape," November 1995, pp. 118–21.

Appendix H   Hospice and Palliative Care

1. Source: WHO <www.who.int>.
2. Material excerpted from the FHSSA's "Draft Strategy Paper for Expansion of Palliative and Hospice Care Services to Africa," August 2003. Reprinted with permission from the FHSSA.

GLOSSARY

Important note: *Information in this glossary was accurate as of early 2004. The state of the art may have changed since the publication date.*

Adherence The degree to which a patient can follow or manage a schedule or mode of treatment or intervention as prescribed.

AIDS (Acquired Immune Deficiency Syndrome) is a progressive immune disorder caused by the HIV virus, which primarily targets immune system cells such as CD4 T-cells that are responsible for fighting infection.

HIV disease progression is usually described in terms of measurements of immune status (CD 4 T-cell counts), or viral activity (viral load), and new or recurring opportunistic infections (OIs).

The **natural history** of HIV infection is divided into stages beginning with:

- **viral transmission** (via blood or bodily fluids): HIV is acquired through unprotected sexual intercourse, exposure to contaminated blood, or perinatal (mother to fetus) transmission.
- **primary or "acute" HIV infection** (also called acute retroviral syndrome): After viral entry and fusion of HIV to CD4 T-cells in the blood or cells lining the vaginal or rectal walls, HIV can infect bystander cells called monocytes and macrophages, producing clusters of infected cells and within 12–24 hours, travels to regional lymph nodes. There HIV

replication speeds up, as immune T-cells are dispatched to fight the virus. Although some infected T-cells die, others are circulated throughout the body, into the brain and lymphatic system.

- **Seroconversion** This marks the brief period of acute exposure when the immune system fights the virus, producing antibodies. HIV replicates very quickly, producing up millions of virus particles (or virions) a day during this acute period, until a balance is achieved with the immune system, usually within six months, something marked by a "**viral set point**." Exposure to HIV particles (called antigens) can be directly measured using a genetic PCR (polymerase chain reaction) or viral load test. The standard HIV antibody tests (Elisa, confirmatory Western Blot) used in most health centers take an indirect measure of exposure and may detect whether seroconversion has occurred as early as 3 weeks, but usually within 6 months after exposure.

- **Asymptomatic "chronic" infection** A period in which HIV may spread but does not produce any outward, or clinical, signs of disease, including persistent generalized lymphadenopathy (PGL), marked by swollen lymph glands). When available, doctors use two laboratory tests, T-cell and viral load, to measure the progress or impact of HIV against the immune system.

  The **rate of progression of HIV disease** varies by individuals. A minority of individuals who have been exposed to HIV have remained free of clinical symptoms for over 10 years and are classified as "**long term survivors**" or "**long term non-progressors**."

  Prior to the arrival of antiretroviral medicines (ARVs), the average period of survival from seroconversion to possible death was 10–12 years in the United States. With the advent of daily ARV therapy, individuals on effective treatment can regain their health and improve immune fuction, but still remain vulnerable to certain opportunistic infections. Current guidelines suggest they remain on "maintenance therapy" or daily treatment for life.

- **Symptomatic HIV infection** Clinical signs (symptoms) of HIV disease. In the early years, this was (and is still) referred to as AIDS Related Complex or ARC, and more recently is called "Stage B": according to the CDC classifications for Staging of HIV Disease. When HIV begins to gain the upper hand, it causes the loss of disease-fighting T-cells, and diminishes the immune system's ability to control infections.

This leaves individuals vulnerable to underlying or latent infections and exposure new "opportunistic" infections (OIs). The most common OI in much of the world is tuberculosis. As HIV spreads, new OIs are cropping up, reflecting the prevalence of diseases common to certain regions.

- **AIDS** A clinical stage of progressive HIV disease marked by a fall of T-cells below 200–250 copies and the emergence of symptoms of one or more opportunistic infections (OIs).

- **Advanced HIV infection, or "late stage" AIDS** A final stage of HIV disease characterized by a severe loss of immune function and and the progressive attack of a range of opportunistic infections on key organs, including the brain. If untreated, diseases such as toxoplasmosis or cytomegalovirus can cause blindness and HIV-related dementia that are hallmarks of late-stage AIDS.

Antibiotic A natural or synthetic substance that inhibits the growth of micro-organisms such as bacteria or fungi. Some antibiotics are used to treat infectious diseases.

Antibody Molecule(s) in the blood or other body fluids that tag, destroy, or neutralize bacteria, viruses, or other harmful toxins (antigens). They are members of a class of proteins known as immunoglobulins, which are produced and secreted by B-lymphocytes in response to stimulation by antigens. An antibody is specific to an antigen.

Antigen Any substance that stimulates the immune system to produce antibodies (proteins that fight antigens). Antigens are often foreign substances such as bacteria or viruses that invade the body.

Antiretroviral (ARV) Drugs A class of medicines designed to block the ability of HIV, a retrovirus, to reproduce itself inside an infected cell. There are several classes of anti-HIV drugs. Each target a key step in the viral life-cycle by blocking or impairing the activity of viral enzymes, or proteins. The first three classes of drugs target the activity of **reverse transcriptase** (RT). **Protease inhibitors** block the activity of the protease enzyme. Fusion inhibitors block a later step called fusion. **Other Entry Inhibitors** block the initial bonding of HIV to a cell surface, by interfering with the activity of CD4, CXCR4 or CCr 5 "docking" co-receptors on the surface of targeted immune T-cells.

Approved HIV drugs include:

- Nucleoside Analog Reverse Transcriptase Inhibitors (NRTIs) or "nukes": These include: Retrovir (AZT), Epivir (3TC), Hivid (ddC), Videx (ddI) , Zerit (d4T), Ziagen (abacavir), Combivir (AZT, 3TC), Trizivir (3TC, AZT, abacavir).
- Non-nucleoside Analog Reverse Transcriptase Inhibitors (NNRTIs) or "non-nukes": Rescriptor (delavirdine), Sustiva (efavirenz), Viramune (nevirapine).
- Nucleotide Analog Reverse Transcriptase Inhibitors (NTTIs): Tenofovir.
- Protease Inhibitors: Agenerase (amprenavir), Crixivan (indinavir), Fortovase (saquinavir), Kaletra (lopinavir/ritonavir), Norvir (ritonavir), Viracept (nelfinavir), Reyataz (atazanavir).
- Fusion Inhibitors: Fuzeon (enfuvirtide, T-20).

Accelerated Approval The process by which the FDA rapidly approves experimental treatments for serious or life-threatening conditions.

ASO AIDS Service Organization.

Bone problems (Osteopenia, Osteopororis, Avascular Necrosis)
Bone cell loss is measured on a scale ranging from mild (osteopenia) to severe (osteoporosis), which indicates the risk of fracture. These conditions are distinct from avascular necrosis, which refers to the death of bone cells and targets the joints of the hips and shoulders in people with HIV on therapy who develop this severe condition. Experts say there may be little clinical evidence of AVN bone loss, and it can be missed by standard X-ray, and even with more sophisticated imaging equipment like a Dexa-Scan. The main syptom of avascular necrosis is acute pain that is not alleviated with anti-inflammatory drugs or painkillers. By the time clinical symptoms appear, some people may require hip replacement surgery.

Diagnosis: A Bone Mineral Density (BMD) test measures bone strength, based on the density of bone cells. A Bone Mineral Content (BMC) test measures which bone cells are affected. (For an overview of emerging HIV-related bone problems, see my April 2002 article in POZ magazine, "Hip To the Future.")

CBO Community-based Organization.

Combination Therapy Using at least two drugs at the same time to treat a disease. With current HIV treatment, combination therapy usually refers to the use of at least three drugs (see HAART).
- **Monotherapy** Treatment consisting of one drug.
- **Dual therapy** Treatment with two drugs.
- **Fixed Dose Combination (FDC)** pills are made by combining more than one drug into a single pill, which makes it easier for patients to adhere to pill regimens.

Compassionate Use A phrase used to describe programs that provide experimental drugs on an individual basis to seriously ill people with few or no treatment options. Often, case-by-case approval must be obtained from the FDA.

Community Advisory Board (CAB) An advisory group formed of members of a community that provide ethical guidance and feedback to researchers or physicians conducting programs or research studies. HIV-positive individuals are increasingly demanding to be part of CABs for new or existing clinical trials, in order to assure that the rights and needs of this community be respected by the medical community. Some CAB's also serve as **TABs – Treatment Advisory Boards** – who provide oversight for proposed treatment protocols and clinical trials.

Diagnostic Tests A number of laboratory tests and markers are used to evaluate HIV's impact on the body and immune system (including T-cells) as well as the amount of HIV particles (antigens) and antibodies in the blood and tissue. HIV tests include:
  Antibody tests:
- **Enzyme-Linked Immunosorbent Assay (ELISA)** antibody test: A type of enzyme immunoassay (EIA) to determine the presence of antibodies to HIV in the blood or oral fluids. Repeatedly reactive (i.e., two or more) ELISA test results should be validated with an independent supplemental test of high specificity.
- **Western Blot** Confirmatory antibody test: A laboratory test for specific antibodies to confirm repeatedly reactive results on the HIV ELISA or

EIA tests. In the US, Western Blot is the validation test used most often for confirmation of these other tests.

T-cell tests measure the amount and ratio of the two primary immune white blood cell types called lymphocytes, **CD4-** and **CD8-T-cells.** As HIV targets these immune soldier cells, their total number and ratio fall, leaving the body vulnerable to infection. As drugs work to stop HIV, T-cell numbers rise again as the immune system restores itself. Many laboratories use **flow cytometry** equipment to measure T-cells (see Immune System).

- **T-cell range** The normal T-cell range in a healthy person is 300 to 1200 T-cells per cubic milliliter of blood. A person with over 500 T-cells is considered at low risk for HIV symptoms. T-cell counts below 500 suggests that HIV may be fighting the immune system and is a warning sign to regularly monitor immune health. A drop below 200 to 300 leave one vulnerable to HIV-related opportunistic infections (OIs).

Alternative Measures of T-cells:

- **Total Lymphocyte Count or TLC** measures the total amount of T-cells. It is considered a less sensitive measure than tests that differentiate between the T-cell families.
- **Syndromic or clinical management** of HIV involves a doctor or trained care provider closely monitoring a patient's health or response to therapy by focusing on signs and symptoms of disease or health, rather than laboratory tests. Basic clinical signs of a positive response to ARV therapy include weight gain, immune status, and resolution of opportunistic infections.
- **Surrogate markers** An alternative or substitute measurement to an accepted standard test or measurement.
- **Viral Load tests** These tests measure the amount of HIV RNA per milliliter of blood that can be detected via existing technologies. A viral load provides a *direct* measurement of HIV particles, or antigens, versus antibody tests which reflect a more *indirect* measurement of the immune system's response to HIV.
- **HIV PCR (Polymerase Chain Reaction) test** A laboratory process that selects a DNA segment from a mixture of DNA chains and rapidly replicates it to create a large, readily analyzed sample of a piece of DNA. As related to HIV: a sensitive laboratory technique that can detect and quantify HIV in a person's blood or lymph nodes (also called RT-PCR). It is an FDA-approved test to measure viral load.

- **Viral load range** An **undetectable** viral load means that the number of copies of HIV RNA is less than the test is able to measure, usually less than 50 or 400 copies, depending on which test is used. In the US, the standard of care calls for getting two initial viral load measurements from the same laboratory to establish baseline viral activity, then measuring 2–4 weeks after therapy or when changing regimens, and repeating these tests every 3–4 months, along with T-cells.
- Note: The WHO's treatment guidelines for resource-limited countries regard T-cell and viral load tests as desirable but not required to start individuals on therapy.

Disease Progression The way that a disease develops, including the specific events involved, bodily tissues or systems affected, mechanisms of damage, and the course of disease over time. HIV disease progression is usually described in terms of CD4 counts, viral load, and new or recurring opportunistic infections.

DNA (deoxyribonucleic acid) A double-stranded molecule that carries genetic information and that makes up the chromosomes in a cell's nucleus.

Double-Blind A method for assigning treatment regimens in a clinical trial that keeps both trial participants and members of the research staff from knowing which participants are on which assigned treatments.

Drug Interaction The effect that can occur when two or more drugs are used together. These include changes of absorption in the digestive tract, changes in rate of the drugs' breakdown in the liver, new or increased side-effects, and changes in the drugs' activity.

Data and Safety Monitoring Board (DSMB) An independent panel of clinical research experts that reviews the results of clinical trials while they are underway. The DSMB can change or close a trial if the early results call for that.

DOT Directly Observed Therapy. An approach to managing patient adherence to treatment first developed for tuberculosis in which a care provider or other individual directly monitors patients to make sure they take their medication on schedule.

Efficacy The effectiveness or ability of a drug to control or cure an illness. The efficacy of an anti-HIV drug usually refers to the drug's ability to lower viral load.

Epidemiology The branch of medical science that deals with the study of incidence and distribution and control of a disease in a population.

Epidemic A disease that spreads rapidly through a demographic segment of the human population, such as everyone in a given geographic area; a military base, or similar population unit; or everyone of a certain age or sex, such as the children or women of a region. Epidemic diseases can be spread from person to person or from a contaminated source such as food or water. The term **pandemic** is also used to describe a disease prevalent throughout an entire country, continent, or the whole world.

Expanded Access A program that distributes experimental drugs to people who are unable to participate in clinical trials and have few or no other treatment options.

FDA (Food and Drug Administration) The agency of the US Department of Health and Human Services that regulates the testing of experimental drugs and approves new drugs and medical products based on evidence of their safety and efficacy. The FDA also regulates the safety of foods, cosmetics, and other products.

First-Line Treatment The most effective starting therapy for someone who has never received therapy before. Because of the potential for the development of cross-resistance by HIV and other microbes, the choice of first-line medication(s) may affect the efficacy of later medications.
- **Second-Line Treatment** A secondary, alternative and often less effective therapy for someone who is responding poorly, has become resistant or cannot tolerate an initial or first-line treatment. Doctors refer to second-line regimens as **"salvage regimens"** and try to choose different classes of drugs from first-line regimens to overcome problems of resistance or side-effects associated with first-line therapy.

Generic drugs A copy of a brandname, patented drug that has been approved for marketing. Generic drugs must show that they work as effectively as the original or "innovator" drugs. Bioequivalence (BE) or comparative efficacy studies are required in order to gain regulatory approval by drug authorities. In India, generic drugs are made through "reverse engineering" in which chemists trace back the chemical steps taken to create the compound or formula.

HAART (Highly Active Antiretroviral Therapy) Anti-HIV treatment that uses a combination of drugs (usually three or more) to reduce viral load to undetectable levels in a patient's blood.

HIV (also HIV-1) Human Immunodeficiency Virus 1. The retrovirus isolated and recognized as the etiologic (i.e., causing or contributing to the cause of a disease) agent of AIDS. HIV-1 is classified as a lentivirus (slow-acting virus) in a subgroup of retroviruses. 2. The genetic material of a retrovirus such as HIV is the RNA itself. HIV inserts its own RNA into the host cell's DNA, preventing the host cell from carrying out its natural functions and turning it into an HIV factory.

HIV-2 A virus closely related to HIV-1 that appears to be endemic to West Africa and has also been found to cause AIDS. Although HIV-1 and HIV-2 are similar in their viral structure, modes of transmission, and resulting opportunistic infections, they have differed in their geographic patterns of infection. HIV-2 causes a slower, less severe form of disease than HIV-1 in most individuals, but may also be transmitted via exposure to blood and sexual body fluids.

HIV Transmission The passing of HIV via blood or sexual body fluids from one person to another via unprotected sex or contaminated blood or from a pregnant HIV-positive woman to a fetus or a nursing HIV-positive mother to a newborn.

Immune System The body's complicated natural or acquired defense against disruption caused by invading foreign agents (e.g., microbes, viruses). There are two aspects of the immune system's response to disease: **innate and acquired**. The innate part of the response is mobilized very quickly in response to infection and does not depend on recognizing specific proteins or antigens foreign to an individual's normal tissue. It includes **complements, macrophages, dendritic cells**, and **granulocytes**. The acquired, or learned, immune response arises when **dendritic cells** and **macrophages** present pieces of antigen to **lymphocytes**, which are genetically programmed to recognize very specific amino acid sequences. The ultimate result is the creation of cloned populations of **antibody-producing B cells and cytotoxic T lymphocytes (T-cells)** primed to respond to a unique pathogen. B-cells produce antibodies that then attack the invader. **White blood cells**, or **leukocytes**, make up the immune system. **Neutrophils, lymphocytes**, and **monocytes** are all leukocytes. Lymphocytes are the primary targets of HIV infection.

- **Immunity** is the natural or acquired resistance to a specific infection or disease by the immune system. Immunity may be partial or complete, long lasting, or temporary.
- **Immunogenicity** is the ability of a vaccine or antigen (a foreign protein particle) to stimulate an immune response.
- A primary **cellular immune response (also called a Type-1 or Th1 response)** is carried out by subset of immune cells including cytotoxic (cell-killing) T-lymphocytes or CTLs (also known as CD8-T-cells.)
- A **secondary (or humoral) antibody immune response (also called a Type-2 response)** involves antibodies that are protein molecules on the surface of immune B-cells that can recognize and bind to specific antigens (foreign proteins) like HIV.
- **Sterilizing immunity** completely prevents the establishment of an infection.
- A **neutralizing antibody (ab) response** prevents infection of a cell by blocking viral entry into the cell.
- **Mucosal immunity** is an immune reponse to an infection by immune cells in the mucosa that line the reproductive, gastrointestinal and nasal tract, and other moist surfaces of the body.

in vitro Latin phrase for "in glass" that refers to lab experiments conducted in cell cultures grown in an artificial environment, for example in a test tube or culture plate.

in vivo Latin phrase for "in life" that refers to studies done in humans or animals.

Institutional Review Board (IRB) An advisory group of experts on a subject topic or field that examines the ethical and other aspects of proposed studies by medical or other researchers. IRB approval is generally required for proposed clinical drug studies, especially involving human or animal subjects.

IVDU Intravenous drug user (or injection drug user): an individual who uses syringes to inject narcotics into their veins.

Lactic Acidosis A buildup of lactic acid in the body. Lactic acid (lactate) is a by-product of the breakdown of carbohydrates. Our bodies usually clear excess lactic acid. Lactic acidosis is a rare side-effect of the nucleoside analogs. Nucleoside analogs can damage the mitochondria (the power plants of cells), making them unable to clear excess lactic acid from the blood. Severe lactic acidosis can be life-threatening. Note: experts stress the importance of distinguishing elevated lactate levels – a common side-effect of HIV therapy – from severe lactic acidosis – a rare event.

Lipids Fats stored in the body and used for energy. Lipids include cholesterol, fatty acids, and triglycerides.

Lipoatrophy The loss of fat stored under the skin, especially in the limbs and cheeks.

Lipodystrophy Changes in body composition. Symptoms include fat loss in the limbs or face, excess fat in the abdomen, breasts, and upper back, increased triglycerides and cholesterol, insulin resistance, and glucose intolerance, possibly leading to a higher risk of heart disease and diabetes. There is no clear definition of lipodystrophy, and there is no one cause, although it is at least partly associated with the use of antiretroviral drugs.

Microbicide Creams, jellies and other products in development that can be used to block vaginal or rectal transmission of HIV.

Mitochondria Structures in human cells that turn nutrients into energy for the cells. Essentially, they are the cells' "power plants."

Mitochondrial Toxicity Damage to the mitochondria caused by factors such as heredity, aging, infections, or certain anti-HIV medications, particularly nucleoside analogs. This toxicity may lead to side-effects such as muscle weakness and muscle loss, peripheral neuropathy, pancreatitis, low platelets, low levels of other blood cells, and lactic acidosis.

MTCT (also PMTCT) Mother-to-child transmission of HIV (also referred to as Prevention of Mother to Child Transmission of HIV) anti-retroviral drug therapy is used to prevent vertical transmission of HIV from a pregnant woman to a fetus or a nursing mother to a newborn. MTCT regimens vary but can include therapy before, during and after delivery.

Myopathy A general term referring to any disease of muscles. Inflammation of muscle tissue, resulting in muscle weakness is a rare side-effect of long-term use of Retrovir (AZT), which is also part of Combivir and Trizivir. Myopathy can also be caused by HIV disease itself.

NGO Non-Governmental Organization.

Off-label A drug prescribed for conditions other than those approved by the FDA.

Opportunistic Infections (OIs) Illnesses caused by various organisms, some of which usually do not cause disease in persons with normal immune systems. Persons living with advanced HIV infection suffer opportunistic infections of the lungs, brain, eyes, and other organs. Opportunistic infections common in persons diagnosed with AIDS include tuberculosis, Pneumocystis carinii pneumonia (PCP); Kaposi's Sarcoma (KS); cryptosporidiosis; histoplasmosis; cytomegalovirus (CMV), and other parasitic, viral, and fungal infections; and some types of cancers.

Phase I Trial The first stage in testing a new drug in humans. The studies are usually done to gather preliminary information on the chemical action and safety of the drug using healthy volunteers. Usually done without a comparison group.

Phase II Trial The second stage in testing a new drug in humans. Performed in patients with the disease or condition being studied. The main purpose is to evaluate the activity of a drug, and to possibly provide information on how well the drug works.

Phase III Trial The third and usually final stage in testing a new drug in humans. Used to collect information about the safety of a drug and how well it works. Once this phase is complete, the drug manufacturers may request permission from the Food and Drug Administration to market the drug.

Phase IV Trial A large trial designed to evaluate the long-term safety and effectiveness of a drug that has been approved by the Food and Drug Administration.

Placebo An inactive agent given as a substitute for an active agent for the purpose of comparison in a clinical trial. A placebo usually looks like the experimental treatment being studied. If a placebo is used in trials of HIV combination therapy, people taking the placebo usually get approved drugs also.

Placebo-controlled A trial in which the effectiveness of an experimental drug is compared to that of a placebo.

PMTCT (see **MTCT**)

Post-Exposure Prophylaxis (PEP) A potentially preventative treatment for HIV that involves using 2 or more antiretroviral drugs to treat individuals within 72 hours of a high-risk exposure (e.g., needlestick injury or other occupational exposure, unprotected sex, needle sharing).

Pregnancy Category The Food and Drug Administration rates drugs in terms of their safety during pregnancy from Category A (safest) to X (least safe – do not use). Most medications have not been studied in pregnant women to see if they cause damage to the fetus. Antiretrovirals are classified as either category B or category C drugs.
- **Category A** Controlled studies in women fail to demonstrate a risk to the fetus in the first trimester (and there is no evidence of a risk in later trimesters), and the possibility of fetal harm appears remote.

- **Category B** Either animal studies have not shown a fetal risk but there are no controlled studies in pregnant women, or animal studies have shown an adverse effect that was not confirmed in controlled studies in women in the first trimester (and there is no evidence of a risk in later trimesters).
- **Category C** Either animal studies have shown adverse effects on the fetus and there are no controlled studies in women, or studies in women and animals are not available. Drugs should be given only if the potential benefit justifies the potential risk to the fetus.
- **Category D** There is positive evidence of human fetal risk, but the benefits from use in pregnant women may be acceptable despite the risk (for example, if the drug is needed in a life-threatening situation or for a serious disease for which safer drugs cannot be used or are ineffective).
- **Category X** Studies in animals or human beings have demonstrated fetal abnormalities, or there is evidence of fetal risk based on human experience, or both. The risk of the use of the drug in pregnant women clearly outweighs any possible benefit.

Protocol The detailed plan for conducting a clinical trial. It states the trial's rationale, purpose, drug or vaccine dosages, length of study, routes of administration, who may participate (inclusion criteria), who is not eligible (exclusion criteria), and other aspects of trial design.

Reagent a substance that takes part in or brings about a particular chemical reaction. Reagents are used to make diagnostic tests, and may include using viral particles, proteins or other substance that will cause such reactions.

Regimen A schedule or plan; a treatment regimen refers to the specific therapeutic intervention, including pill or nutritional program or health plans.

Resistance The ability of a virus (or other germ) to become less sensitive to a drug, usually by genetic mutation. In HIV, the viral enzymes and proteins (genes) mutate, or change, so that an antiretroviral drug cannot attach to them.
- **Cross-Resistance** The phenomenon by which HIV (and other disease-causing organisms) that develops resistance to one drug also becomes resistant to other drugs. For example, HIV that develops resistance to

one of the non-nucleoside reverse transcriptase inhibitors will also likely have resistance to other drugs in the same class.

- **Multi-drug resistance (MDR)** resistance to more than one drug or class of drugs. MDR HIV strains are harder to treat.

There are different types of HIV **drug resistance tests** used primarily for research purposes and by some clinicians:

A phenotypic test (or assay) A procedure in which sample DNA of a patient's HIV is tested against various antiretroviral drugs to see how well the virus can grow in the presence of the drugs — if the virus is susceptible or resistant.

A genotypic test (or assay) determines if HIV has become resistant to the antiviral drug(s) a patient is taking. The test analyzes a sample of the virus from the patient's blood to identify any mutations in the virus that are associated with resistance to specific drugs. Also known as GART (Genotypic Antiretroviral Resistance Test).

Retrovirus A type of virus that, when not infecting a cell, stores its genetic information on a single-stranded RNA molecule instead of the more usual double-stranded DNA. HIV is an example of a retrovirus. After a retrovirus penetrates a cell, it constructs a DNA version of its genes using a special enzyme called **reverse transcriptase**. This DNA then becomes part of the cell's genetic material.

RNA (ribonucleic acid) A single-stranded molecule composed of nucleotides. It is similar in basic structure to half of the double-stranded DNA. In healthy cells, RNA is used to copy portions of the cell's DNA in order to produce other cell components. HIV's RNA stores the viral genes that are later converted to DNA.

SARS Sudden Acute Respiratory Syndrome, caused by a coronavirus, is characterized by acute flu-like symptoms, fever, and difficulty breathing.

Side-Effect (or adverse event) The action or effect of a drug beyond what it is supposed to do. The term usually refers to negative effects, such as headache, nausea, or liver damage. Side-effects can be expected or unexpected, desired or undesired. Experimental drugs are studied for both short- and long-term side-effects.

SIV (Simian Immunodeficiency Virus) An HIV-like Simian virus that infects monkeys, chimpanzees, and other non-human primates. Some SIV viruses are virtually identical in structure to HIV viruses, providing an evolutionary picture of how these viruses crossed the species barrier into humans. Recent studies suggest some humans carry hybrid SIV viruses or animal viral sequences, though these animal viruses have not been found to cause active infection or disease in these humans.

Suboptimal An inadequate or ineffective response (as in not optimal). Suboptimal treatment means a given therapy is not strong enough to prevent HIV replication, compared to the gold standard of a 3-drug combination. ARV monotherapy and 2-drug regimens are considered suboptimal.

Subtype HIV is a constantly evolving virus that has generated several sub-types. The main HIV types are Groups M, N and O; Group M viruses are broken down into subtypes A, B, C, etcetera. Subtype B viruses are preva-lent in the United States and Western Europe; subtype C viruses are common to Africa and Asia.

Toxicity The extent, quality, or degree of being poisonous or harmful to the body.

TRIPs Trade Related Aspects of Intellectual Property agreement is a set of World Trade Organization rules adopted in 1994 by WTO-member nations that govern patents and copyrights of products and processes for industries that include pharmaceuticals. The TRIPs agreement contains a number of legal clauses that provide governments with means to seek access to generic drugs. They include:
- **Compulsory Licensing** A legal trade mechanism in which a govern-ment agency, different company or third party gains the right to man-ufacture and distribute a patented drug, and pay a royalty to the patent holder.
- **Parallel Importing** A legal trade mechanism that involves buying a drug at low cost in one country and reselling or distributing it in another country where the price was originally higher.

Vaccine Vaccines work by introducing particles of an infectious agent like a virus or bacteria to the immune system, which mounts an immune defense using an army of immune cells that can recognize the invader and kill it, or prevent cells from being infected.

- **Priming** involves giving vaccines in timed doses in order to generate initial immune responses that may be enhanced by follow-up immunizations with the same vaccine or another type of vaccine.

Viral replication The ability of a virus to infect cells and reproduce or copy itself and continue to spread in the body.

Viral suppression The ability of drugs to kill or effectively cripple a virus' ability to infect cells and reproduce itself.

VCT (Voluntary Counseling and Testing): This involves offering pre-test and post-test counseling to clients who are voluntarily seeking an HIV test.

Wasting A clinical description of severe weight loss associated with HIV disease that is exacerbated by chronic diarrhea, poor absorption of food, and nausea related to treatment.

This glossary was compiled and adapted from numerous public sources, including the US National Institutes of Health online AIDS glossary (www.aidsinfo.nih/ gov/ed_glossary) and US federal guidelines for HIV treatment. Reprinting of the ACRIA Update glossary, the CPCRA Glossary of Medical, Statistical, and Clinical Trials Terminology by Carlton Hogan, University of Minnesota was made with ACRIA's permission.

LIST OF ACRONYMS AND
INTERNET ADDRESSES

ACT UP: AIDS Coalition to Unleash Power (www.actupny.org)
AFEW: AIDS Foundation East–West (www.afew.org)
amfAR: American Foundation for AIDS Research (www.amfar.org)
ANAC: Association of Nurses in AIDS Care (www.anacnet.org)
AMD: Alliance for Microbicide Development (www.microbicide.org)
AFB: Association Francois-Xavier Bagnoud for orphans (www.fxb.org)
AVAC: AIDS Vaccine Advocacy Coalition (www.avac.org)
CDC: US Centers for Disease Control (www.cdc.gov)
CPT: Consumer Project on Techology (www.cptech.org)
CRIN: Child's Rights Information Network (www.crin.org)
CHANGE: Center for Gender and Health Equity (USA)
(www.change.org)
DATA: Debt AIDS Trade Africa (www.data.org)
FDA: Food and Drug Administration (www.fda.gov)
EGPAF: Elizabeth Glaser Pediatric AIDS Foundation (www.pedaids.org)
GAA: Global AIDS Alliance (www.globalaidsalliance.org)
GFATM: Global Fund for AIDS, TB, and Malaria (www.theglobalfund.org)
GHC: Global Health Council (www.globalhealth.org)
GNP+: Global Network of People Living with HIV/AIDS
(www.gnpplus.net)
Health GAP: (Global AIDS Project) (www.healthgap.org)
HAI: Harvard AIDS Institute (www.hsph.harvard.edu)

IAPAC: International Association of Physicians in AIDS Care (www.iapac.org)

IAS: International AIDS Society (www.ias.se)

IAVI: International AIDS Vaccine Initiative (www.iavi.org)

ICASO: International Coalition of AIDS Service Organizations (www.icaso.org)

ICW: International Community of Women Living with HIV/AIDS (www.icw.org)

IHA: International HIV/AIDS Alliance, UK (www.aidsalliance.org)

MDM: Médecins Du Monde or Doctors of the World (www.medecinsdumonde.org)

MSF: Médecins Sans Frontières or Doctors Without Borders (www.msf.org)

NAPWA: National Association of People Living with HIV/AIDS (www.napwa.org)

NCAN: National Catholic AIDS Network (www.ncan.org)

NMAC: National Minority AIDS Counciil (www.nmac.org)

PIH: Partners In Health (www.pih.org)

PPFA: Planned Parenthood Federation of America (www.plannedparenthood.org)

NIH: National Institutes of Health (www.nih.gov)

SWAA: Society of Women and AIDS in Africa (www.maxpages.com/swaauganda)

TAC: Treatment Action Campaign of South Africa (www.tac.org.za)

USAID: US Agency for International Development (www.usaid.gov)

WTO: World Trade Organization (www.wto.org)

United Nations Agencies

ILO: International Labor Organization (www.ilo.org)

UNICEF: United Nations Children's Fund (www.unicef.org)

UNAIDS: Joint United Nations Programme on HIV/AIDS (www.unaids.org)

UNFPO: United Nations Population Fund (www.unfpa.org)

UNIFEM: UN Development Fund for Women (www.genderandaids.org)

UNESCO: (UN Educational, Scientific and Cultural Organization (www.unesco.org)

WFP: World Food Program (www.wfp.org)
WHO: World Health Organization (www.who.int)

Key Internet resources, journals and databases for HIV treatment information

AEGIS: AIDS Educational Global Information System(www.aegis.org)
AID FOR AIDS: medicine recycling project (www.aidforaids.org)
AIDS In Africa: global coalition of NGOs (www.aidsinafrica.com)
AIDS In Asia: website clearinghouse
(www.growthhouse.org/asianhiv.html)
AIDS: medical journal of International AIDS Society
(www.aidsonline.com)
AIDSETI HIV: medicines recycling project (www.aidseti.org)
AIDSMAP: British HIV AIDS site (www.aidsmap.org)
African-American AIDS Policy and Training Institute
(www.blackaids.org)
Africa Action: site for African affairs (www.africaaction.org)
All Africa (www.allafrica.com/AIDS)
ATN: AIDS Treatment News (www.atn.org)
The Body: (www.thebody.org)
CATIE: Canadian AIDS Treatment Information Exchange
(www.catie.org)
Critical Path AIDS Project: website on treatment access programs
(www.critpath.org)
DAAIR: Complimentary therapies website (www.daair.org)
GMHC: Gay Men's Health Crisis (www.gmhc.org)
GTT: Grupo del Trabajo sobre Tratamientos del VIH (espanol)
(www.gtt.vih-org)
HIV and Hepatitis.com (www.HIVandhepatitis.com)
HIV InSite: U of California at San Francisco site (hivinsite.ucsf.edu)
Johns Hopkins AIDS Service: Johns Hopkins University site
(www.hopkins-aids.edu)
Henry J. Kaiser Family Foundation: (www.kff.org)
HIV ATIS: federal aids website (hivatis.org)
I-base: UK-based treatment journal in English, French (www.i-Base.org.uk)

LACCASO: Latin American and Caribbean Council of Organizations working with HIV/AIDS (www.laccasso.org)

Medscape – HIV/AIDS (www.medscape.com)

NATAP: National AIDS Treatment Advocacy Project (www.natap.org)

PATAM: Pan African Treatment Action Movement (www.patam.org)

One World International: A global portal "AIDS Channel" (www.oneworld.net)

POZ: magazine for HIV-positive community (www.poz.org)

Positive Nation: (www.positivenation.co.uk)

Project Inform: (www.projectinform.org)

REDLA: Latin American Association of People Living with HIV/AIDS (www.redla.org)

SAATHI: Southern Indian AIDS group (www.saathi.org)

SAFAIDS: Southern African AIDS site (www.safaids.org)

Stop AIDS UK (www.stopaidscampaign.org.uk)

TTAG: Thai Treatment Action Group (www.ttag.org)

TAG: Treatment Action Group (www.tag.org)

UN IRIN Plus news: UN African regional AIDS news (www.irinnews.org)

WE-ACT: Women's Equity in Access to Care and Treatment – a global HIV/AIDS initiative (www.we-actx.org).

The Well Project: for women with HIV (www.thewellproject.org)

ACKNOWLEDGMENTS

Much of the core material for the country field reports was originally published as part of a global AIDS feature series during 2001–2003 in amfAR's *Treatment Insider*, a medical newsletter aimed at HIV professionals and affected communities that is published by the American Foundation for AIDS Research. Other pieces were derived from reporting for the *IAVI Report*, a vaccine newsletter published by the International AIDS Vaccine Initiative. Other information came in part from reporting for other media, including *POZ* magazine. For this book, I greatly expanded on my initial amfAR articles by reporting on events up to December 2003 and extensively interviewing key subjects I had met about their experience and insights to date. I also included new material on the social, political, and economic dimensions of the treatment access picture that I gathered during my field visits and afterward.

I would like to thank amfAR for its support of my work, including David Gilden, my editor there, and Kevin Frost, director of clinical research, who gave the green light to the global series. At IAVI, Patricia Kahn was a responsive editor. Finally, it's been pleasure to work with my editor at Verso, Amy Scholder, and the rest of the Verso Team, including Charles Peyton, Niels Hooper, and Tim Clark.

I would also like to thank the many people who helped me carry out my field inquiries, including Anand Grover and Vivek Diwan in India, Ilya Kolmanovsky, Alexander Tsekhanovitch, and Masha Gessen in Russia, Paul Farmer, Loune Viaud, Michael Goff, and Jean Pape in Haiti, Gustavo

Reyes-Teran and Tim Horn for Russia, Paolo Teixiera, Jacques and Noemia d'Adesky in Brazil. I also benefited from the insights of activists and advocates in the global treatment access movement, including: Asia Russell, Sharon Ann Lynch, Paul Davis, John Iversen and Brook Baker of Health GAP; Donna Rae Palmer of Mobilization Against AIDS; Eric Sawyer of Act Up; Zackie Achmat of TAC; John James of ATN; Jamie Love of CP-Tech; Richard Stern of Agua Buena; Emily Bass of IAVI; Gregg Gonsalves of Gay Men's Health Crisis; Rebecca Denison of WORLD; Keith Cylar of Housing Works; Rebecca Schleifer of Human Rights Watch; Craig McClure of IAS; Dr. Kathryn Anastos of the Women's HIV Interagency HIV Study; the women of NACWOLA and WTAG in Uganda; and HIV-positive women in South Africa.

A special word of thanks goes to Shanti Avirgan and Ann T. Rossetti, my colleagues on "Pills, Profits, Protest: Voices of Global AIDS Activists," a related documentary film about the global access to drugs movement; to my family and my daughter Lucy Blue Brady and Kathy Brady, to Hannah Taylor, Judy Sisneros, Larin Sullivan, Marisa Cardinale, Kate Sorensen, Richard Jefferys, Sophie Russell, Ann Maniglier, Angela Garcia, Angelique Von Halle, Davy Walter, Selby Schwartz and Romy Suskin for their personal support; and to my *companeras en la lucha*, Cindra Feuer and Megan McLemore.

INDEX